Advanced Research in Electronic Devices for Biomedical and mHealth

Advanced Research in Electronic Devices for Biomedical and mHealth

Edited by

Rajesh K. Kesharwani, PhD, MTech

Upendra Kumar, PhD

Raj K. Keservani, PhD, MPharm

AAP | APPLE ACADEMIC PRESS

First edition published 2025

Apple Academic Press Inc.
1265 Goldenrod Circle, NE,
Palm Bay, FL 32905 USA

760 Laurentian Drive, Unit 19,
Burlington, ON L7N 0A4, CANADA

CRC Press
2385 NW Executive Center Drive,
Suite 320, Boca Raton FL 33431

4 Park Square, Milton Park,
Abingdon, Oxon, OX14 4RN UK

Library and Archives Canada Cataloguing in Publication

Title: Advanced research in electronic devices for biomedical and mHealth / edited by Rajesh K. Kesharwani, PhD, MTech, Upendra Kumar, PhD, Raj K. Keservani, PhD, MPharm.
Names: Kesharwani, Rajesh Kumar, 1978- editor. | Kumar, Upendra, 1979- editor. | Keservani, Raj K., 1981- editor.
Description: First edition. | Includes bibliographical references and index.
Identifiers: Canadiana (print) 2024034927X | Canadiana (ebook) 2024034930X | ISBN 9781774915165 (hardcover) | ISBN 9781774915172 (softcover) | ISBN 9781003424666 (ebook)
Subjects: LCSH: Medical informatics. | LCSH: Medical electronics. | LCSH: Machine learning. | LCSH: Wearable technology.
Classification: LCC R858 .A38 2025 | DDC 610.285—dc23

Library of Congress Cataloging-in-Publication Data

CIP data on file with US Library of Congress

ISBN: 978-1-77491-516-5 (hbk)
ISBN: 978-1-77491-517-2 (pbk)
ISBN: 978-1-00342-466-6 (ebk)

About the Editors

Rajesh K. Kesharwani, PhD, MTech
Associate Professor, Department of Computer Application,
Nehru Gram Bharati (Deemed to be University), Prayagraj, India

Rajesh K. Kesharwani, PhD, MTech, is Associate Professor, Department of Computer Application, Nehru Gram Bharati (Deemed to be University), Prayagraj, India. He has more than 11 years of research and nine years of teaching experience at various institutes of India, imparting bioinformatics and biotechnology education. He has received several awards, including the NASI-Swarna Jayanti Puruskar by the National Academy of Sciences of India. He has supervised one PhD and more than 20 undergraduate and graduate students for their research work. Dr. Kesharwani has authored over 49 peer-reviewed articles, 49 book chapters, and 35 edited books with international publishers. He has been a member of many scientific communities as well as a reviewer for many international journals. He has presented many papers at various national and international conferences. Dr. Kesharwani received his PhD from the Indian Institute of Information Technology, Allahabad, and worked at NIT Warangal for two semesters. He has been a recipient of a Ministry of Human Resource Development (India) Fellowship and a Senior Research Fellowship from the Indian Council of Medical Research, India. His research fields of interest are medical informatics, protein structure and function prediction, computer-aided drug designing, structural biology, drug delivery, cancer biology, nanobiotechnology, and biomedical sciences.

Upendra Kumar, PhD
Assistant Professor, Institute of Engineering & Technology, Lucknow, Uttar Pradesh, India

Upendra Kumar, PhD, is Assistant Professor in the Department of Computer Science and Engineering at the Institute of Engineering and Technology, Dr. A.P.J. Abdul Kalam Technical University, Uttar Pradesh,

Lucknow, India. He has around four years of industrial experience at Tata Consultancy Services, where he worked on many corporate projects as a JAVA/J2EE developer. He also has more than 10 years of teaching and research experience. His areas of research interest include digital image processing, machine learning, medical informatics, biomedical signal processing, fractal and chaos analysis, embedded systems and robotics with embedded C, medical imaging and diagnostic system, big data analytics, etc. He has published many papers in international and national journals and conferences. He has also published books and book chapters with international publishers and filed one Indian patent with the collaboration of IIIT Allahabad, India. He supervises research scholars for their PhD thesis work. Dr. Kumar has delivered expert lectures at various international and national conferences, workshops, and seminars and is a member of several review committees of national and international journals, conferences, and professional bodies. Apart from teaching and research work, he has held an administrative role working as Deputy Dean of Students Welfare at the Institute of Engineering and Technology. Dr. Kumar has an MTech in IT from IIIT Allahabad and a PhD in Computer Science and Engineering from Dr. A.P.J. Abdul Kalam Technical University, Uttar Pradesh, Lucknow, India.

Raj K. Keservani, PhD, MPharm
Associate Professor, Faculty of B. Pharmacy, CSM Group of Institutions, Prayagraj, India

Raj K. Keservani, PhD, MPharm, is working as Associate Professor in the Faculty of B. Pharmacy at the CSM Group of Institutions, Prayagraj, India. He has more than 12 years of academic (teaching) experience from various institutes of India in pharmaceutical education. He has supervised more than 25 undergraduate students for their research work. He has published over 50 peer-reviewed papers in the field of pharmaceutical sciences in national and international journals, six patents, over 70 book chapters, three co-authored books, and over 40 edited books. He is also active as a reviewer for several international scientific journals. His research interests include nutraceutical and functional foods, novel drug delivery systems (NDDS), transdermal drug delivery/drug delivery, health science, cancer biology, and neurobiology. Dr. Keservani graduated with a pharmacy degree from the Department of Pharmacy, Kumaun University, Nainital, Uttarakhand, India. He received his Master of Pharmacy (MPharm) (specialization in pharmaceutics) from the School of Pharmaceutical Sciences, Rajiv Gandhi Proudyogiki Vishwavidyalaya, Bhopal, India. He earned his PhD degree from IKG Punjab Technical University, Jalandhar, Punjab, India. Dr. Keservani is a life member of the Society of Pharmaceutical Education and Research (SPER).

Contents

Contributors

Deepika Agrawal
Department of Information Technology, NIT Raipur, Chhattisgarh, India

Amit Bage
Department of Electronics and Communication Engineering, National Institute of Technology, Hamirpur, India

Manju Devi
Deenbandhu Chhotu Ram University of Science and Technology, Murthal, Haryana, India

Abhinav Dubey
V.B.S.P.U. Jaunpur, Uttar Pradesh, India

Adarsh Dubey
National Institute of Technology, Hamirpur, Himachal Pradesh, India

R. K. Jarial
National Institute of Technology, Hamirpur, Himachal Pradesh, India

Rajesh Kumar Kesharwani
Nehru Gram Bharati (Deemed to be University), Prayagraj, Uttar Pradesh, India

Aman Kumar
Department of Electronics and Communication Engineering, National Institute of Technology, Hamirpur, India

Saurabh Kumar
Department of Electrical Engineering, Engineering Degree Division, Institute of Engineering and Rural Technology, Prayagraj, India

Upendra Kumar
Department of Computer Science and Engineering, Institute of Engineering & Technology, Lucknow, Uttar Pradesh, India

Puneeta Marwaha
Department of Electronics and Communication Engineering, National Institute of Technology Karnataka, Surathkal, India

Tulika Narang
Institute of Engineering and Technology, Lucknow, India

Manoj Kumar Pal
Indian Institute of Information Technology, Allahabad, Prayagraj, Uttar Pradesh, India

Sudhakar Pandey
Department of Information Technology, NIT Raipur, Chhattisgarh, India

Harshita Rai
Analytics and Insights Unit, Tata Consultancy Services, Pune, India

Badavath Mohan Rao
Department of Electronics and Communication Engineering, National Institute of Technology, Hamirpur, India

Himanshu Kumar Shukla
Department of CSE, BBDITM, Lucknow, Uttar Pradesh, India

Narendra Kumar Shukla
Department of ECE, University Of Allahabad, Prayagraj, Uttar Pradesh, India

Shubham Shukla
Department of ECE, Kiet Ghaziabad, Uttar Pradesh, India

Ashutosh Singh
Department of CSE, BBDITM, Lucknow, Uttar Pradesh, India

Sukhdip Singh
Deenbandhu Chhotu Ram University of Science and Technology, Murthal, Haryana, India

Rohit Srivastava
Department of CSE, BBDITM, Lucknow, Uttar Pradesh, India

Nitesh Tiwari
Department of Electrical Engineering, Madan Mohan Malaviya University of Technology Gorakhpur, Uttar Pradesh, India

Esha Tripathi
Pranveer Singh Institute of Engineering, Kanpur, Uttar Pradesh, India

Abhay Kumar Tripathi
Pranveer Singh Institute of Engineering, Kanpur, Uttar Pradesh, India

Shailendra Tiwari
Thapar Institute of Engineering and Technology (TIET), Patiala, Punjab, India

Kamal Kishor Upadhyay
Department of Information Technology, NIT Raipur, Chhattisgarh, India

Neevatika Verma
Department of Electrical Engineering, Delhi Technological University, New Delhi, India

Diwakar Yagyasen
Department of CSE, BBDITM, Lucknow, Uttar Pradesh, India

Abbreviations

ACE	angiotensin-converting enzyme
ADC	apparent diffusion coefficient
AF	atrial fibrillation
AFE	analog front end
AFL	atrial flutter
AHA	American Heart Association
AI	artificial intelligence
AI	avian influenza
ANN	artificial neural network
AoV	angles and direction of retinal views
AR	augmented reality
ASPP	atrous spatial pyramid pooling
ASR	automatic speech recognition
BP	blood pressure
BPM	blood pressure management
BraTS	brain tumor segmentation challenge
BSN	build a body sensor network
CACTUS	clustering categorical data using abstracts
CAD	computer-aided design
CAM	class activation
CART	regression trees and classification tree
CCPA	California Consumer Privacy Act
CDSSs	clinical decision support tools
CHF	congestive heart failure
CI	confidence interval
CKD	chronic kidney disease
CLB	clenbuterol
CLIQUE	clustering in quest
CMOS	complementary metal oxide semiconductor
CMRR	common-mode rejection ratio
CNN	convolution neural network
COVID-19	Coronavirus Disease 2019

CR	compression ratios
CRF	conditional random fields
CRISPR	clustered regularly interspaced-based short palindromic repeats
CT	computed tomography
CT	coronary thrombosis
CVD	cardiovascular disorders
CXR	chest X-ray
DA	discriminant analysis
DBP	diastolic BP
DBSCAN	density-based spatial clustering of applications with noise
DCCA	discriminant canonical correlation analysis
DENCLUE	density-based clustering
DL	deep learning
DLP	digital light processing
DNNs	deep neural networks
DR	diabetic retinopathy
DT	decision tree
DWT	discrete wavelet transformation
ECG	electrocardiogram
EDM	entropy degradation technique
EEG	electroencephalogram
EEH	environmental bio-energy harvesting
EHR	electronic healthcare records
EMEH	electromagnetic energy harvesters
EMG	electromyography
FBP	filtered back projection
FC	fully connected
FCIA	flow cytometric immunoassay
FL	federated learning
FPGA	field programmable gate arrays
GA	genetic algorithm
GBCVDS	global burden of cardiovascular disease survey
GDPR	general data protection regulation
GLCM	gray level co-occurrence matrix
GNB	Gaussian Naive Bayes
GPU's	graphics processing units
GUID	globally developed unique identifier

HA	heart arrhythmia
HCA	hierarchical cluster analysis
HDRS	human dynamic reporting service
HF	heart failure
HIOT	Healthcare IOT
HIPAA	Health Insurance Portability and Accountability Act
HIV	human immunodeficiency virus
HR	heart rate
HTA	hypertensive arteriopathy
ICT	information communication technology
ICU	intensive care unit
ILSVRC	ImageNet Large Scale Visual Recognition Competition
IoT	Internet of Things
IoU	Intersection over Union
IR	infrared
IRB	Institutional Review Board
ISODATA	iterative self-organizing data
KNN	K-nearest neighbor
KPCA	Kernel Principal Component Analysis
LAMP	loop-mediated isothermal amplification
LASSO	least absolute shrinkage and selection operator
LED	light-emitting diode
LDA	linear discriminant analysis
LGG	low-grade gliomas are included
LPS	local positioning system
LR	logistic regression
LSI	large-scale ICs
LSTM	long short-term memory
LUNA	lung nodule analysis
MBPNN	multilayer backpropagation neural network
MCM	multichip module
MCODE	molecular complex detection
MEMS	microelectromechanical systems
mHealth	mobile health
ML	machine learning
MLC	Markov cluster algorithm
MLP	multilayer perceptions
MLPNN	multilayer perception neural network

MRI	magnetic resonance imaging
mRMR	minimal redundancy maximal relevance
MS	macrovesicular steatosis
MSD	medical segmentation decathlon
MSI	medium-scale ICs
NB	Naive Bayes
NLP	natural language processing
OCD	obsessive compulsive disorder
OM	optical microscopy
OPNET	optimized network engineering tool
OPTICS	ordering points to discover the clustering structure
OVO	one-versus-one rule
PCA	principal component analysis
PD	Parkinson's disease
PDAs	personal digital assistants
PDMS	polydimethylsiloxane
PET	positron emission tomography
PNA	peptide nucleic acid fluorescent-labeled
POC	point of care
PPG	photoplethysmography
PPV	positive predictive value
PRODIGI	portable real-time-based optical detection, identification based, and guidance for intervention
PSVT	paroxysmal super ventricular tachycardia
PUS	portable ultrasound scanners
qPCR	polymerase chain reaction
QUASR	quenching of unincorporated-based amplification signal reporters
rbST	recombinant bovine somatotropin
ReLU	rectified linear unit
RFA	random forest algorithm
RFID	Radio Frequency Identification technology
RNN	recurrent neural network
RNSC	restricted neighborhood search cluster
RTLS	real-time location system
RTPCR	real-time reverse transcriptase polymerase chain reaction test
SBP	systolic BP

SCLC	small-cell lung cancer
SFTA	segmentation-based fractal texture analysis
SIDs	smartphone-based imaging devices
SIFT	scale-invariant feature transform
SIP	system in package
SMOTE	synthetic minority oversampling technique
SOC	system-on-chip
SPC	superparamagnetic clustering
SPCE	screen-printed carbon electrode
SPECT	single-photon emission computed tomography
SPIHT	set partitioning in hierarchical trees
SRIS	smartphone-based retinal imaging system
SURF	speeded-up robust feature
SVM	support vector machine
TB	tuberculosis
UID	unique identifiers
UUID	universally unique identifier
UWB	ultra-wideband
VF	ventricular fibrillation
VLSI	very large-scale ICs
VR	virtual reality
WHO	World Health Organization
WLAN	wireless local area network
WMS	wearable medical sensor
WSN	wireless sensor network
YOLO	you only look once
3D	three-dimensional

Acknowledgments

This book is based on the research conducted on applications of electronic devices in biomedical and mHealth. We are very grateful to our parents and friends for encouraging us to start the work, preserve it, and finally publish it. We would like to sincerely thank our Head of the Department, Prof. D. S. Yadav, IET Lucknow, for providing wonderful academic culture and environment in our department. We would like to extend our heartfelt thanks to our mentors Prof. Krishna Misra and Prof. Tapobrata Lahiri, IIIT Allahabad, India, for their continuous guidance and encouragement. We would also like to acknowledge those authors whose research have been referred to in this book chapter and all those who were involved directly or indirectly in the preparation of this book.

Foreword

It gives me immense pleasure to write the foreword for this book, *Advanced Research in Electronic Devices for Biomedical and mHealth.* This book provides detailed information on research done in the development of electronic devices for biomedical and mHealth applications. It introduces the most recent developments in electronics, informatics, and telecommunications applications in healthcare. Various cutting-edge technologies are in use and have helped improve the biomedical and mHealth services day by day. This book mainly focuses on the design and development of new technological solutions for low-cost, more efficient devices, circuits, and systems for biomedical and mHealth applications. It also covers the application of machine learning in combination with IoT devices in biomedical and healthcare/mHealth field, which in turn produces overwhelming responses in terms of low cost, efficient, and fast healthcare solutions.

The main driving force for editing this research is the transformation of the current healthcare system with a growing aging population, sharp rising healthcare costs, and frequent occurrences of chronic diseases. Today, it is the need of the day to deliver healthcare services in more cost-effective and responsive ways. The traditional hospital-centered healthcare system is in the transformation phase to provide personalized advanced healthcare facilities for early diagnosis, treatment, and long-term digital monitoring. This book is aimed at mainly attracting graduate students and researchers in biomedical engineering and medical informatics, medical device designers, and researchers all over the world. All the contributing authors demonstrate an exceptional expertise in the field of research in electronic devices for biomedical and mHealth applications and provide a global perspective on current and future advances in the same.

I congratulate the editors for bringing together experts in the field of research in electronic devices for biomedical and mHealth applications and the authors for their excellent contributions.

Neelendra Badal, PhD, Director,
Rajkiy Engineering College, Bijnor, UP, India;
Professor, KNIT Sulatnpur, UP, India

Preface

The book *Advanced Research in Electronic Devices for Biomedical and mHealth* is a compilation of advanced empirical knowledge of current e-healthcare system and its use in medical sciences. Cumulative research findings and various advanced technologies available based on diversified hybrid medical and engineering strategies are acknowledged in this book. This present book comprises 10 chapters, attempted to acknowledge the current thrust in biomedical and in mHealth care system. The main driving causes for the transformation of current healthcare system are the growing aging population, sharp rising healthcare costs, and frequent occurrences of chronic diseases. Today, we need to deliver healthcare services in more cost-effective and responsive ways. The medical-expert centric hospital-centered healthcare system, which mainly focuses on diagnosis and treatment, is now ready to transform into individual-center-based healthcare system, which in turn focuses on early detection, early diagnosis, and long-term monitoring.

The role of portable, wearable, and networked electronic medical devices has become an important and essential component for future biomedical and mHealth applications. Furthermore, the development of biomedical and mHealth instrumentations should be done in a cost effective manner with affordable transportation, and with power consumption as low as possible. Therefore, integrated circuits (ICs) design-based biomedical devices should be developed in these biomedical and mHealth applications.

The recent biomedical IC design technologies with low power, low noise, and low frequency which have been used in multiparameter applications, monitoring of human body signal and processing are need of today's biomedical and mHealth applications. These are widely used in acquisition of physiological signals.

Smartphone-based applications have revolutionized biomedical practices with artificial intelligence. However, for various reasons like the need of presence of experts in the cloud, continuous data connectivity to the device, rising demand for high-quality medical services, telemedicine, etc. mHealth applications suffer from its inherent limitations. The present book is a compilation of various chapters to describe major design challenges and research potential in biomedical systems and, cover the fundamental principles underlying biomedical engineering and its advancement in health care/mHealth system.

CHAPTER 1

Machine Learning in the Healthcare Domain

TULIKA NARANG[1] and HARSHITA RAI[2]

[1]*Institute of Engineering and Technology, Lucknow, India*

[2]*Analytics and Insights Unit, Tata Consultancy Services, Pune, India*

ABSTRACT

Machine learning is a domain of computer science that facilitates the computers to think, learn, and take decisions like human beings. There are a vast variety of implementation of machine learning techniques in different fields. Machine learning in healthcare domain is extensively useful in clinicians and patient care. It is useful in clinical decision support and the development of clinical care guidelines. Machine learning methods automatically analyze and identify patterns and analyses of reasons about data. A machine learning algorithm for instance can help radiologists make intelligent decisions by reviewing images such as conventional radiographs, MRI, CT, and radiology reports. A machine learning algorithm can detect breast cancer and achieve results which are comparable to the human counterpart. Machine learning algorithms can be employed to optimize hospital resources. The demand of resources such as beds and IC use can be predicted in advance. Machine learning in healthcare sector is thus proving useful and valuable.

1.1 INTRODUCTION

Machine learning is the domain of computer science that gives computers the capability to learn and make decisions without being explicitly programmed (Arthur L. Samuel, AI pioneer, 1959).

Advanced Research in Electronic Devices for Biomedical and mHealth.
Rajesh K. Kesharwani, Upendra Kumar, Raj K. Keservani (Eds)

Machine learning uses an algorithm to apply statistical operations against inputs. The inputs are converted to outputs without much interference from humans. Machine learning implements artificial intelligence and computers are programmed to learn information without human intervention.

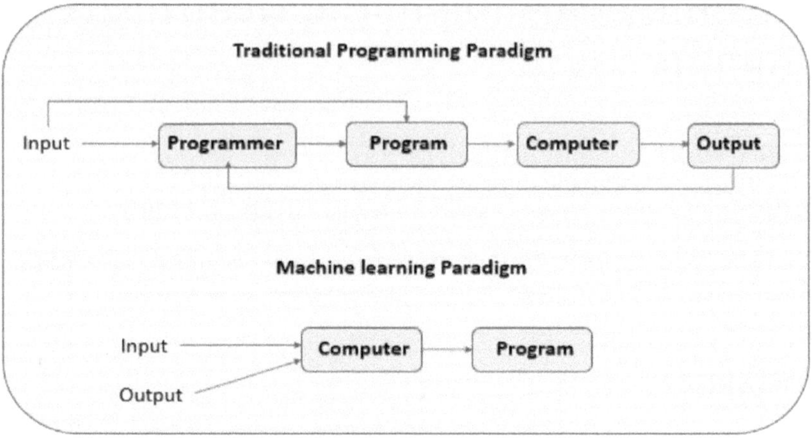

FIGURE 1.1 Traditional vs machine learning paradigm.

Source: Adapted from Sebastian Raschka (2020). https://sebastianraschka.com/blog/2020/intro-to-dl-ch01.html

In words of Tom Mitchell (Machine Learning Professor at Carnegie Mellon University), "A computer program is said to learn from experience E with respect to some class of tasks T and performance measure P, if its performance at tasks in T, as measured by P, improves with experience E."

The essential components of Machine Learning algorithms are:

- Representation. This component refers to the hypotheses that can be represented given a certain algorithm class.
- Optimization. It is the optimization metric that is used to test the model.
- Evaluation. The evaluation component is the phase to compute the performance of the model after training phase.

A machine learning algorithm defines the following steps of approaching a machine learning application:

1. Problem statement definition.
2. Collection of labeled data.
3. Selection of an algorithm.

4. Selection of an optimization metric.
5. Selection of a metric for evaluating the model.

Machine learning processes and finds useful and valuable patterns in data sets. The resulting patterns are used for decision-making.

The machine learning applications comprise various algorithms. The algorithms are a specific set of instructions for accomplishing objectives of different domains. The algorithms are designed in such a manner that tasks are performed without or very least human intervention. With time and experience the prediction accuracy of machine learning algorithms improves without explicit programming.

Machine learning is the area in artificial intelligence that is attributed to focus on the utilization of data and drawing inferences from this data through various algorithms to mimic human understanding and show steady improvement in the accuracy of the model with the availability of more and more data.

IBM is one of the organizations that has played an important role in the advancement in machine learning. Arthur Samuel from IBM is the one who came up with the term "machine learning." In his research that focused on the game of checker, the computer program run on the IBM 7094 for the first time defeated the human opponent Robert Nealey in the year 1961. When compared to the variety of operations the machine learning programs can perform today, the game may appear to be trivial, but it can be considered the initial stage or prototype for what was to come including everything from self-driven car to powerful recommendation systems.

Within various fields of data science such as data mining and statistical analysis, business intelligence and strategy-making machine learning plays an essential role in understanding and extracting vital insights using statistical methods and algorithms which are designed to handle various tasks such classification and prediction to assist in businesses' decision-making. The advancement in the application of computer systems in handling various tasks had led to the generation of large volume of data known as "big data" which is a very crucial and underutilized resource in many business domains and with advancement in machine learning algorithms data scientists will see increase in the number of businesses that want to leverage this technology.

Machine learning algorithm consists of three essential modules:

1. **A Decision Process**: Machine learning algorithms work by identifying hidden patterns in the input data which can be either

labeled, unlabeled, or a combination of the two; the algorithm uses an optimization function to perform tasks such as prediction and classification and make predictions about the patterns in the data.

2. **An Error Function**: The prediction of any machine learning model needs to be evaluated and this is where the error function comes into picture; it compares the model output with the known examples to assess the accuracy of the model.
3. **A Model Optimization Process**: Once the initial training iterations are completed the model needs to be optimized. In order to reduce the difference between the actual value and predicted values the feature weights are adjusted on the training data. The optimization cycle is repeated, and the feature weights are readjusted until the desired accuracy is achieved.

1.2 MACHINE LEARNING METHODS

Machine Learning algorithms can be categories into the following groups:

- Supervised
- Unsupervised
- Semi-supervised
- Reinforcement Learning

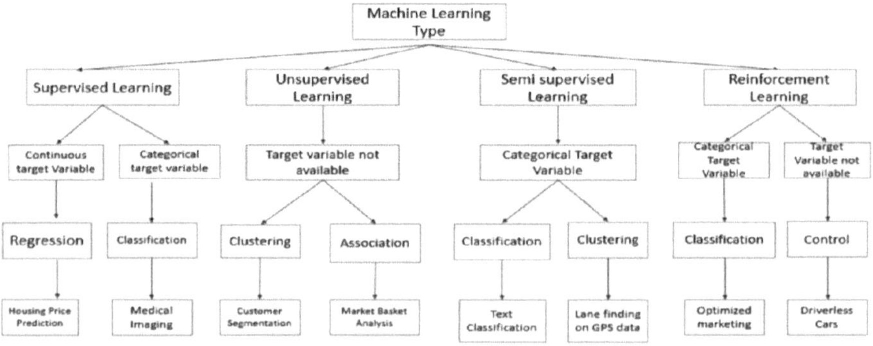

FIGURE 1.2 Classification of machine learning algorithms.

Source: Reprinted from Fumo, 2017.

Figure 1.2 shows the different categories in the machine learning approaches.

1.2.1 SUPERVISED MACHINE LEARNING

The models in supervised learning are trained to optimize a function to predict values for input samples looking at other input and output samples (labeled data) (Singh et al., 2016).

The function utilizes the training samples to update and optimize its weights until they are adapted to wanted precision. This happens as a feature of the cross-validation process to guarantee that the model keeps away from overfitting or underfitting. Supervised learning assists organizations with addressing for an assortment of real-world issues at scale, for example, classification spam in a different folder from your inbox. A few techniques utilized in supervised learning include support vector machine (SVM), neural networks, decision tree, naïve bayes, logistic regression, random forest, linear regression, and more. The Supervised approach can be classified into two subcategories:

- **Continuous Target Variable:** Numeric variables that have an infinite number of values between any range can be referred to as continuous variables. These types of variables can either have a numeric value or a date/time related data. For example, the weight of children or the date and time of a maximum sale.
- **Categorical Target Variable:** Instead of numerical values the variables are represented by label values, which can be utilized to categorize the data. The label values are part of an identified set of values or categories. Categorical variables can be referred to as nominal. Some examples include: A "vehicle" variable with the values: "car" and "bike."

In case of supervise learning the target values are available for all the sample data points in the data set.

1.2.2 UNSUPERVISED LEARNING

The models in unsupervised learning (Gentleman and Carey, 2008) are trained on unlabeled data to identify patterns and generate predictions. The models group the data points into clusters. The model is responsible for identifying hidden patterns in the data set to associate similar categories of data together. The algorithms involved in unsupervised learning are K-mean clustering, Association Rule Mining, Topic Modeling, and Dimensionality Reduction Techniques.

- **Target Variable not Available:** In case of unsupervised learning the target variable is not available for any of the data points in the data set.

1.2.3 SEMI-SUPERVISED LEARNING

Semi-supervised learning is an approach based on a combination of features of supervised learning and unsupervised learning. In case of supervised learning which works with labeled data and unsupervised learning which works on unlabeled data, some information is missed which can be derived from the labels.

Semi-supervised learning is a mix of both which takes both labeled and unlabeled data; the thought behind this is that data a smaller set of labeled data will result in considerable improvement in the accuracy, thus reducing the effort spent in annotation in case of supervised learning while adding the information that is conveyed through the label information. In the training phase a smaller labeled data set is used to guide classification and feature extraction from a larger, unlabeled data set.

- **Categorical Target Variable:** Semi-supervised learning approaches use categorical label for the data points in the dataset.

1.2.4 REINFORCEMENT LEARNING

This is an iterative process which is mostly dependent on the feedback from the environment. The algorithm is designed in such a way that it improves and performs based on the feedback it has received from the environment without requiring any external intervention. These models are like supervised learning, only difference being that the model does not need to be trained on the sample data; instead the model learns by reinforcing a sequence of successful outcomes to identify the best strategy for a given problem.

The IBM Watson® system became a great example for this system when it won the *Jeopardy!* challenge in 2011. Reinforcement learning was used by the system to decide whether to attempt a question or not, which square to play from the board, and how much to wager in each round.

- **Categorical Target Variable:** In reinforcement learning the data with categorical target labels are used in classification problems. The label for the data points in the dataset is known for all.
- **Target Variable not Available:** For datasets which do not have target values available in reinforcement learning those cases can be done through control approaches.

1.3 APPLICATION OF MACHINE LEARNING

AI applications are widely used in a variety of fields of the present world. Different applications, for example, email spam detection, face identification and matching (e.g., iPhone X), Web search (e.g., DuckDuckGo, Bing, Google, Stock predictions, Smart colleagues (Apple Siri, Amazon Alexa, **etc.**), Product suggestions (e.g., Netflix, Amazon), Self-driving vehicles (e.g., Uber, Tesla), Medical analyses are simply to name not many of them.

- **Speech Recognition:** Speech recognition applications apply natural language processing (NLP) to process human speech and convert it to a written format. Various mobile applications include speech recognition feature into their use-cases and facilitate speech-based features like voice search. Examples such as Siri or OK Googleor provide more accessibility around texting or notes taking.
- **Customer Service:** Chatbots can be utilized to answer frequently asked questions and provide assistance to the end client for a better user experience. The chatbots can help the user in fetching information related to their previous order or activity or even act as a help to guide and facilitate then with targeted recommendations, modifying the way we think about client commitment across sites and web-based media stages. These models have access to all of the user data that is captured by the business to improve on the results the user is presented with.
- **Computer Vision:** The application of AI in the field of computer vision enables us to tape into data sources like video recording, computerized pictures, and other visual data sources to derive insights. Powered by convolutional neural organizations, computer vision finds its application in various fields including applications in radiology imaging in medical care, photograph labeling in online

media, self-driving vehicles in the motor vehicle business, and even in surveillance and security.

- **Recommendation Engines:** Based on the past behavior information of a user AI algorithms can predict and assist with finding information drifts in a user's queries and this can be utilized to establish more viable strategically recommended methodologies. This is utilized to make targeted suggestions to clients during the checkout for online stores and retailers.
- **Automated Stock Trading:** Designed to automatically implement trading strategies on multiple stock portfolios without any human intervention, AI-driven trading strategies execute thousands or even a large number of exchanges each day after capturing and processing various data points.
- **Healthcare Sector**: In the healthcare domain different AI systems find their applications in various applications. Computer vison and image processing can be used in radiology imaging in medical care. There is a huge volume of data that is generated as part of patient intake and treatment; the processing and management of this data is important for signal detection and providing better solutions and treatment to the patients. AI system is designed to make the complete process faster and more efficient.

1.4 HEALTHCARE APPLICATION FOR MACHINE LEARNING

Machine learning, artificial intelligence, and deep learning algorithms are extensively used in the field of Healthcare to diagnose diseases and generate results and reports with accuracy and precision. An example is, neural networks are applied to identify and examine carcinogenic injuries from radiology images.

With the quicker processing speed, distributed architecture and consistent result machine learning application are enabled to detect anomalies in radiology images which are otherwise missed by human eyes and facilitate the diagnostic process.

The authors in the paper Kumardeep et al. (2018) based the work on a dataset of 271 patients where 204 patients have positive samples for estrogen receptor and 67 with negative samples for estrogen receptor. After normalizing the data using K nearest neighbor a combination of deep learning and machine learning algorithms such as support vector machine, random forest, LDA, partitioning tree, regression trees, and generalized boosting model among others is used to predict the status of the estrogen receptor. On comparison the deep learning approach resulted in the best accuracy of AUC value of 0.93.

Researchers (Gurovich et al., 2019) have framed their work in applying deep learning to the problem of identification of facial phenotypes of genetic disorders. The dataset used comprised 1700 patient samples with 200 syndromes covered. The trained model has an accuracy of 91%. They have proposed a framework DeepGestalt based on deep learning which applies deep convolutional neural network, after which the image is normalized by cropping and converting it to grayscale, Gestalt model uses this normalized image to predict the syndromes.

Researchers in their work in Marcus et al. (2018) analyze XGBoost a machine learning algorithm to predict minimum antimicrobial concentration among patient data sample. Dataset of 5278 patients consists of non-typhoidal Salmonella genomes samples. Using gradient boosting to minimize the error XGBoost was applied. The results suggested that among the models compared the bet results of 95% accuracy were achieved using the XGBoostmodel.

Another stream of healthcare informatic that has seen a lot of applications for machine learning is Transcriptomic data. This is the data collected for various mRNA transcripts data consisting within a sample. Different datasets and samples can be formed by analyzing and extracting these samples. The following authors have worked with and based their research on Transcriptomic data: Carly et al. (2019) proposed a framework for the diagnosis of tuberculosis using integrated multiple gene expression. From the results, random forest was identified as the best performing model with an average accuracy of 95%. The authors of the paper (Suhas et al. 2020) proposed a model with 96% accuracy for profiling of single-cell RNA sequencing data; the model is based on an approach that uses a combination of an unsupervised clustering for single cell and the feature generated by deep learning model used to profile single-cell RNA sequencing datapoints. The approach in Marin et al. (2018) developed a machine learning model with 80% accuracy for marking age-related changes in the human muscle. The neural network model identifies aging biomarker by analyzing the signature data from patients of different age groups.

Representation of proteins in the form of tissues, cells, or an organism forms the Proteomic data. The work on proteomic datasets is applied by various authors. The authors in their work in Christine et al. (2019) proposed deep learning algorithms with best performance accuracy of 97% for the analysis of leukemia patients for FLT3-ITD. Babita et al. (2021) proposed a hybrid model for the identification of protein structure class. The result shows that the proposed approach has accuracies of 85.36%, 84.2%, 94.3%, 95.9%, 94.9%, and 93.1% independent of whether the dataset is small or large in size.

A lot of data in healthcare is captured from various sensory devices; this includes time series signals which are an ordered sequence of pairs in sensor data. The data from these sensors can range from simple numerical data to more complicated data. The following authors have based their work on such data. Researchers in Luca et al. (2018) proposed utilizing data collected from wearable device to detect Parkinson's disease with the help of machine learning models. The model training data set comprised data collected from 20 patients, while performing 13 different tasks and being monitored by 6 sensors. The total set of 41,802 data clips generated over the period of data collection process was used to train convolutional neural networks and random forest classifier. The performance of the random forest exceeds that of the CNN as it generated results with AUROC values of 0.73 and 0.79 for the two sub-tasks in the problem.

The authors in the paper David et al. (2018) have worked on the area of detection of risk developmental AD and TD in infants. In the experiment the infants are divided into two groups based on their age, group one with infants between the age group of 0–6 months and the other with infants from 6 to 12 months. The movements are recorded using an Opal sensor attached to the ankles of infants. A set of 19 movements as features in the form of count duration and other features were selected as univariate feature selection. The paper presents a comparison of three machine learning approaches including support vector machine, logistic regression, and adoboost for prediction. Different approaches have better accuracy for the two data groups. The SVM has an accuracy of 90% for the 0–6 months data and adaboost has an accuracy of 83% accuracy on the 6–12 months data.

The authors (Sota et al., 2018) have proposed a 90% accurate method for the classification approach for the detection of assisted motion. The data was captured from five patients during two variations in the experiment short set and long step. Eight Flexiforce sensors were used with the shoe to capture the required data; these data pints then were used to build the features for the classification model training.

The authors in Prabhjot et al. (2019) compared and analyzed a hybrid approach for the detection of stress using the Heart rate and Blood presser of the individuals. The sensor in this experiment is mobile phones which are readily available. A combination of Bayesian network and neural network resulted in an accuracy of 92.86% for (Blood Pressure Management) BPM and 85.71% for (Heart Rate) HR which is better than the other approaches considered.

In the research in Shamsul et al., (2018) the authors have worked on a model for the detection of human activities. The data used for experiment was collected using body sensors; these data points then were used to create features based on the Kernel Principal Component Analysis (KPCA) and Linear Discriminant Analysis (LDA). The model itself was trained on the deep-belief network which consists of 40 hidden layers. The accuracy of the trained model is higher than any other counterpart with the accuracy of 97.5%.

The researchers in Elimen et al. (2019) have designed an approach for human emotion detection; the approach is based on a combination of Convolutional Neural Network and Long Short-term Memory Recurrent Neural Network.

The data collection through sensors is done by using mobile devices; some of the data are captured through sensors and some through direct input from the user. A group of 40 females were part of the study and around 550,432 sensor data points were captured in total. The data include biometric parameters, environmental data points, and self-reported inputs for the subjects. The model has shown best accuracy of 95%.

Researchers in Diana et al. (2018) did a comparative analysis of four classification techniques including decision trees, regression Deepnets, and ensemble for diction of fall in elders. The data points were collected using a 3D-axis accelerometer fitted in 6lowPAN wearable device. Sliding window feature extraction was used to extract the features from the data points collected. The performance of the ensemble algorithm was better than the others as it performed at an accuracy of 94%.

The authors of the paper (Jessica et al., 2018) have worked with a sample collected from 64 children to detect depression and anxiety under stress. Wearable sensors were used to measure motions of the participants while performing 90 sec fear-induced tasks. The authors have used machine learning algorithm of k nearest neighbor model with an accuracy of 75%.

Research work in Patrick et al. (2019) proposed an approach for risk assessment in hazard characterization. Availability of high dimensionality of genomics data makes the problem suitable to apply machine learning. DNA data sets for isolation and sequencing are collected and features extracted. A variety of classification approaches such as random forest, support vector machine, and logic boost were applied. An accuracy of 75% was detected for logic boost classification approach.

1.5 IMPACT OF MACHINE LEARNING IN HEALTH INFORMATICS ON HEALTHCARE

The accompanying segments talk about three regions in which AI in health informatics impacts medical services.

- **Recordkeeping**: Record keeping and maintaining is an integral part of healthcare informatics; this includes electronic health record and patient information. The use of natural language processing is to identify and extract relevant information for the HER so that the physician can derive insight. Another application is that of image processing which works with radiological images to support medical decision-making.
- **Data Integrity:** The primary data source for machine learning algorithms in healthcare is EHRs; this data is mostly in the form of natural language, and the data needs to be pre-processed and cleaned before it can be used for training models. Any irregularity in the healthcare information can result in machine learning algorithms making incorrect predictions, which can adversely impact clinical decision-making.
- **Predictive Analytics:** Predictive analysis along with the data from healthcare informatics enables us to improve upon the existing healthcare processes. The development of clinical decision support tools can help improve the patient outcome. The improvement in the healthcare practices lies in the ability to derive insights from the data to predict patient outcome though predictive analytics.

Machine learning can also help in automating certain business processes to generate better outcomes.

- **Disease Identification and Diagnosis:** Machine learning algorithms can distinguish pattern related to disease and ailments by concentrating on a huge number of medical care records and other patient information. Ongoing improvements in AI can assist with expanding medical care access in emerging nations and advance disease analysis and therapy. Various models developed through different research programs can now help in the detection of breast cancer and skin cancer by analyzing medical images.
- **Medical Imaging Diagnosis:** Machine learning based image processing helps in analyzing high-resolution CAT scans, MRIs. AI has exhibited its worth in assisting clinical experts with working on their efficiency and accuracy. Normal use cases for AI in clinical imaging incorporate recognizing cardiovascular irregularities, distinguishing musculoskeletal wounds, and evaluating malignancies.
- **Robotic Surgery and Patient Support Tasks:** AI can utilize the data from previous surgeries and medical records of patients to derive insights that may help in getting favorable results. These procures will not only reduce the chances of human error but also develop minimal invasive surgeries. Robots can assist with increasing patient capacities. These supports could include robot-assisted surgeries and bionics to help patients with physical disabilities.
- **Personalized Medicine:** The ability of machine learning to process huge volume of data from various sources such as EHRs and genetic data, which will help in the advancement of personalized care.

1.6 TYPES OF DATA IN MEDICAL DOMAIN

Data mined from various data sources such as clinical trial records, Omics data along with literature and research articles from sources like PubMed.

- **Clinical Data:** The data generated and recorded during various stages of a clinical trial including electronic healthcare records

(EHR). These would include information regarding the lab test, drug information, and adverse drug reaction data.

- **Omics Data:** Collection of large volume of high dimensional and complex data with information regarding gene, transcriptomic, and proteomics data. Such a large volume of data can be better handled by machine learning approaches.
- **Transcriptomic Data:** The data is an assortment of numerous mRNA records information inside a natural example. These examples are examined and removed to create distinctive datasets.
- **Proteomic Data:** Proteomic information is an assortment of proteins expressed in the structure cell, tissue, or an organic entity. It is the portrayal of genuine practical atoms in the cell.
- **Literature and Research Articles:** With all the research and development in the field of drug developments and the study of the impacts of these drugs on patients and population, it is important to generate insights from these research papers and articles for signal detection.

1.7 CHALLENGES OF MACHINE LEARNING

As AI innovation progresses, it has surely made our lives simpler. In any case, carrying out AI inside organizations has additionally raised various moral concerns encompassing AI advancements. Some of these include:

1. **Ethics in Healthcare**
   Machine learning solution has minimum to no human intervention due to which automated processing has its own set of ethical issues, some of which are listed below:
   - ***Sharing Patient Information***: The personal information that can be used to identify a patient is protected by laws and legislation step by the government. Any part of the patient's personal identification information cannot be shared unless it is for medical reason.
   - ***Patient Safety and Outcomes***: For any machine learning model to perform well, the model needs a very good quality data set for the training. Training dataset quality is dependent on the noise and variation that are covered by the data. In

case of health care domain there are various data generation sources due to which there is a lack of standardization and variations in the data resulting in the model generating incorrect predictions. The training data when imbalanced may not have enough data points to properly represent the minority population and can lead to bias result for the data points that the model was trained on. To summarize, the reliability and effectiveness of a machine learning model is dependent on the data used for training. Such a model when used in a healthcare setup can have adverse impact on the patient health due to incorrect predictions.

2. **Technological Singularity:** Though this topic attracts a great deal of public eye, various analysts and researchers are not bothered by the idea of a machine learning system outperforming its counterpart humans in the future. When we start talking about independent frameworks such as self-driving vehicles where AI systems are to work in close proximity with humans, it brings up some fascinating issues in terms of the ethical implications that this interaction may result in. With the social, legislative, and moral impact of highly intelligent system still not completely explored or understood, it forms a gray area when we are talking about the ethical impact of using such systems in close interaction with common public. And a call needs to be made on whether this system can become part of the public arena or are they only good as research areas.
3. **Impact of AI on Jobs:** There has been a great deal of public focus regarding AI based on employment cutback; the situation needs to be reassessed and restructured. With the mass implementation of any technology there is always a shift in the market demand in the domain. The demand of the market is never gone; it just moves from one form to another, as in the case of automobile industry more and more of the market is moving toward sustainable solution from the existing solution. A similar trend can be observed in case of AI where it will shift the focus from one type of jobs and tasks to another. The data keeps on developing on a daily basis and there will always be need for people to assist in dealing with this

data. The focus of the future job will be on working and resolving more complicated issues that are part of the business process.

4. **Privacy:** Digital data and identity of people and measures to secure and protect this information is talked about when information security and data privacy, data protection, and the concerns regarding the same have enabled the policymakers and legislators to take more steps to ensure the same. In the year 2016, GDPR enactment was made to secure the information of individuals in the European Union and European Economic Area, providing people more control of the personal information they share with different organizations. In the United States, many states have come up with arrangements with organization to ensure that they notify the end user regarding what data is being collected from them and the possible use that the data will/can be put to, like the California Consumer Privacy Act (CCPA). The new constraints and guidelines have helped the organizations to reassess how they store and utilize by and by recognizable information (PII). Moreover, other security concerns have turned into an expanding need for organizations as they identify and eliminate any weak spots or vulnerabilities and openings for hacking, surveillance, and cyberattacks.

5. **Bias and Discrimination:** Diverse implementations of AI/ML frameworks in different domains have, from time to time, reported cases of bias and discrimination which raise many ethical and moral issues with the utilization of these frameworks. The biased results from the models are mostly due to the bias in the training data. While organizations mostly have benevolent goals around their AI/ML automation framework design, this may sometimes also lead to some unexpected and discriminating results. In their effort to automate and improve on an interaction, Amazon unexpectedly biased potential applicants by sexual orientation for an open technical profile, and they at last needed to scrap the project. With more such observations surfacing, Harvard Business Review has also highlighted other aspects and issues around the usage of AI in employment process, for example, what data should you utilize while assessing a possibility for a job. The human resource use case is one of the many use cases where the impact of bias

and discrimination has been observed; some of the other common applications to show impact of bias include social media applications and facial recognition.

6. While organizations have become more mindful of the impact with AI, they have likewise become more flexible and dynamic in their conversation around AI morals and ethics. For instance, Arvind the CEO of IBM has said that they have paused their facial recognition and analysis products, stating that "IBM firmly against and will not condone uses of any technology, including facial recognition technology offering available, for racial profiling, mass surveillance, violations of basic human rights and freedoms, or any purpose which is not consistent with our values and Principles of Trust and Transparency."
7. To further read and have more information regarding the same, look at IBM's strategy blog, transferring its perspective on "A Precision Regulation Approach to Controlling Facial Recognition Technology Exports."
8. **Accountability:** The AI/ML frameworks are very new as compared to the counterpart business processes and because of this there is a lack of significant legislation and legal framework to regulate ML/AI practices. The enforcement of ethics in AI has no real monitoring or enforcement; it is more often than not left to the organization that handles the framework to maintain the ethical aspect as well. As of right now, the prime objective of these AI enabled organizations is to abide by the above said rules that have negative consequences due to malpractice in the AI framework. To reduce this gap, efforts from ethicists and researchers have been directed toward designing ethical frameworks. As of right now, these mainly serve to guide, and research indicates that the blend of distributed liability and absence of premonition into potential results is not helpful for forestalling adverse impact on the society.

1.8 FUTURE OF HEALTHCARE WITH ADVANCED TECHNOLOGY

Healthcare informatics experts remain at the entrance of chance, assuming a key part in empowering AI's combination into medical care and clinical cycles. Their detailed understanding on innovation and how it tends to be applied to work on understanding consideration and results offers tremendous worth to a developing medical services industry progressively dependent on information. The turnaround time of clinical data and patient audit can be reduced by using deep learning algorithms, thus ensuring quicker patient recuperation.

AI has as of now demonstrated to be helpful in the current worldwide pandemic. As HealthITAnalytics reports, a deep learning device can anticipate COVID-19 floods in U.S. provinces with almost 65% precision. As medical services associations look to incorporate AI into medical care and clinical cycles, an essential obligation of Healthcare informatics experts—to guarantee that medical care information is dependable—turns into a high need. Different innovation-driven medical services ideas show guarantee in further developing consideration conveyance in the coming years. These advancements will likewise change the wellbeing informatics expert's job.

- **Virtual Reality:** VR is changing medical services by changing patients' lives and making it simpler to prepare specialists.
- **Augmented Reality:** AR applications in medical services can help better plan clinical understudies. AR advancements can furnish understudies with freedom to gain straightforwardly from specialists performing genuine medical procedures.
- **Wearable Tech:** From counting steps to checking heart rhythms, different sorts of customer wearable advancements give data that can assist individuals with turning out to be more fit. Other wearable advances can furnish specialists with essential data about tolerant wellbeing, including heart cadence, circulatory strain, temperature, and pulse. As per Pew Research Centre, around 21% of Americans utilize wearable advances, like wellness trackers and smartwatches. As more individuals embrace wearable advancements, healthcare data experts can assist with working on the correspondence and exactness of information divided among these gadgets and healthcare data frameworks that specialists use.

- **Genome Sequencing:** Genomic data can assist specialists with making customized treatment plans for their patients. AI in wellbeing informatics empowers hereditary transformations to be examined a lot quicker and helps in diagnosing conditions that can prompt illness. Genome sequencing, made conceivable through AI applications, can affect malignancy conclusion and treatment, and relieve the effect of irresistible infection.
- **Nanotechnology:** As indicated by the National Nanotechnology Initiative, nanotechnology is characterized as "the arrangement and control of issue at the nanoscale." Nanotechnology application in medical services is alluded to as nanomedicine. Nanotechnology can assist with executing undertakings, for example, drug conveyance in which particles, cell designs, and DNA are working. For instance, future nanotechnology medication incorporates drug conveyance techniques that "empower site-explicit focusing to stay away from the gathering of medication compounds in solid cells or tissues," as indicated by Engineering.com.
- As such, medications can be conveyed to designated locales bypassing regions in the human framework that are not influenced by diseases.
- **3D Printing:** According to review published in the Journal of Polymers and the Environment, 3D imprinting in biomedicine offers open doors in the wellbeing area. 3D printing measures consider the proficient production of medication details, inserts, prostheses, biosensor gadgets, and surprisingly human tissues and organs. It sets out open doors for customizing clinical medicines, further develops medical services' quality, diminishes costs, and limits creation chances.

1.9 CONCLUSIONS

With the vast volume of electronic data that is generated now, design and development of faster, more effective, and efficient frameworks to deal with various problems in the health care domain will not only improve the quality of human life but also help us move our focused toward new area. Different machine learning approaches and algorithms such as supervised learning, reinforcement learning, and unsupervised learning can be used to improve the prediction of the models. The results of the model can be analyzed for performance parameters like precision, F1 score, accuracy, and Area under Curve. Different models and approaches have different performance in different use cases. In the sections above we have discussed various approaches for feature creation, extraction, and model training for data from healthcare domain; these include data from clinical trials, genetic data DNA sequences data.

KEYWORDS

- **healthcare informatics**
- **supervised learning**
- **unsupervised learning**
- **semisupervised learning**
- **reinforcement learning**

REFERENCES

Alakwaa, F. M.; Chaudhary, K.; Garmire, L. X. Deep Learning Accurately Predicts Estrogen Receptor Status in Breast Cancer Metabolomics Data. *J. Proteome Res.* **2017,** *17* (1), 337–347.

Bobak, C. A.; Titus, A. J.; Hill, J. E. Comparison of Common Machine Learning Models for Classification of Tuberculosis Using Transcriptional Biomarkers from Integrated Datasets. *Appl. Soft Comput.* **2019,** *74*, 264–273.

Fumo, J. Types of Machine Learning Algorithms You Should Know. Published in Towards Data Science. Jun 15, **2017**. https://towardsdatascience.com/types-of-machine-learning-algorithms-you-should-know-953a08248861

Goodfellow, D.; Zhi, R.; Funke, R.; Pulido, J. C.; Mataric, M.; Smith, B. A. *Predicting Infant Motor Development Status using Day Long Movement Data from Wearable Sensors*. arXiv preprint; 2018, arXiv,1807.02617.

Gurovich, Y.; Hanani, Y.; Bar, O.; Nadav, G.; Fleischer, N.; Gelbman, D.; et al. Identifying Facial Phenotypes of Genetic Disorders Using Deep Learning. *Nat. Med.* **2019,** *25* (1), 60.

Hassan, M. M.; Huda, S.; Uddin, M. Z.; Almogren, A.; Alrubaian, M. Human Activity Recognition from Body Sensor Data Using Deep Learning. *J. Med. Syst.* **2018,** *42* (6), 99.

Kanjo, E.; Younis, E. M.; Ang, C. S. Deep Learning Analysis of Mobile Physiological, Environmental and Location Sensor Data for Emotion Detection. *Inf. Fusion* **2019,** *49*, 46–56.

Kaur, P.; Malhotra, S. Improved SLReduct Framework for Stress Detection Using Mobile Phone-Sensing Mechanism in Wireless Sensor Network. In *Advanced Computing and Intelligent Engineering*, 2019; pp 499–507.

Kitagawa, K.; Uezono, T.; Nagasaki, T.; Nakano, S.; Wada, C. In *Classification Method of Assistance Motions for Standing-up with Different Foot Anteroposterior Positions using Wearable Sensors*, 2018 International Conference on Information and Communication Technology Robotics (ICT-ROBOT), 2018; pp 1–3.

Liang, C. A.; Chen, L.; Wahed, A.; Nguyen, A. N. Proteomics Analysis of FLT3-ITD Mutation in Acute Myeloid Leukemia Using Deep Learning Neural Network. *Ann. Clin. Lab. Sci.* **2019,** *49* (1), 119–126.

Lonini, L.; Dai, A.; Shawen, N.; Simuni, T.; Poon, C.; Shimanovich, L.; et al. Wearable Sensors for Parkinson's Disease: Which Data are Worth Collecting for Training Symptom Detection Models. *Npj Digit. Med.* **2018,** *1*, 64.

Mamoshina, P.; Volosnikova, M.; Ozerov, I. V.; Putin, E.; Skibina, E.; Cortese, F.; Zhavoronkov, A. Machine Learning on Human Muscle Transcriptomic Data for Biomarker Discovery and Tissue-Specific Drug Target Identification. *Front. Genet.* **2018,** *9*, 242.

McGinnis, R. S.; McGinnis, E. W.; Hruschak, J.; Lopez-Duran, N. L.; Fitzgerald, K.; Rosenblum, K. L.; et al. In *Wearable Sensors and Machine Learning Diagnose Anxiety and Depression in Young Children*, 2018 IEEE EMBS International Conference on Biomedical & Health Informatics (BHI), 2018; pp 410–413.

Nguyen, M.; Long, S. W.; McDermott, P. F.; Olsen, R. J.; Olson, R.; Stevens, R. L.; Tyson, G. H.; Zhao, S.; Davis, J. J. Using Machine Learning to Predict Antimicrobial Minimum Inhibitory Concentrations and Associated Genomic Features for Nontyphoidal Salmonella. *J. Clin. Microbiol.* **2018,** *57* (2), e01260–18.

Njage, P. M.; Leekitcharoenphon, P.; Hald, T. Improving Hazard Characterization in Microbial Risk Assessment using Next Generation Sequencing Data and Machine Learning: Predicting Clinical Outcomes in Shigatoxigenic Escherichia coli. *Int. J. Food Microbiol.* **2019,** *292*, 72–82.

Panda, B.; Majhi, B. A Novel Improved Prediction of Protein Structural Class Using Deep Recurrent Neural Network. *Evol. Intell.* **2021,** *14* (2), 253–260.

Srinivasan, S.; Johnson, N. T.;Korkin, D. A Hybrid Deep Clustering Approach for Robust Cell Type Profiling Using Single-Cell RNA-seq Data. *BioRxiv.* **2019,** 511–626.

Yacchirema, D.; de Puga, J. S.; Palau, C.; Esteve, M. Fall Detection System for Elderly People Using IoT and Big Data. *Procedia Comput. Sci.* **2018,** *130*, 603–610.

CHAPTER 2

Emerging Trends in IoT with Machine Learning Techniques for Biomedical and Healthcare Systems

ESHA TRIPATHI[1], UPENDRA KUMAR[2], and ABHAY KUMAR TRIPATHI[1]

[1]*Pranveer Singh Institute of Engineering, Kanpur, UP, India*

[2]*Institute of Engineering & Technology, Lucknow, UP, India*

ABSTRACT

This era of Internet of Things (IoT) with machine learning algorithms enables the advancement of healthcare from face-to-face interaction to telemedicine. Machine Learning Techniques in healthcare make use of growing amounts of health information from the Internet of Things to improve patient outcomes with real-time monitoring of patients which brings out tremendous possibilities for several areas of biomedical and healthcare system. The major areas of machine learning in IoT environment include medical imaging, biomedicine, biomedical event extraction, disease prediction, and detection. Commonly, use of various machine learning techniques in biomedical system is to retrieve information from various medical reports which is used for the prediction and diagnosis of a disease. Meanwhile, new difficulties and issues have been arisen as a result of the technologies. Though the concerns increase, it is being redirected toward treatment of patients not just depending on the type of illness they have, as well as on their genetics, a process known as precision medicine. Medical image processing with IoT-enabled machine learning algorithms is used to diagnose a variety of diseases nowadays. Additionally, machine

Advanced Research in Electronic Devices for Biomedical and mHealth.
Rajesh K. Kesharwani, Upendra Kumar, Raj K. Keservani (Eds)

learning-based prediction is also used in patient care, allocating resources and investigation of therapies for several diseases. Throughout this research article involves various IoT-based machine learning algorithms used for decision-making in a wide area of healthcare and biomedical system in the current scenario.

2.1 INTRODUCTION

Hospitals can use biomedical and healthcare technologies to quickly allocate patients to less congested medical centers. It increases a number of people who obtain proper health-related care. Though healthcare prediction system deals with the problem of unexpected changes in the treatment of a patient in clinics, the request for healthcare-related services in hospitals is driven through emergency works, for example, arriving ambulance during natural disasters, various accidents through motor vehicle, and regular outpatient request (Mtonga et al., 2019). Sometimes medical clinics have missed real-time data on patient flow; often it may create stress for meeting patient's demand, while nearest services may have less patients. Therefore, IOT provides a link between virtual machines and physical objects for smooth communication. It permits the immediate gathering of information through innovative microprocessor chips.

Healthcare is defined as the enhancement and maintenance of health through the analysis and prevention of illness. Diagnostic technologies such as MRI (magnetic resonance imaging), SPECT (single-photon emission computed tomography), CT (computed tomography), and PET (positron emission tomography) can be used to look for anomalies or ruptures beneath the skin's periphery. Similarly, abnormal illnesses such as heart attack and epilepsy can be tracked (Mosenia et al., 2017). The rapid growth of the population, as well as the irregular development of chronic diseases, has put pressure on modern healthcare services. Overall, there is a strong demand for medical resources, such as nurses, doctors, and hospital beds (Iqbal et al., 2021). Therefore, it is necessary to minimize strain on healthcare programs while sustaining the best quality and suitable standards of health-related facilities (Wu et al., 2017). The Internet of Things (IoT) offers potential solutions for reducing the pressure on healthcare systems. RFID technologies, for example, are utilized in medical facilities to reduce medical costs and improve healthcare delivery. Doctors can quickly monitor patients' cardiac impulses through healthcare monitoring networks, which helps them provide an appropriate diagnostic (Birje and Hanji, 2020). Various wearable appliances have been created to provide stable wireless data transmission. Despite the benefits of IoT in healthcare, data security is a concern for both IT specialists and medical practitioners (Shahbazi and Byun, 2020). As a result, several research has looked into combining machine learning with IoT for monitoring patients having medical illnesses as a means to maintain integrity.

2.1.1 BIOMEDICAL AND HEALTHCARE SYSTEM

The Internet of Things has entered a new era in healthcare, allowing professionals to interact with patients in real time. When the Internet of Things is combined with the machine learning, it evaluates demands for emergency care to devise a plan for dealing with problem throughout specific periods. The problem of overpopulation in waiting rooms creates difficulty for many outpatient departments (Kumar et al., 2018). Patients who attend hospitals have a variety of illnesses, some of which necessitate immediate medical attention. When people in need of emergency care are enforced to wait in a long line, the condition becomes even worse. In developing countries, when hospitals are understaffed, the problem becomes even worse. Due to hospital overpopulation, many patients are compelled to return home without getting medical treatment.

Yuvaraj et al. (2017) proposed a platform for wearable medical sensor (WMS) which made up of several applications and utilities. They conducted a thorough examination of the use of WMSs and their advancements, as well as a comparison of their performance to that of other platforms. The authors emphasized the benefits of using these devices to monitor the health of people suffering from illnesses including Alzheimer’s disease and cardiac arrest. However, Miotto et al. (2018) suggested a structure having a fuzzy logic and wireless sensor network (WSN) for monitoring. The researchers combined micro-electromechanical systems (MEMS) with WSN to build a body sensor network (BSN) which detects aberrant alters in patients’ health in a regular period. The researchers (Shahbazi and Byun, 2021) created a measurement method for clinical data that included a microcontroller system, a pulse sensor, and a temperature sensor. Furthermore, the proposed model was connected with base station appliances for remotely managing the temperature and pulse of patients and transferring the data to the medical physician's phone. In emergencies, biomedical and healthcare system can send a message to both medical specialists and the patient's relatives (Iqbal et al., 2021). After that, patients can receive remote medical treatment from medical practitioners by using this technology.

Furthermore, the Internet of Things application has IOT-enabled hospitals to track the critical signs of patients having chronic illnesses (Sohaib et al., 2017; Gao et al., 2020). The IOT system makes use of this variety of data in various ways to anticipate a patient's health status. IoT sensors are attached to the patient's body to detect and recognize their behavior as well as to anticipate their health status. The IoT sensors system, for example, monitors diabetic patients to forecast disease trends and any aberrant state. Patients might receive recommendations for alternative hospitals to seek treatment through the health prediction system. Rajkomar et al. (2018) suggested Zigbee Technology-based and BSN-based healthcare surveillance systems for remote patient monitoring using clinical sensor data. To analyze the health status of patients, they used efficient measures like Zigbee IEEE 802.15.4 protocol, spirometer data, temperature signals, electrocardiogram, and heart rate (Jamil et al., 2020). The data is subsequently transferred across radio frequencies that are visible on visual devices such as desktop computers or mobile phones. As a result, the proposed framework may track patient characteristics such as temperature, glucose, EEG (electroencephalogram), respiration, BP (blood pressure), and ECG (electrocardiogram), and then send data to a database via GPRS or Wi-Fi. After being given to Zigbee, the sensor data is sent to a different network, allowing viewing on several appliances like emergency devices and doctors' and relatives' mobile phones (Shahbazi and Byun, 2021). As a result, by strengthening the link between patients and doctors, the integration of IoT with machine learning simplifies the administration of healthcare in case of patients.

The Internet of Things (IoT) provides methods for supervising and monitoring patients through sensor networks that combine software and hardware. The Raspberry Pi board, temperature sensors, heart rate sensors, and blood pressure sensors are among latter. The model procedure comprises sensor data recording, storing data in the cloud, and analyzing data saved in the cloud to look for health anomalies (Jadhav et al., 2019). Anomalies, on the other hand, frequently arise when anonymous activities occur in unidentified body segments. Whenever the seizure takes place in the brain, for example, the heartbeat tends to be higher (Ahmad et al., 2018). The Raspbian Pi and Raspberry Jessi boards are compatible with a variety of open-source cloud computing systems (Jamil et al., 2019). Machine learning techniques are used by these devices to analyze the recorded data and detect any irregularities (Wiens and Shenoy, 2018). Therefore, the utilization of machine learning with IoT aids in the prediction of anomalies caused by unacknowledged actions in various bodily areas.

It is important to remember that machine learning is a branch of artificial intelligence (AI). Machine learning's main goal is to learn from previous experiences and paradigms. In contrast to traditional methods of just generating code, large data is fed into a generic algorithm, and analysis is done with the data available (Hung et al., 2017). Since big data enables machine learning and IoT systems to rapidly train a model for identifying medical anomalies using simple data, prediction accuracy is directly dependent on the quantity of large trained data (Ngiam and Khor, 2019). As a result, big data enhances the predictive potential of machine learning systems used by healthcare prediction platforms.

Patient load prediction techniques, fortunately, are relied on machine learning, allowing hospitals to quickly share patient load information. In a hospital, past data is collected and utilized to forecast future patient loads so that suitable planning may be made. IoT devices with integrated machine learning methods are utilized to develop a classifier that can identify certain health occurrences in older people, such as falls. The clustering techniques are capable of detecting problematic patterns of behavior in patients and alerting healthcare providers. Similarly, daily habit modeling with IoT microchips is used to track a patient's everyday behavior. The information is used to identify anomalies in older persons.

The purpose of this study is to examine a well-known machine learning algorithm for IoT data classification and prediction in the healthcare business. This article shows that how they worked and compared them based on a variety of factors. To pick acceptable algorithms for developing an efficient prediction model, the study evaluates literature, highlights their merits and drawbacks, and elaborates possible gaps in each existing approach. Based on our findings, K-Nearest Neighbor (KNN) appears to be the most popular prediction and classification technique. In real-time applications, however, predicting the result could take a lengthy time. As a result, some researchers believe that merging Long Short-Term Memory

Neural Networks (LSTM) and recurrent neural networks (RNN) can rise prediction performance. The following question is addressed in this study: How can IoT data be used with machine-learning algorithms to create more accurate healthcare and biometric-based prediction system? The remaining paper is laid out as follows: The ML models and classification are discussed in Section 2. Section 3 goes through the most well-known machine learning techniques that are utilized in prediction and variety applications. The applications of machine learning algorithms are discussed in Section 4. The vast use of IoT and machine learning in healthcare is discussed in Section 5. Finally, Section 6 brings the work to close by outlining future research scenarios.

2.1.2 MACHINE LEARNING FOR THE BIOMEDICAL AND HEALTHCARE SYSTEM

Machine Learning is a subdiscipline of artificial intelligence that concerns about the capability of computer systems to fetch solutions for given problems on their own by identifying patterns in databases. But machine learning allows model to spot patterns and then build appropriate solution concepts based on current algorithms and data sets. As a result, artificial knowledge is developed based on experience in machine learning. After learning through data sets, mathematical and statistical methods are utilized in machine learning. Since subsymbolic approaches and symbolic approaches are two main systems, subsymbolic systems are basically an artificial neural network; on the other hand, symbolic systems are the system in which the knowledge content is explicitly represented. Commonly knowledge content is induced rules and examples. This research is based on the implicit representation of knowledge contents in the human brain. Large amount of input data and several types of input data, streaming data with high speed, and ambiguous and incomplete data are all key concerns in machine learning for big data (Birje and Hanji,2020). Supervised, unsupervised, and reinforcement learning are the types of machine learning. Figure 2.1 shows various types of machine learning, including categories and examples.

2.2 MACHINE LEARNING ALGORITHMS

Machine learning concept is defined as a scientific study concerned with how a computer learns from data and improves learning significantly.

Primarily, it is based on probability and statistics approach. When it comes to decision-making, however, it outperforms more established statistical methods. The information acquired from a dataset and fed to the algorithm is referred to as features. The quality features provided to the algorithm determine the accuracy of the model's predictions. The job of the developer is to find a subset of feature vectors which accurately meet the purpose, enhancing model's accuracy. It is not a simple task. Experiments can be carried out on a regular basis in order to identify the feature subset for the algorithm. Often, it comes to applying a machine-learning approach to an application, then three essential processes are required: training, testing, and validation. The accuracy of the output is dependent on the training dataset; hence training is vital. The algorithm's performance will be evaluated using the test dataset. When using test data to assess performance, it is also essential to minimize bias and increase variance during the testing time. The bias-variance trade-off must be optimized by a suitable machine learning method. Throughout the validation period, the validation dataset is utilized to assess the final machine learning algorithm's performance (Calamuneri et al., 2017). To begin with, it is a good idea to familiarize yourselves with the numerous methodologies used in machine learning, as well as many algorithms that are frequently used for clustering and classification in machine learning.

2.2.1 SUPERVISED LEARNING METHOD

In this approach, training set with acceptable objectives is required. In supervised learning, there are two categories: classification and regression. The trained model assigns input data into distinct classes using classification methods in classification. But the input sources in regression are continuous rather than distinct. Regression predictions are evaluated using root-mean-squared error, while classification predictions are evaluated using accuracy (Bharat et al., 2018). The purpose of supervised learning is to estimate a known output based on the collective dataset. Most tasks that are accomplished by supervised learning can also be completed by a qualified individual. Supervised learning emphasizes on classification technique that requires selecting a subgroup to best define a new set of input data, and prediction, that requires predicting an unidentified parameter. It is frequently used to evaluate and model risk while uncovering links that people cannot see (Deo, 2015). Below are a few supervised learning approaches that are commonly used in computational biology and biomedicine.

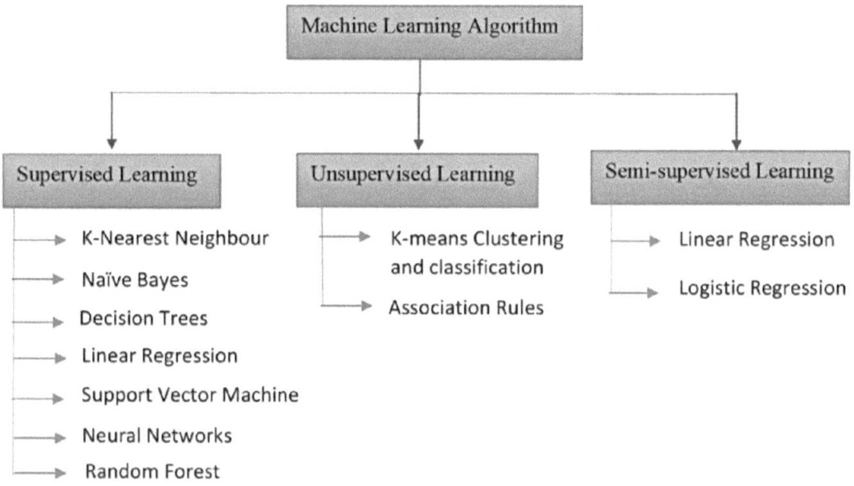

FIGURE 2.1 Classification of machine learning algorithms.

2.2.1.1 K-NEAREST NEIGHBOR (KNN)

KNN is a well-known supervised classification technique that is applicable in a variety of applications, including pattern recognition and intrusion detection. KNN is an easy-to-understand and simple algorithm. Although KNN has a high level of accuracy, it is computationally expensive and requires a lot of memory because both testing and training data must be saved (Mishra et al., 2019). Finding the most comparable cases first and afterward summarizing output variable based on similar instances yields predictions for a new instance. The mean value can be used in regression, and the mode value can be used in classification. The distance measure is used to determine a similar instance. The most common way of calculating distance is the Euclidean distance, i.e., the training dataset should comprise several vectors in a multidimensional feature space, each labeled as a class (Bharat et al., 2018).

2.2.1.2 SUPPORT VECTOR MACHINE (SVM)

Support Vector Machine, a supervised machine learning technique that is often utilized to solve classification problems, may also be used to solve regression problems. The data items in this approach are first plotted as points in an n-dimensional space, with the feature value corresponding to a specific coordinate. It locates the hyperplane that divides the data into two groups. The marginal distance between the selection hyperplane and close-to-the-boundary instances can thus be maximized (Bharat et al., 2018). SVM features fundamental functions that can map points to additional dimensions utilizing nonlinear relationships, which put it ahead of other algorithms (Erickson et al., 2017). SVM is also known as the non-probabilistic binary classifier since it separates data points into two classes. When compared to many other algorithms, SVM is more accurate. However, it is best suited to problems with small datasets, as the training becomes more complex and time-intensive as the dataset grows larger. It is impossible to perform efficiently when data contains noise. SVM uses a subset of training points to improve classification efficiency. SVM can solve both linear and nonlinear problems, although nonlinear SVM is preferable to linear SVM since it performs better (Mishra et al., 2019).

2.2.1.3 DECISION TREES (DTS)

It is a supervised algorithm that uses a tree-like model to examine decisions, their likely implications, and their outcomes. Each branch represents an outcome, and the leaf nodes known as class labels. Once a sample data reaches a leaf node, the label of the matching node is assigned to the sample. When the problem is simple and the dataset is small, this strategy works well. Even though the technique is simple to learn, it has some shortcomings, such as overfitting and biased results when working with unbalanced datasets. However, DT can map both linear and nonlinear relationships (Mishra et al., 2019).

2.2.1.4 REGRESSION TREES AND CLASSIFICATION TREES (CARTS)

It is a predictive model that predicts the output value based on the values already present in the generated tree. A binary tree illustrates the CART model, with each root representing a single input and a fragmented point on that variable. The output of the leaf nodes is used to make predictions (Bharat et al., 2018).

2.2.1.5 *LOGISTIC REGRESSION (LR)*

In the field of machine learning, LR is a prominent mathematical modeling approach for epidemiologic datasets. It starts by utilizing the logistic function to calculate. It learns the logistic regression model's coefficients and then uses that logistic regression model to generate predictions (Radhika et al., 2019). This is a generalized linear model with two components: a linear part and a link function, The linear component is in terms of handling the classification model's calculations, while the link function is in charge of providing the calculation's outcome (Al-Zebari and Sengur, 2019). A hypothesis and a cost function are required for LR, which is a supervised machine learning algorithm. It is worth mentioning that improving the cost function is vital (Al-Hadidi et al., 2016).

2.2.1.6 *RANDOM FOREST ALGORITHM (RFA)*

It is a prevalent machine learning method that can perform both regression and classification (Yarabarla et al., 2019). It is a supervised learning algorithm that uses recursion as its foundation. A group of decision trees is generated in this algorithm, and the bagging approach is utilized for training (Sharma et al., 2018). RFA is noise-insensitive and can be applied to unbalanced datasets. The issue of overfitting is also missing in RFA (Mishra et al., 2019).

2.2.1.7 *NAIVE BAYES (NB)*

The Bayes theorem is used to classify binary and multiclass issues, and NB classifiers are a set of classifying algorithms built on the Bayes theorem. However, they all follow the same rule: every pair of attributes being classed must be independent of one another (Bharat et al., 2018). It is similar to SVM, but it makes use of statistical approaches in the process. When a new input is introduced, the probabilistic value for the given input is calculated among the classes, and the data is labeled with the class that has the highest probability value for the given input (Radhika et al., 2019).

2.2.1.8 ARTIFICIAL NEURAL NETWORK (ANN)

It is a well-known supervised machine learning approach for image recognition issues. Artificial neurons are the underlying principle of ANN in machine learning, and they are analogous to biological neural networks. In an ANN, there are three layers, and each layer's nodes are associated with the nodes in the other layers. A deeper neural network can be built by increasing the number of hidden layers (Ahmed et al., 2018). There are three sorts of functions in neural networks. For a specified set of inputs, the error function will determine how effective or awful the result was. The search function will find the adjustments that will make the error function smaller. According to the search function, the update function will regulate how the changes will be prepared. This is an iterative process that would increase the algorithm's performance (Erickson et al., 2017).

2.2.2 UNSUPERVISED LEARNING

It is impossible to label the data and present them as the training dataset when a developer does not have wide-ranging knowledge of the data linked with the system. Machine learning techniques are used to find similarities and dissimilarities between data objects in these situations. This is an unsupervised approach of machine learning. The existing patterns will be recognized in this procedure, and the data will be grouped according to the patterns found (Calamuneri et al., 2017). As a result, the system creates decisions without being trained by a dataset because the system is not given labeled data that may be used to make predictions (Bharat et al., 2018). Unsupervised learning, it should be mentioned, is an effort to uncover naturally occurring patterns or clusters within data. The difficult element is determining whether or not the recognized patterns or clusters are beneficial in any manner. This is why unsupervised learning plays such an important role in precision medicine. For instance, when individuals are grouped based on their genetics, environment, and medical history, unsupervised machine learning algorithms may identify previously undiscovered links between them (Deo, 2015). Unsupervised techniques include K-means, mean shift, affinity propagation, density-based spatial clustering of applications with noise (DBSCAN), Gaussian mixture modeling, Markov random fields, iterative self-organizing data (ISODATA), and fuzzy C-means (Erickson et al., 2017). Clustering is an unsupervised learning strategy that can be used to divide inputs into groups. However, these clusters are not detected at first but rather clustered together based on their similarities (Bharat et al., 2018). The root techniques are differentiated in clustering based on the distinct features they have. They can be partitioning (k-means), hierarchical, grid-based, density-based, or model-based, using numerical, discrete, and mixed data types within an approach; inheritance links between clustering algorithms indicate shared qualities and advances that they make on each other. The desired clustering qualities that are essential in a clustering method to be implemented inside a biomedical application are speed, minimal parameters, robustness to noise, outliers, redundancy handling, and object order independence. When datasets are too complicated for manual examination, clustering techniques are used; as a result, they must be fast and unaffected by redundant arrangements. It is critical to examine a clustering algorithm to determine whether it is appropriate for the task at hand, like

1. Scalability: When working with huge datasets, the runtime and memory requirements must not be exceeded.
2. Robustness: the capacity to distinguish outliers from the respite of the samples.
3. Order insensitivity: the order in which the inputs are presented should have no bearing on the final result.
4. User-specified minimal input: minimum of constraints that must be provided.
5. Mixed data types: the given objects may have a variation of data types.
6. Arbitrary-shaped cluster: the capability to find clusters of any shape.
7. Admissibility of point proportions: duplicating objects and reclustering should not affect the outcome (Andreopoulos et al., 2009).

When considering the aforementioned variables, it is worth noting that, as a result of the usage of unsupervised machine learning in healthcare, when a patient is being detected for a given condition, the patient will be identified for extra disease as well, if one exists. The purpose for this is that the algorithm has learned facts that must be measured for various sorts of diseases, and it examines the data and categorizes them as diseases based on those data. Furthermore, even though different reports used to identify diseases may contain different types of data, this method allows all of this data to be analyzed at the same time, which is very convenient and time-saving. Concerning the aforementioned features, there is no doubt that the unsupervised machine learning technique greatly benefits healthcare decision-making.

2.2.2.1 PARTITION CLUSTERING

Objects are partitioned and may change clusters based on dissimilarity in partition clustering. It helps a lot in bioinformatics when deciding on the number of clusters to select, such as when working with a limited gene expression dataset. The disadvantage is that the number of clusters must be manually set as an input. However, this method is widely utilized in Bioinformatics. Partition clustering algorithms include clustering big applications (CLARA), fuzzy k-means, COOLCAT, and clustering large applications based on randomized search (CLARANS) (Andreopoulos et al., 2009).

2.2.2.2 GRAPH-BASED CLUSTERING

In interactomes, graph-based clustering is used to make sophisticated predictions and sequence networks. However, this method is slow and sensitive to user-specified parameters. Graph-based clustering methods include molecular complex detection (MCODE), superparamagnetic clustering (SPC), Markov cluster algorithm (MCL), and restricted neighborhood search cluster (RNSC) (Andreopoulos et al., 2009).

2.2.2.3 HIERARCHICAL CLUSTERING

Objects are partitioned into a tree of nodes in hierarchical clustering, and these nodes are referred to as clusters. There are two types of nodes: parent and child. Each node can have one or more child nodes, and each node can have one or more parents. Because clusters may be traversed at many degrees of granularity, this strategy is popular in bioinformatics. The disadvantages are that they are frequently slow, that errors made when merging clusters cannot be undone although they affect the result, and that even if big clusters are merged, interesting local cluster structures may be lost. This method is used to depict protein sequence family relationships, but it might also be used to depict gene relationships based on gene similarity. Hierarchical clustering algorithms include Chameleon, ROCK (robust clustering using links), LIMBO (scalable information bottleneck), and spectral (Andreopoulos et al., 2009).

2.2.2.4 DENSITY-BASED CLUSTERING

The clusters in density-based clustering are subspaces in which the items are dense and divided by low-density subspaces, while the clusters are subspaces in which the objects are dense and separated by low-density subspaces. It is a bioinformatics technique for locating the densest subspaces in interactome networks, which usually involve cliques. The advantages of this strategy are its speed and ability to locate clusters of various forms. User parameters are accepted by some of these algorithms, but not the number of clusters. Density-based clustering techniques include ordering points to discover the clustering structure (OPTICS), density-based clustering (DENCLUE), clustering in quest (CLIQUE), and clustering categorical data using abstracts (CACTUS).

2.2.2.5 MODEL-BASED CLUSTERING

Objects are supposed to match a model, which is generally a statistical distribution, in model-based clustering. A parameter can be used to specify the model, and the model can even be altered throughout the process. In bioinformatics, this method is used to incorporate contextual knowledge into gene expressions, interactomes, and sequences. This approach has a disadvantage in that it takes a long time to process large datasets. If the user's assumptions are incorrect when defining the models, the results will be incorrect as well. Model-based clustering methods include SVM-based clustering, COBWEB, and AutoClass (Andreopoulos et al., 2009).

2.2.3 SEMISUPERVISED LEARNING

A partial training set of data is provided for semisupervised learning. This sort of training is employed when some missing results can be focused on by training data. Semisupervised learning techniques are designed for both labeled and unlabeled data. As a result, it has properties of both supervised and unsupervised machine learning algorithms (Latif et al., 2019).

2.2.4 EVOLUTIONARY LEARNING

In biology, evolutionary learning is mostly used to learn about biological species and estimate their survival rates. The level of correctness of a result can also be anticipated using this method (Latif et al., 2019).

2.2.5 ACTIVE LEARNING

The system only receives the training tags for a limited set of occurrences in active learning. It can be used to improve the optimality of substances to get tags for the desired objective. The advantage of this strategy is that the algorithm not only learns continually but also has the facts it has self-learned validated by querying a user or an information source interactively. It is a modern machine learning method for decision-making that is analogous to budget functions in an organization.

2.2.6 DEEP LEARNING

It is a type of machine learning that revolves around the use of neural networks to learn and predict data. Complex generalized systems capable of accepting any sort of problem and making predictions can be developed using this method (Latif et al., 2019).

2.2.7 REINFORCEMENT LEARNING

The training data is only provided as a response to the program's activity in a self-motivated setting in reinforcement learning. It has an iterative continuous learning mechanism from the surroundings (Sharma et al., 2018).

It would be advisable to include a few examples of machine learning applications in the field of biomedicine after describing numerous machine learning methodologies so that this review is intriguing from the start. Machine learning classifiers are being used in neuroscience to investigate the functional and structural dynamics of the brain.

In cancer prediction and prognosis, machine learning approaches are applied. Prostate cancer is detected using SVM classifiers. Alzheimer's disease has been studied using hierarchical clustering. Different subtypes of psychogenic nonepileptic seizures have been classified using ANN (Calamuneri et al., 2017). With the knowledge gained on numerous machine learning approaches and algorithms, most of which are related to computational biology and biomedicine, it is now time to go deeper into the subject and identify the applications of these algorithms in the topic under discussion.

To begin with, supervised learning refers to a set of problems in which a model is used to learn a mapping between input samples and the target variable, necessitating the use of labeled data with inputs and outputs. Second, unsupervised learning refers to a set of issues in which a model is used to characterize or extract correlations in data without the use of labeled training data or the presence of desired goals in the environment. Third, reinforcement learning refers to a set of issues in which an agent must learn to operate in a given environment utilizing feedback.

2.3 MACHINE LEARNING IN DISEASE PREDICTION AND DETECTION

Various machine learning algorithms have been deployed to forecast or detect a disease in its early stages so that treatment is less complicated and the patient's chances of being cured are higher. Different sorts of diseases have been recognized as a result of these approaches, although with varying degrees of accuracy depending on aspects like the algorithm utilized, feature set, training dataset, and so on. A few diseases will be addressed as examples in this section, along with the necessity of detecting disease as soon as possible, the machine learning algorithms used to diagnose the condition, and the features examined when making predictions.

2.3.1 CANCER

The human body contains the appropriate number of cells of each type. The onset of cancer is marked by sudden alterations in cell arrangement.

The regulation and division of cells are determined by the signals generated by cells. When these signals are disrupted, cells multiply excessively, resulting in a lump known as a tumor. Thermography is more reliable nowadays because it is noninvasive and nonionizing. It has been delivering efficient and positive results with emerging technology, making it superior to other technologies. The manifestation of cancer cells can be detected from thermographic pictures using feature extraction techniques and machine learning techniques. To extract features from images, scale-invariant feature transform (SIFT) and speeded-up robust feature (SURF) approaches can be utilized. The features could be further filtered using principal component analysis (PCA) to make better explanations (Mishra et al., 2019).

2.3.2 BREAST CANCER

Breast cancer is a kind of cancer that affects predominantly women and is the greatest cause of mortality in women. However, early diagnosis of malignant cells by procedures such as magnetic resonance imaging (MRI), mammography, ultrasound, and biopsy can help to lower this risk. The tumor is classified to diagnose breast cancer. Tumors are classified as benign or malignant. It is worth noting that cancerous tumors are more dangerous than benign tumors. However, distinguishing between different tumors is difficult for clinicians. This makes machine learning algorithms useful since they may learn and improve without being explicitly programmed (Bharat et al., 2018).

Many machine learning algorithms for breast cancer diagnosis and classification have been developed in recent years. Preprocessing, feature extraction, and classification are the three stages of their process that can be examined. The feature extraction stage is critical because it aids in the malignant tumors and differentiation of benign. Segmentation is used to extract image attributes such as smoothness, thickness, depth, and regularity (Dhahri et al., 2019). Images are usually converted into binary to extract meaningful information. However, it was discovered that by doing so, several significant elements in the image vanished, omitting crucial information, leading to the decision to leave the photographs in grayscale format. Discrete wavelet transformations can be used to convert images from the time domain to the frequency domain (DWT). The wavelet decomposition is made up of four matrices: the approximation coefficient matrix, the horizontal detailed coefficient matrix, the vertical detailed coefficient matrix, and the diagonal detailed coefficient matrix. These are the values that will be employed in machine learning methods (Al-Hadidi et al., 2016).

2.3.3 LUNG CANCER

The windpipe, major airway, or lungs are all possible places for lung cancer to start. Lung cancer is more likely to be diagnosed in those who have emphysema and have had previous chest difficulties. Lung cancer can be caused by a variety of causes, including tobacco, smoking, and air pollution. The initial stage of lung cancer begins in the lungs and progresses to other organs in the second stage. Lung cancer symptoms do not appear until the disease has progressed to a point when it is extremely threatening (Radhika et al., 2019). When compared to MRI and X-ray findings, computerized tomography (CT) reports are quieter. Techniques such as grayscale conversion, noise reduction, binarization, and segmentation are critical for obtaining the image in the desired format with minimal noise and distortion. The average of RGB is utilized to convert to a gray scale, and a median filter is employed to reduce noise. Segmentation cleans up the images by removing extraneous features and locating objects and boundaries. Features including area, perimeter, and eccentricity are taken into account during the feature extraction step (Rahane et al., 2018).

Small-cell lung cancer (SCLC) identification is exceedingly difficult for humans since it looks almost identical to a healthy lung. This is where machine learning techniques, such as CNN-based deep learning approaches, could be utilized to detect SCLC. Deep learning techniques typically necessitate big training datasets, which is a problem. To get around the problem, you can employ the entropy degradation technique (EDM). High-resolution lung CT scans must be used for both training and testing. EDM uses a shallow neural network to convert vectorized histograms to scores, which are then turned into probability using a logistic function. SCLC detection is treated as a binomial problem in this technique, with only two groups: healthy people and lung cancer patients. As a result, both of these sorts of data are originally provided. While this approach is reasonably accurate, it is far from perfect, and there is much room for improvement. However, it is suggested that it be improved further by supplying a larger training set and a deeper network. Because CNN is utilized in many CT imaging applications (Wu et al., 2017), combining it with image processing improves image processing for better detection.

2.3.4 DIABETES

Diabetes is a chronic disease that must be detected early to receive proper treatment. Diabetes is produced when the sugar ratio in the blood rises, and it makes life difficult for sufferers for a variety of reasons. Diabetes is divided into three categories: diabetes 1, diabetes 2, and gestational diabetes. Discriminant analysis (DA) is a method for determining an input's class label using a set of equations derived from input data. DA typically has two goals: establishing a relevant equation for classifying test samples and interpreting the prediction equation to better understand the link between features.

Pregnancy, the patient's weight, blood pressure, glucose concentration, insulin ratio in the blood, diabetes pedigree function (PDF), skinfold thickness, and the patient's age are all factors to consider when classifying the patient (Al-Zebari and Sengur, 2019). Prediction of type 2 diabetics was possible using machine learning algorithms such as LR, Gaussian Naive Bayes (GNB), KNN, RFA, CART, and SVM, as well as variables from electronic medical records such as BMI, age, serum-glucose1, serum-glucose2 levels, creatinine level, race, gender, etc. (Mani et al., 2012). Various machine learning approaches were applied from time to time to try to increase the accuracy of the forecasts. Neural networks were used in one technique. A backpropagation technique was used to train a feed-forward neural network in this method. Even with this technique, the number of births, skinfold thickness, serum insulin, BMI, PDF, and age were all taken into account, with the plasma-glucose level being the most important factor. When compared to other machine learning techniques, predictions made using neural networks were found to have a better accuracy (Priya and Rajalaxmi, 2012). Deep neural networks (DNNs) have also been used for diabetic prediction, with fivefold and tenfold cross-validation being used to train the DNN. It is worth noting that both of the aforementioned neural network-based techniques have exhibited near-97 percent accuracy in diabetes prediction (Ayon and Islam, 2019).

2.3.5 HEART DISEASES

Heart disease is a serious condition caused by a blockage in the arteries of the heart. The build-up of plaque inside the coronary arteries causes chronic heart disease, which progresses slowly and can lead to a heart attack. Several risk factors for major heart illnesses have been found, including abnormal glucose metabolism, dyslipidaemia, high blood pressure, smoking, aging, and lack of physical activity. Shortness of breath, physical body weakness, swollen feet, and exhaustion, among other symptoms, are all markers of heart disease (Ahmed et al., 2018).

Diagnostics and therapies in several subfields of cardiology are among the tasks that precision medicine has completed. Precision medicine in cardiology has accomplished jobs in interventional cardiology, individualized therapy choices for rectifying heart rhythms, certain gender variations affecting the outcome of cardiovascular diseases, and various genomes studies, to name a few. In today's healthcare informatics, services like patient monitoring and clinical decision support tools are available (CDSSs).

Machine learning has advanced to the point where complicated issues that could previously only be handled by humans may now be solved by machines. The CDSS might be developed to make difficult clinical judgments, recognize newer phenotypes, and create person-oriented specific treatment options using these precision medicine methodologies.

Blood tests are popular among the several research procedures in precision medicine in cardiology. AGES is a precision medicine test that avoids ischemic heart disease by combining other factors with blood tests. Precision medicine is primarily concerned with genetics, and several research studies are being conducted to identify genetic reasons for disease. Precision cardiology has special areas of study in cardiac genetics, cardiac oncology, and ischemic heart disease. When it comes to precision medicine in cardiology, methods like blood testing, genetic tests, imaging tests, or even a mix of these could be employed for diagnostic and therapeutic purposes.

Genetics has a role in a lot of cardiovascular disorders. As a result, precision medicine-based solutions are thought to be more effective, particularly in certain types of disorders. A few machine learning approaches that could be utilized to build exact CDSS utilizing deep learning are Convolution Neural Network, natural language processing (NLP), recurrent neural network (RNN), SVM, and long short-term memory (LSTM) (Niazi et al., 2020).

A machine learning strategy for identifying cardiologic disorders includes preprocessing, feature selection, cross-validation methods, machine learning classifiers, and classifier performance evaluation. Missing value removal, standard scalar, and MinMax scalar are some of the preprocessing techniques available. In machine learning, feature selection is crucial since irrelevant features might skew the classification results of the algorithm. Implementing feature selection before classification reduces execution time and improves classification accuracy. There are a variety of feature selection algorithms available. Relief, Minimal Redundancy Maximal Relevance (mRMR), and Least Absolute Shrinkage and Selection Operator (LASSO) are a few common feature selection strategies (Haq et al., 2018).

2.3.6 CHRONIC KIDNEY DISEASE (CKD)

CKD is a kind of kidney disease that impairs kidney function over time and eventually leads to renal failure. Clinical data, blood testing, imaging scans, and biopsy can all be used to diagnose CDK. However, biopsy has several drawbacks, such as being intrusive, costly, time-consuming, and sometimes dangerous. This is where machine learning can help overcome these drawbacks. SVM was a common classifier in many illness predictions utilizing machine learning. However, when it comes to CKD, there is not much study that employs SVM to classify patients. The main machine learning classifiers utilized in this domain were ANN, DT, and LR. When comparing ANN to DT and LR for CKD diagnosis, the results showed that ANN performed considerably better (Amirgaliyev et al., 2018).

2.3.7 PARKINSON'S DISEASE (PD)

Parkinson's disease (PD) is a progressive and persistent movement disorder. There are no known causes, no cure, and only a few treatment options are available. Parkinson's disease is thought to be caused by a decline in dopamine production, a neurotransmitter that controls movement and coordination. Tremors, rigidity, delayed movement, and postural instability are just a few of the signs of Parkinson's disease. A key characteristic of this condition is abnormal writhing movement. Machine learning techniques and computer vision have been used by some researchers to distinguish healthy controls from PD patients using video recordings and computer vision. Voice samples have also been utilized by some researchers to distinguish healthy controls from PD patients (Shetty and Rao, 2016). PCA and a genetic algorithm can be used to generate a feature set for classification (GA). Darwin's theory of evolution inspired GA. A variable can be thought of as a gene. A chromosome is a gene sequence. The quality of a chromosome is assessed using a present function, and the best-performing chromosome is used to make the offspring. To develop the offspring, genetic operations such as mutation and crossover are employed. It is the concept that will be underlying the feature extraction utilizing the GA (Aich et al., 2019). It is essentially a fight between the chromosomes in which the fittest will live to the end. PCA is a statistical technique for identifying new patterns in high-dimensional data that uses an unsupervised linear conversion technique. Face recognition and picture compression are two common PCA uses (G¨unaydin et al., 2019).

2.3.8 DERMATOLOGICAL DISEASES

Dermatological illnesses are complex and diverse, and few people are knowledgeable about them. Early detection is usually preferable because it can prevent significant consequences. Dermatological illnesses such as eczema, herpes, melanoma, and psoriasis should all be diagnosed early to save lives. The first phase of one technique for diagnosing dermatological illnesses comprised data collecting and data augmentation using photographs. Phase 2 is critical since it is during this phase that the model is developed and trained. The image is turned to an array in the last phase, and the features are broken down using the trained model that was produced. Synthetic minority oversampling technique (SMOTE) and computer vision techniques such as gray scaling, blurring, enhancing contrast, altering the color channel, sharpening, decreasing noise, and smoothing are some of the augmentation techniques available. The model should be trained when there are more examples in the database. Overfitting is avoided by training the CNN using a large dataset. An SVM classifier is used to make the prediction, and the features from the final convolutional layer can be directly fed into the SVM. However, the SVM must first be trained by feeding it the final convolutional layer's trained features as the training dataset. The features will subsequently be transformed into vectors and stored by the SVM (Hasija et al., 2017).

2.4 IOT AND MACHINE LEARNING APPLICATIONS IN HEALTHCARE SYSTEMS TO PREDICT FUTURE TRENDS

As previously mentioned, IoT and machine learning AI have enhanced the health sector by consenting people to wear equipment such as quality jackets and smart bands that monitor their situation and provide regular reports to a database that doctors can access (Vanani and Amirhosseini, 2021). The gadgets can track a patient's vital signs and tissues, as well as provide a progress report to a database. Pathogen presence and symptoms are also collected and reported by the system (Wang et al., 2018). This is a significant development that will aid the healthcare sector in delivering optimal practices. In healthcare, the availability of smart medications, sensors, and wearable monitoring provides value. These techniques aid in the monitoring and prediction of illness patterns as well as future developments. The goal of automating patient and disease monitoring chores is to save time and step in when all doctors are busy, such as during a medical emergency (Shahzad et al., 2018).

Smart technology is critical in this industry for saving lives during pandemics like COVID-19. The wearable monitoring gadgets collect data and transfer it to a database, where a doctor can review it and diagnose the patient or write a treatment. During pandemics, patients can be implanted with smart medicines and smart bands (Internet of Things) that keep track of and collect exact data in order to feed a database. These technologies assist doctors and additional machines in understanding illness patterns and symptoms, allowing doctors to better understand and analyze symptoms in order to produce quick and safe diagnostics (Mocnik et al., 2020). During periods of quarantine, such tactics can improve patient and healthcare provider safety by preventing physical contact with patients contaminated with dangerous airborne viruses using machine learning technologies.

Cloud computing is an important component of the Internet of Things. It enables the connection of a wide range of machine learning AI devices in order to analyze and store data. Another essential element of cloud computing is its ability to store large amounts of data, allowing it to meet the healthcare system's needs. Cloud computing's data-sharing capabilities allow diverse devices to access the same information. Cloud computing, on the other hand, is currently confronted with a number of challenges that must be addressed. These issues could open up new research opportunities for scientists and academics interested in improving the usability of machine learning and the

Internet of Things in the healthcare industry. Data privacy and security is one of these issues. Medical records, which contain individuals' protected health information, are extremely sensitive and must be carefully secured in the healthcare industry (PHI). As a result, severe laws have been enacted to control the process of obtaining and analyzing these data, such as the Health Insurance Portability and Accountability Act (HIPAA). This poses a huge barrier for modern data mining and machine learning (ML) methods like deep learning, which require a substantial amount of training data. Patient privacy may be endangered by sharing this type of sensitive information in order to improve care quality. ML technology has been used to develop a number of solutions for protecting patient privacy.

Federated learning is one solution (FL). In this new ML paradigm, deep learning is utilized to train and enable mobile devices and servers to develop a shared, robust ML model without transferring data (Xu et al., 2021). Researchers can also use FL to solve important concerns like data security, data access rights, and heterogeneous data access. The complexity of machine learning is increased by storing data in a centralized cloud computing environment, because using the same server to collect shared data from several devices while maintaining a generic model exposes the server-to-server failure and bias. This may lead to an improperly trained model, which will have a detrimental impact on the accuracy of the projected outcome. As a result, one of the best practices at the moment is decentralized data storage. Blockchain is a technology that allows for decentralized data storage.

Blood pressure, body temperature, and heart rate can all be monitored using equipment. They are excellent for gathering and storing information about patients, and hence can aid in diagnosis. IoT and machine learning can assist healthcare practitioners in staying current with developments, which is critical for a healthy society. Because keeping track of diagnostic data and COVID-19 symptoms is critical to eradicating a disease or discovering a vaccine, and data can be maintained in a central database and accessed by scientists and medical practitioners for cross-examination, analysis, and real-time exchange of results.

2.5 CONCLUSIONS AND FUTURE SCOPE

Big data's function in healthcare is to help us create better health profiles and predictive models for individual individuals, allowing us to better detect and treat disease. Understanding the biology of disease is one of the major difficulties in today's healthcare and pharmaceutical industries. Big data is used to gather more and more information on what constitutes a disorder at many sizes, from DNA, proteins, and metabolites via cells, tissues, organs, species, and ecosystems. Those are the biological scales we need to model with big data integration. The applications, processing, and handling of huge data utilizing various machine learning approaches were covered in this study. Furthermore, the metrics used to assess the machine learning models' success are based on large data. Machine learning also aids in effective decision-making by employing various strategies to forecast diseases and diagnoses in a timely manner, which can have a favorable impact on a patient's health. Information may be predicted ahead of time, and diseases can be avoided early on. Machine learning allows you to create models utilizing various methods to assist and forecast variables while maintaining flawless accuracy. The rapid implementation of EHR has resulted in a plethora of fresh patient data, which is a gold mine for bettering our understanding of human health. We will witness quick, widespread application and utilization of big data employing machine learning in the healthcare business and healthcare organizations in the future.

As big data analytics becomes more popular, issues including ensuring security, setting standards, ensuring privacy, and governance, as well as continually developing tools and technology, will gain traction. Big data analytics and applications in healthcare are still in their infancy, but significant advancements in platforms and technologies can hasten the process.

KEYWORDS

- **Internet of Things**
- **machine learning**
- **healthcare**
- **medical image**
- **biomedical**

REFERENCES

Ahmad, M. A.; Eckert, C.; Teredesai, A. In Interpretable Machine Learning in Healthcare, Proceedings of the 2018 ACM International Conference on Bioinformatics, Computational Biology, and Health Informatics; Washington, DC, USA, 2018; vol 24–29, pp 559–560.

Ahmed, M. R.; Hasan Mahmud, S. M.; Hossin, M. A.; Jahan, H.,; Haider Noori, S. R. In *A Cloud Based Four-Tier Architecture for Early Detection of Heart Disease with Machine Learning Algorithms*, Proceedings of the IEEE 4th International Conference on Computer and Communications; Chengdu, China, 2018.

Aich, S.; Kim, H.; Younga, K.; Hui, K. L.; Al-Absi, A. A.; Sain, M. In *A Supervised Machine Learning Approach Using Different Feature Selection Techniques on Voice Datasets for Prediction of Parkinson's Disease*, Proceedings of the 21st International Conference on Advanced Communication Technolog, PyeongChang Kwangwoon_Do, Korea (South), 2019.

Aich, S.; Younga, K.; Hui, K. L.; Al-Absi, A. A.; Sain, M. In *A Nonlinear Decision Tree Based Classification Approach to Predict the Parkinson's Disease Using Different Feature Sets of Voice Data*, Proceedings of the 20th International Conference on Advanced Communication Technology; Chuncheon-si Gangwon-do, Korea South, 2018.

Alharbi, R.; Almagwashi, H. In *The Privacy Requirments for Wearable IoT Devices in Healthcare Domain*, Proceedings of the 2019 7th International Conference on Future Internet of Things and CloudWorkshops (FiCloudW), Istanbul, Turkey; IEEE: Piscataway, NJ, USA, 2019; pp 18–25.

Al-Hadidi, M. R.; Alarabeyyat, A.; Alhanahnah, M. In *Breast Cancer Detection Using K-nearest Neighbor Machine Learning Algorithm*, Proceedings of the 9th International Conference on Developments in eSystems Engineering, Liverpool, UK, 2016.

Al-Zebari, A.; Sengur, A. In *Performance Comparison of Machine Learning Techniques on Diabetes Disease Detection*, Proceedings of the 1st International Informatics and Software Engineering Conference; Ankara, Turkey, 2019.

Amirgaliyev, Y.; Shamiluulu, S.; Serek, A. In *Analysis of Chronic Kidney Disease Dataset by Applying Machine Learning Methods*, Proceedings of the IEEE 12th International Conference on Application of Information and Communication Technologies, Almaty, Kazakhstan, 2018.

Andreopoulos, B.; An, A.; Wang, X.; Schroeder, M. A Roadmap of Clustering Algorithms: Finding A Match for a Biomedical Application. *Brief. Bioinformatics* **2009,** 10 (3), 297–314.

Ayon, S.; Islam, M. Diabetes Prediction: A Deep Learning Approach. Int. J. Inf. Eng. Electron. Bus. **2019,** *7* (6), 21–27.

Bharat, A.; Pooja, N.; Reddy, R. A. In *Using Machine Learning Algorithms for Breast Cancer Risk Prediction and Diagnosis*, Proceedings of the 3rd International Conference on Circuits, Control, Communication and Computing; Bangalore, India, 2018.

Birje, M. N.; Hanji, S. S. Internet of Things Based Distributed Healthcare Systems: A Review. *J. Data Inf. Manag.* **2020,** *2*, 149–165.

Calamuneri, A.; Donato, L.; Scimone, C.; Costa, A.; Angelo, R. D.; Sidoti, A. On Machine Learning in Biomedicine. *Life Saf. Secur.* **2017,** 5 (12), 96–99.

Deo, R. C. Machine Learning in Medicine. *Circulation* **2015,** *132* (20), 1920–1930.

Dhahri, H.; Maghayreh, E. Al..; Mahmood, A.; Elkilani, W.; Nagi, M. F. Automated Breast Cancer Diagnosis Based on Machine Learning Algorithms. *J. Healthc. Eng.* (2019)vol. 2019, Article ID 4253641.

Dike, H. U.; Zhou, Y.; Deveerasetty, K. K.; Wu, Q. In *Unsupervised Learning Based on Artificial Neural Network: A Review*, Proceedings of the 2018 IEEE International Conference on Cyborg and Bionic Systems (CBS); Shenzhen, China, 2018; pp 322–327.

Erickson, B. J.; Korfiatis, P.; Akkus, Z.; Kline, T. L. Machine Learning for Medical Imaging. *RadioGraphics* **2017,** *37* (2), 505–515.

Gao, H.; Qin, X.; Barroso, R. J. D.; Hussain, W.; Xu, Y.; Yin, Y. Collaborative Learning-Based Industrial IoT API Recommendation for Software-Defined Devices: The Implicit Knowledge Discovery Perspective. *IEEE Trans. Emerg. Top. Comput. Intell.* **2020,** 1–11.

G¨unaydin, O.; G¨unay, M.; Sengel, O. In *Comparison of Lung Cancer Detection Algorithms*, Proceedings of the Scientific Meeting on Electrical-Electronics & Biomedical Engineering and Computer Science, Istanbul, Turkey, 2019.

Haq, A. U.; Li, J. P.; Memon, M. H.; Nazir, S.; Sun, R. A Hybrid Intelligent System Framework for the Prediction of Heart Disease Using Machine Learning Algorithms. *Mob. Inf. Syst.* **2018,** *2018*, 3860146.

Hasija, Y.; Garg, N.; Sourav, S. In *Automated Detection of Dermatological Disorders Through Image-Processing and Machine Learning*, Proceedings of the International Conference on Intelligent Sustainable Systems, Palladam, India, 2017.

Hung, C. Y.; Chen, W. C.; Lai, P. T.; Lin, C. H.; Lee, C. C. In *Comparing Deep Neural Network and Other Machine Learning Algorithms for Stroke Prediction in a Large-Scale Population-Based Electronic Medical Claims Database*, Proceedings of the 2017 39th Annual International Conference of the IEEE Engineering in Medicine and Biology Society; Jeju Island, Korea, July 11–15, 2017; pp 3110–3113.

Iqbal, N.; Jamil, F.; Ahmad, S.; Kim, D. A Novel Blockchain-Based Integrity and Reliable Veterinary Clinic Information Management System Using Predictive Analytics for Provisioning of Quality Health Services. *IEEE Access* **2021,** *9*, 8069–8098.

Jadhav, S.; Kasar, R.; Lade, N.; Patil, M.; Kolte, S. Disease Prediction by Machine Learning from Healthcare Communities. *Int. J. Sci. Res. Sci. Technol.* **2019,** *2019*, 29–35.

Jamil, F.; Ahmad, S.; Iqbal, N.; Kim, D. H. Towards a Remote Monitoring of Patient Vital Signs Based on IoT-Based Blockchain Integrity Management Platforms in Smart Hospitals. *Sensors* **2020,** *20*, 2195.

Jamil, F.; Hang, L.; Kim, K.; Kim, D. A Novel Medical Blockchain Model for Drug Supply Chain Integrity Management in a Smart Hospital. *Electronics* **2019,** *8*, 505.

Kumar, P. M.; Gandhi, U. D. A Novel Three-Tier Internet of Things Architecture with Machine Learning Algorithm for Early Detection of Heart Diseases. *Comput. Electr. Eng.* **2018,** *65*, 222–235.

Latif, J.; Xiao, C.; Imran, A.; Tu, S. In *Medical Imaging Using Machine Learning and Deep Learning Algorithms: A Review*, Proceedings of the 2nd International Conference on Computing, Mathematics and Engineering Technologies; Sukkur, Pakistan, 2019.

Mandal, S.; Daivajna, V. In *Machine Learning Based System for Automatic Detection of Leukemia Cancer Cell*, Proceedings of the IEEE 16th India Council International Conference; Rajkot, India, 2019.

Mani, S.; Chen, Y.; Elasy, T.; Clayton, W.; Denny, J. Type 2 Diabetes Risk Forecasting from EMR Data Using Machine Learning, 2012; pp 606–615.

Miotto, R.; Wang, F.; Wang, S.; Jiang, X.; Dudley, J. T. Deep Learning for Healthcare: Review, Opportunities and Challenges. *Brief. Bioinform.* **2018,** *19*, 1236–1246.

Mishra, V.; Singh, Y.; Kumar Rath, S. In *Breast Cancer Detection from Thermograms Using Feature Extraction and Machine Learning Techniques*, Proceedings of the IEEE 5th International Conference for Convergence in Technology; Bombay, India, 2019.

Mocnik, F. B.; Raposo, P.; Feringa, W.; Kraak, M. J.; Köbben, B. Epidemics and Pandemics in Maps–the Case of COVID-19. *J. Maps* **2020,** *16*, 144–152.

Mosenia, A.; Sur-Kolay, S.; Raghunathan, A.; Jha, N. K. Wearable Medical Sensor-Based System Design: A Survey. *IEEE Trans. Multi-Scale Comput. Syst.* **2017,** *3*, 124–138.

Mtonga, K.; Kumaran, S.; Mikeka, C.; Jayavel, K.; Nsenga, J. Machine Learning-Based Patient Load Prediction and IoT Integrated Intelligent Patient Transfer Systems. *Future Internet* **2019,** *11*, 236.

Ngiam, K. Y.; Khor, W. Big Data and Machine Learning Algorithms for Health-Care Delivery. *Lancet Oncol.* **2019,** *20*, e262–e273.

Niazi, S.; Khattak, H. A.; Ameer, Z.; Afzal, M.; Khan, W. A. In *Cardiovascular Care in the Era of Machine Learning Enabled Personalized Medicine*, Proceedings of the International Conference on Information Networking; Barcelona, Spain, 2020.

Panch, T.; Szolovits, P.; Atun, R. Artificial Intelligence, Machine Learning and Health Systems. *J. Glob. Health* **2018,** *8*, 020303.

Priya, S.; Rajalaxmi, R. In *An Improved Data Mining Model to Predict the Occurrence of Type-2 Diabetes Using Neural Network*, Proceedings of the International Conference on Recent Trends in Computational Methods, Communication and Controls: Kochi, India, 2012.

Radhika, P.; Nair, R.; Veena, G. In *A Comparative Study of Lung Cancer Detection Using Machine Learning Algorithms*, Proceedings of the IEEE International Conference on Electrical, Computer and Communication Technologies; Coimbatore, India, 2019.

Rajkomar, A.; Hardt, M.; Howell, M. D.; Corrado, G.; Chin, M. H. Ensuring Fairness in Machine Learning to Advance Health Equity. *Ann. Intern. Med.* **2018,** *169*, 866–872.

Rahane, W.; Dalvi, H.; Magar, Y.; Kalane, A.; Jondhale, S. In *Lung Cancer Detection Using Image Processing and Machine Learning Healthcare*, Proceedings of the International Conference on Current Trends towards Converging Technologies; Coimbatore, India, 2018.

Shahbazi, Z.; Byun, Y. C. Towards a Secure Thermal-Energy Aware Routing Protocol in Wireless Body Area Network Based on Blockchain Technology. *Sensors* **2020,** *20*, 3604.

Shahbazi, Z.; Byun, Y. C. Improving Transactional Data System Based on an Edge Computing–Blockchain–Machine Learning Integrated Framework. *Processes* **2021,** *9*, 92.

Shahzad, A.; Lee, Y. S.; Lee, M.; Kim, Y. G.; Xiong, N. Real-Time Cloud-Based Health Tracking and Monitoring System in Designed Boundary for Cardiology Patients. *J. Sens.* **2018,** *2018*, 1–15.

Sharma, S.; Aggarwal, A.; Choudhury, T. In *Breast Cancer Detection Using Machine Learning Algorithms*, Proceedings of the International Conference on Computational Techniques, Electronics and Mechanical Systems; Belgaum, India, 2018.

Shetty, S.; Rao, Y. S. In *SVM Based Machine Learning Approach to Identify Parkinson's Disease Using Gait analysis*, Proceedings of the International Conference on Inventive Computation Technologies, Coimbatore, India, 2016.

Sohaib, O.; Lu, H.; Hussain, W. In *Internet of Things (IoT) in E-commerce: For People with Disabilities*, Proceedings of the 2017,12th IEEE Conference on Industrial Electronics and Applications (ICIEA); Siem Reap, Cambodia, 2017; pp 419–423.

Vanani, I. R.; Amirhosseini, M. IoT-Based Diseases Prediction and Diagnosis System for Healthcare. In *Internet of Things for Healthcare Technologies*; Springer: Berlin/Heidelberg, Germany, 2021; pp 21–48.

Wang, M. H.; Chen, H. K.; Hsu, M. H.; Wang, H. C.; Yeh, Y. T. Cloud Computing for Infectious Disease Surveillance and Control: Development and Evaluation of a Hospital Automated Laboratory Reporting System. *J. Med. Int. Res.* **2018,** *20*, e10886.

Wiens, J.; Shenoy, E. S. Machine Learning for Healthcare: On the Verge of a Major Shift in Healthcare Epidemiology. *Clin. Infect. Dis.* **2018,** *66*, 149–153.

Wu, T.; Wu, F.; Redoute, J. M., Yuce, M. R. An Autonomous Wireless Body Area Network Implementation towards IoT Connected Healthcare Applications. *IEEE Access* **2017,** *5*, 11413–11422.

Wu, Q.; Zhao, W. In *Small-Cell Lung Cancer Detection using a Supervised Machine Learning Algorithm*, Proceedings of the International Symposium on Computer Science and Intelligent Controls; Budapest, Hungary, 2017.

Xu, J.; Glicksberg, B. S.; Su, C.; Walker, P.; Bian, J.; Wang, F. Federated Learning for Healthcare Informatics. *J. Health Inform. Res.* **2021,** *5*, 1–19.

Yarabarla, M. S.; Ravi, L. K.; Sivasangari, A. In *Breast Cancer Prediction via Machine Learning*, Proceedings of the 3rd International Conference on Trends in Electronics and Informatics; Tirunelveli, India, 2019.

Yuvaraj, N.; SriPreethaa, K. R. Diabetes Prediction in Healthcare Systems Using Machine Learning Algorithms on Hadoop Cluster. *Cluster Comput.* **2017,** *22*, 1–9.

CHAPTER 3

Machine Learning Techniques Used for Diagnosing Cardiac Abnormalities using Electrocardiogram

BADAVATH MOHAN RAO[1], AMAN KUMAR[1], PUNEETA MARWAHA[2], and AMIT BAGE[1]

[1]*Department of Electronics and Communication Engineering, National Institute of Technology, Hamirpur, India*

[2]*Department of Electronics and Communication Engineering, National Institute of Technology Karnataka, Surathkal, India*

ABSTRACT

Atrial fibrillation (AF) damages around 1–2% of the human body and is the most serious heart arrhythmia in human healthcare. As per the guidelines of World Health Organization (WHO), coronary thrombosis (CT) is the main cause of mortality throughout world and in India. As a consequence of coronary artery disorder, high blood pressure, alcoholic abuse, and a life in emotional stress, heart arrhythmias, or irregular heartbeats, are among the most prevalent CTs. In addition to the CTs described, an irregularity in heart rhythm is produced by mental stress in long duration, which is a difficult problem for researchers to solve. One of the most important areas of study after the development of the electrocardiogram (ECG) and robust machine learning algorithms is the early detection of cardiac arrhythmia using automated electronic methods. As a gold standard for studying heart function, cardiologists and researchers rely on the ECG because it records changes in electrical activity connected to the cardiac cycles. The research was conducted on ECG

Advanced Research in Electronic Devices for Biomedical and mHealth.
Rajesh K. Kesharwani, Upendra Kumar, Raj K. Keservani (Eds)

analysis and categorization utilizing classic and novel artificial intelligence (AI) methods. As a result of the research, a detailed report is expected. Recent years have seen a rise in the use of AI methods to detect arrhythmia signs automatically and early. This chapter examines the literature of the past few years to assess the performance of artificial intelligence and other computer-based systems for processing ECG data for the detection of heart problems. Performance measurements such as specificity, sensitivity, accuracy, positive predictive value (PPV), etc. are used to evaluate machine learning (ML) and deep learning (DL) methods for detecting the AF from ECG signal analysis and categorization. These are crucial in the early detection of AF because accurate detection of heart problems can reduce mortality.

3.1 INTRODUCTION

Every heartbeat acts as a pump. It supplies oxygenated and nutritious blood to the whole body. The electrical signals that direct contraction and expansion are called heartbeats. Cardiac arrest, acclamation, and heart rhythmus are all examples of cardiovascular disorders (CVDs) and are caused by any irregularity in the heart's operation. Scientists and academics have long been concerned about using automatic algorithms to predict CVDs because many of them can be cured if recognized and treated at an early stage (Thomas et al., 2018). Through an ECG, the sinoatrial node produces electrical impulses at each heartbeat that are recorded. A cardiac arrhythmia is a condition in which the heart beats irregularly compared to the usual range. Cardiac arrhythmia is defined as a violation of abnormality in the rhythm of the heart waveform. Heart arrhythmia is characterized by abnormal heartbeat electrical recordings. This leads to irregular heartbeats, such as those that are too slow, too fast, or disorder in their rhythm. Rhythm of the heartbeat includes paroxysmal super ventricular tachycardia (PSVT), atrial flutter (AFL), atrial fibrillation (AF), and ventricular fibrillation (VF). Hypertensive arteriopathy (HTA), congestive heart failure (CHF), alcoholism, bad food habits, and today's life in modern lifestyle are the most prevalent cause of the cardiac arrhythmia disorder's. CVDs are the most popular causes of mortality rate in worldwide, according to the WHO it account for more than 17.3 million deaths per year (Thomas et al., 2018). Similarly, 17.9 million populations are died in 2016 as a result of cardiovascular disease, according to the latest WHO information sheet ("cardiovascular diseases" 2017). CVD is a reason for death in India, according to the global burden of cardiovascular disease survey (GBCVDS), accounting for around 24.8% of all CVD-related deaths. India has a higher CVD mortality rate (272 per lakh people) than the rest of the world (235 over one lakh people). Furthermore, between 1990 and 2010, the number of CVD-related deaths in India grew by 59% proposed by Prabhakaran et al. (2016).

The prevalence of heart arrhythmia (HA) and heart failure (HF) in CVD patients in India was examined by Vora et al. (2017). Heart failure affected 58% of patients, while supra-ventricular tachyarrhythmia's affected 15% and ventricular tachycardia or fibrillation affected 4% (Vora et al., 2017). AF is one of the most frequent CVDs in India, and it is developed at an increased effect as a function of the modern lifestyle. Long-term AF can be fatal and raises the risk of heart failure (HF). According to the realized AF survey, 1–2% of CVD patients have AF (Narasimhan et al., 2016). The study found that 28% of 301 people in India with heart problems had paroxysmal AF, 26% had persistent AF, and 34.35% had permanent AF. In 14.3%, the condition was discovered for the first time. Even though most arrhythmias are controllable, if they are not detected early and preventative actions are not followed, they can advance to a critical stage and cause stroke and other cardiac disorders. ECG is a great tool for capturing electrical cardiac activity in the heart because it records the signal as it changes in space and time. The numbers above emphasize the necessity for an effective, accurate, and automatic method of recognizing arrhythmia symptoms early. Wearable technologies for acquiring physiological signals, as well as electricity wireless connectivity methods such as mobile, may clear the way for this strategy (Longoni et al., 2018).

Many academics and scientists have researched this problem, and they have developed several artificial intelligence (AI)-based methods to diagnose the type of arrhythmia and provide appropriate treatment at an early stage. A "multilayer back propagation neural network (MBPNN)" with ECG is represented in a minimalistic manner and parameters were used to present a novel technique for diagnosing ECG abnormalities, which is widely used in AI (Andrysiak, 2016; Dua et al., 2019). The neural network model used to validate the method was trained and tested using the well-known MIT-BIH database. The NN model's detection accuracy was 98.66%, with 40 neurons in each of the three hidden layers. Based on weighted fuzzy membership functions, a neuro-fuzzy system was created by Lee et al. (2017) to establish an automatic approach for detecting ventricular fibrillation (VF). The accuracy of the categorization approach was tested using 48 arrhythmia recordings from the MIT-BIH collection. Normal sinus rhythm and VF were appropriately diagnosed, according to the simulation results (99.5% classification accuracy). Manogaran et al. (2018) described a strategy based on a neuro-fuzzy inference system for identifying cardiac disease. To better understand heart disease, they developed a multilevel neural network structure with positive nodes in the hidden layers. IF-THEN rules are used to train the model on a variety of clinical indications such as high blood pressure, pulse rate, skin temperature, cholesterol, and more. The mean square error of 0.01 with the parameters connected to the model cardiac arrest symptoms and the parameters used to test the network for better cardiac disease diagnosis. Researchers have used the ML and DL neural networks, and they had worked out to extract and classify features from ECG data for continuous processing and assessment.

El Attaoui et al. (2020) classified normal and diseased heart rhythms based on "wireless sensor networks (WSN) and the internet of things (IoT)." The MIT-BIH database's ECG signals are fed into a "multilayer perception neural network (MLPNN)" that has been competent to capture R-R intervals appearance. A real-time electrocardiogram signals recording prototype of the suggested method has also been created. Myocardial infarction is a serious cardiac condition that causes abnormal heart rhythm and early death due to a shortage of oxygenated blood supply to the cardiac muscle. According to the WHO, heart attacks cause 85% of cardiovascular disease (CVD) mortality (El Attaoui et al., 2020).

Cervigón et al. (2021) proposed a primary aim of this article to calculate the influence of ECG signal compression and automated identification of AF. To decompose the data, the researchers utilized wavelet transforms, followed by the "set partitioning in hierarchical trees (SPIHT)" method to compress the ECG signal. To determine the existence or absence of AF, R-R interval statistics were utilized to calculate Shannon entropy. There is evidence to suggest that compression ratios (CRs) accuracy of up to 90% is achieved while retaining a detection ROC of at least 0.9. In Chen et al. (2021) by our estimating criteria, we propose to use multi-feature extraction from ECG signals, cluster analysis, one-versus-one rule (OVO), and support vector machine (SVM) to identify AF based on CNN. Using the proposed method 98.92% accuracy, 97.04% specificity, 97.19% sensitivity, and 96.47% true positive rate were achieved. The accuracy of this algorithm is 23.25% better than the existing methods. In Shi et al. (2021), in this study, ECG signals with just one lead are screened for the presence of atrial fibrillation (AF). "Discriminant canonical correlation analysis (DCCA) feature fusion" is used in the proposed technique. They got experimental results accuracy, sensitivity, specificity, and F1-score as 91.7%, 90.4%, 93.2%, and 88%, respectively. Because of the emergence of wearable and implanted sensing technologies (Yang et al., 2019), there is much potential to develop solutions for the collection of biomarkers including ECG that are low-cost, low-energy, and efficient. Instead, cutting-edge machine learning and deep learning algorithms can use ECG data acquired from smart sensing devices to harness the intelligence needed for AF's automatic decisions. Although the possibilities are unlimited and both industries continue to grow, currently, the idea of having an electronic sensor system with AI for automatic evaluations or AF assessment is unrealistic. To satisfy the demands of "always online" conditions and true diagnostic requirements, thus a system should be low-power and low-cost. To eliminate unnecessary in-clinic visits and false alarms that can lead to stress, acceptable identification accuracy along with high computing capacity is required. This study analyzes and exposes relevant concepts and important processes in an organized manner, as illustrated in Figure 3.1, to create a machine learning-based AF detection solution.

The following are the main contributions of this chapter:

1. It summarizes the most common causes of AF and the related risks.
2. For those who do not know anything about AF, this is a great starting point.
3. It covers a list of common AF data collection methods and equipment.
4. Key biomarkers essential for the creation of machine learning-driven AF detection algorithms are identified, reviewed, and discussed.

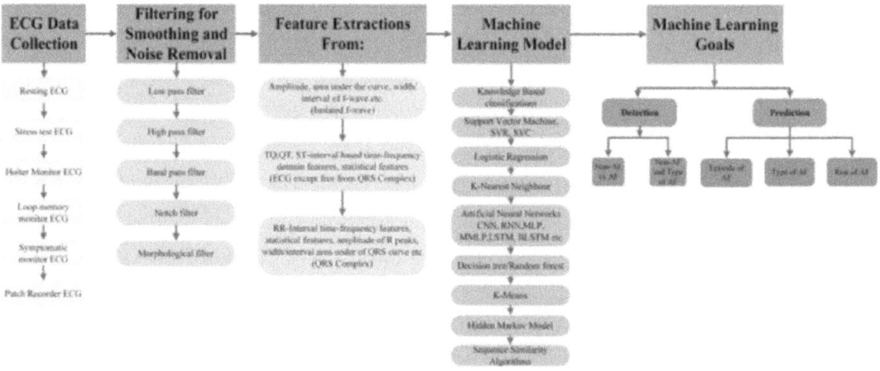

FIGURE 3.1 AF detection process based on ECG data and important characteristics.

We need to find detailed explanations of all the essential steps involved in data preprocessing and the creation of ML models to detect and identify AF.

This chapter contains a brief overview of current technology and electronic system used for AF diagnosis, how to record ECG signal and collection of dataset. This chapter provides a comprehensive discussion of all these aspects of AF self-determination in one place, which has never been done before. Researchers wanting to create ML-based methods for early detection and prediction of AF might use this paper as a thorough guide.

3.2 ELECTROCARDIOGRAM

A noninvasive electrocardiogram (ECG) is recorded using skin electrodes and processed by an ECG device. ECG reveals a voltage between electrode pairs as well as the heart's muscular activity monitored from different angles. Each arrhythmia has its unique heartbeat pattern. It is feasible to identify these patterns and kinds of patterns in a variety of situations. An electrocardiogram is the basic diagnostic tool for analyzing ECG signals. With every heartbeat, the atrial depolarization ventricular depolarization, and ventricular repolarization occur successively and represented by ECG waves. Electrical activity and heartbeats are recorded by an ECG machine. Due to their complexity, these complexes can be used to diagnose a wide spectrum of heart issues.

3.2.1 CARDIAC CYCLE AND ECG SIGNAL

In the human body, the circulatory system ensures that the blood, which contains oxygen and nutrients, reaches the whole body. Four chambers work together to form the cardiovascular system. The upper two chambers of the heart, the left and right atriums, receive blood and transmit it to the lower chambers via a pair of valves. The left and right ventricles, the lower chambers of the heart, are responsible for supplying oxygenated blood to other organs and tissues in the body (Athanasiou et al., 2017). Deoxygenated blood is stored on the right side of the heart, while oxygenated blood is stored on the left side (Calvert et al., 2012). Figure 3.2 depicts the heart's atria, ventricles, lungs, and other major organs as they change over the cardiac cycle.

The heartbeats are separated by the cardiac cycle, which is a set of mechanical movements that occur in the heart muscles between one pulse and the following heartbeat. Diastole and systole are the two primary phases of the

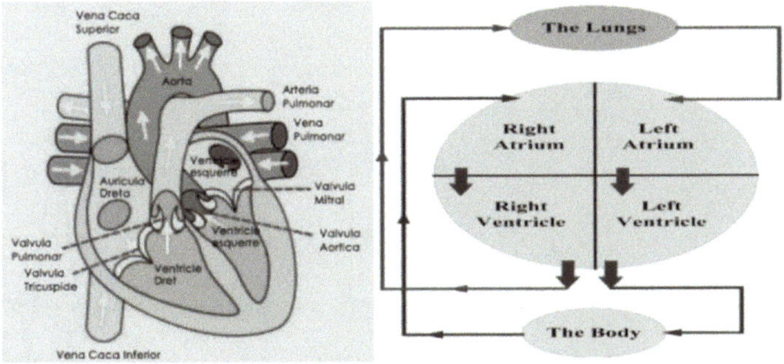

FIGURE 3.2 (a) Human heart structure; (b) blood flow in chambers and other body parts.

Source: Reprinted with permission from Saini et al., 2021. Copyright © 2021, The Author(s), under exclusive license to Springer Nature B.V.

heart cycle. During diastole, heart chambers relax to allow blood to fill them, whereas during systole, heart chambers contract to allow blood to exit. Diastole and systole phases are defined by cyclic changes in heart volume and pressure (Calvert et al., 2012). While in diastole, as seen in Figure 3.3, the volume and pressure of the left ventricle fluctuate. Electrical impulses are generated under the supervision of the sinoatrial node; it works like a biological pacemaker to promote regular contraction and relaxation of the cardiovascular system. As the heart rate (HR) and stroke volume (SV) are multiplied, we get cardiac output. Cardiovascular output is calculated by multiplying the stroke volume (70 mL) by the usual heart rate of 72 beats per minute (bpm).

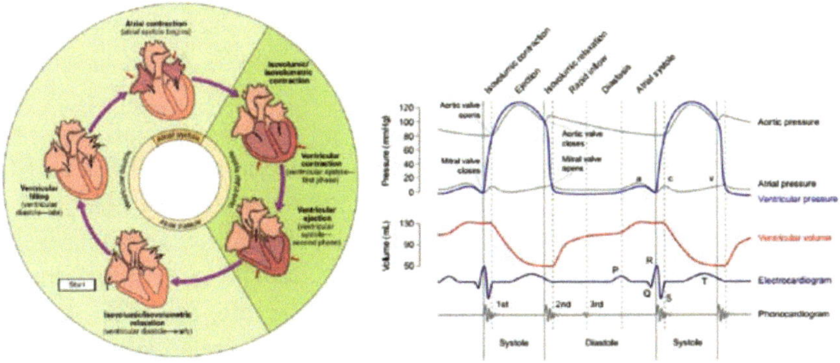

FIGURE 3.3 (a) Various steps of cardiac cycle; (b) diastole and systole steps variations in pressure and volume.

Source: (a) Access for free at https://openstax.org/books/anatomy-and-physiology-2e/pages/1-introduction. https://creativecommons.org/licenses/by/4.0/

(b) adh30 revised work; Redrawn as SVG by xavax. https://creativecommons.org/licenses/by/4.0/

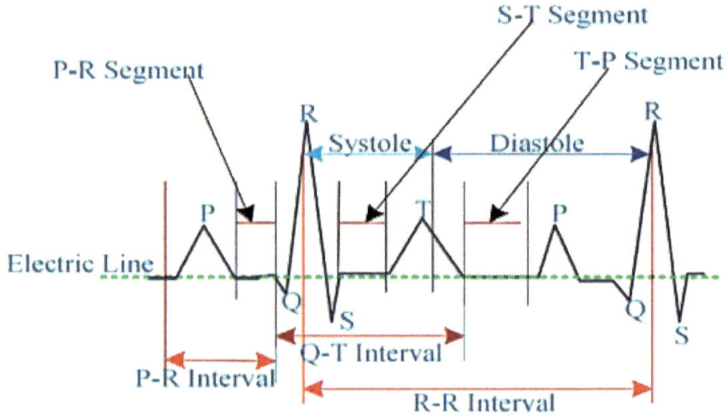

FIGURE 3.4 ECG waveform indicating important events.

TABLE 3.1 ECG Wave Components (Chinchkhede et al., 2011).

ECG segments	Heart functions
P-wave	Atrial Systole (Atrial Depolarization and Contraction)
QRS-Complex	Ventricular Systole (Ventricular Depolarization and Contraction)
T-wave	Ventricular Diastole (Ventricular Repolarization and Relaxation)
U-wave	After Depolarization in ventricular

As shown in Figure 3.4, an electrocardiogram, commonly known as an EKG, is a graphical representation of bio-potentials formed based on electrical stimulation connected with a cardiac functioning. It is widely used by physicians and researchers to diagnose a range of heart dysfunction (Chinchkhede et al., 2011; Trahanias et al., 1990). An ECG recording consists of five important waveforms, P, Q, R, S, and T (Trahanias et al., 1990). An ECG graph is shown in Figure 3.4 as bio-potentials (mV) over time (seconds). Atrial systole occurs when the P wave appears on an ECG. As the function of depolarization of the ventricles, the "QRS complex" (Q, R, and S points) appears. Ventricular diastole, or ventricular repolarization, is shown by the T wave (Mahmoud et al., 2006). The ECG signal does not record atrial repolarization. During the heart's cycle, the ECG wave has several portions, as shown in Table 3.1. Since it has a relatively high amplitude compared to other electrocardiogram segments, the "QRS complex" is employed as the most important segmentation in EKG signal for the diagnosis of the heart disease. 5–25 hertz (Hz) is the time-frequency bands of the QRS waveform (Subramanian, 2017). A collection of ECG segments important for studying and diagnosing disorders is provided in Table 3.2.

TABLE 3.2 Normal ECG Wave Duration (Subramanian, 2017).

ECG segments	Time duration (S)
PR-Segment	0.12–0.2
QRS-Complex	0.08–0.12
QT-Interval	0.35–0.44
ST-Segment	0.05–0.15
P-Complex	0.08–0.11

3.2.2 ECG SIGNAL ACQUISITION

Electrical impulses from the sinoatrial node are transmitted to the heart muscle to coordinate the rhythmic activity of each heart chamber. Electrical events on the skin's surface generate potentially, which can be detected utilizing noninvasive procedures, appropriate electrodes, and digital components. Working electrode on the body surface records bio-potentials, which are converted into weak electrical signals and processed through several steps of a data acquisition circuit to produce a digital ECG record. Figure 3.5 shows the data acquisition of the primary bio-potentials required to acquire the digital version of the ECG signal. The signal must be filtered between 0.05 and 150 Hz before digitalization at a sample rate of 500 samples per second.

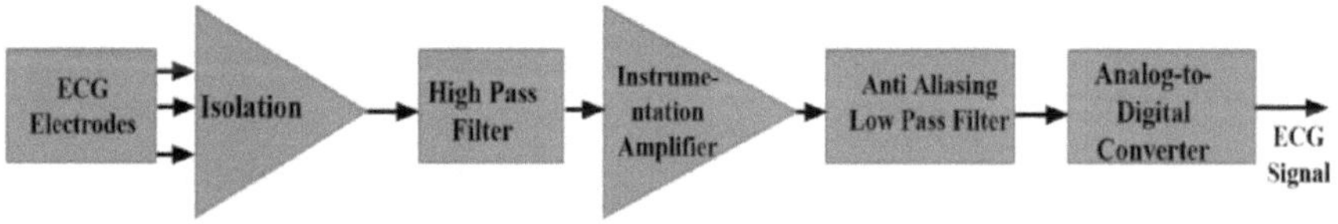

FIGURE 3.5 ECG signal recording for all stages.

While much progress has been made since 1887, the great majority of ECG recordings are still restricted to healthcare center observation and full-length ECG recordings are not prevalent. A variety of ECG signal capture methods are currently available. An ECG recording is morphologically affected by the positioning of electrodes (Silva et al., 2015). In hospitals, bedside monitors and Holter monitoring systems use the standard 12-lead electrode placement approach, where electrodes are inserted at particular locations on the chest, arms, and legs. For the 12-lead ECG standard, Figure 3.6 shows the different sites at the chest and limbs of the subject.

3.2.3 ECG LEADS

Electrocardiography, for example, uses electrodes (sensors) attached to the chest, limbs, wires, and hardware to connect them to a processing and recording device to store the potentially connected cardiac electrical events as it spreads throughout the body's surface. The precise positioning of electrodes is essential for the electrocardiograph's morphology and accuracy, as well as for preventing muscular artifacts (Hornick et al., 2019). Various ECG lead systems are available, for example, motionless systems, mobile healthcare devices, and many of these biomarkers relate to our mental wellness and physical health, and there is new *wearable technology* that picks up on our emotions (Trahanias et al., 1990).

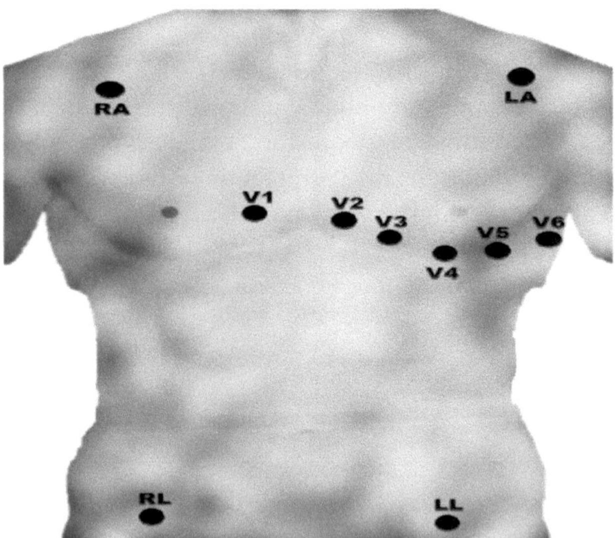

FIGURE 3.6 12-leads ECG electrodes placement.

The difference in electrical potential between two electrodes is referred to as a "lead." Conventional ECG cardiographs use 12-electrode devices (via 10 leads) that record every electrical wave marked by the heart functioning from various phases to graphically fully classify the cardiac movement (Luz et al., 2016). Each lead causes the heart to beat in a unique pattern. The ECG signal formed by the 12 leads is shown in Figure 3.7. The 12-lead system has four electrodes on each right and left limb, as well as six additional electrodes on different areas of the chest. Figure 3.6 depicts a configuration of ten electrodes. The system's electrical ground is provided by the RL electrode. The extremity or limb leads come from the limb electrodes, whereas the precordial or chest leads come from the chest electrodes.

The two types of extremity leads are bipolar limb leads and enhanced unipolar limb leads. Enhanced unipolar limb leads are measured by combining leads aVR, aVL, and aVF. Standard limb leads are measured by combining leads I, II, and III. Einthoven's triangle was named after the Dutch cardiologist and scientist that came up with the concept of recording the ECG in 1895 utilizing bidirectional wires to assess the electrical potential at one electrode for another (Goldberger et al., 2017).

To achieve almost zero potential, three (RA + LA + LL) end electrodes are connected in one place. Unipolar leads were discovered in the 1930s, years after bipolar leads were used to measure bio-potential at a single-limb electrode.

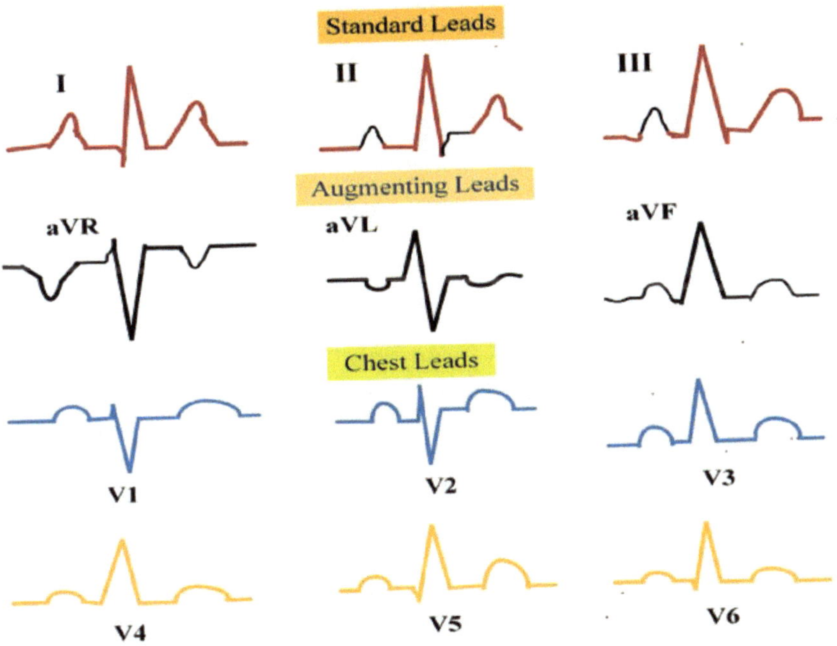

FIGURE 3.7 Normal ECG recording from the 12 surface leads.

Source: Adapted from Washington Heart Rhythm Associates LLC. https://www.washingtonhra.com/ekg-monitoring/12-lead-electrocardiogram-ekg.php

The electrical potential of a particular electrode is measured for precardial leads (V1–V6). Preset points on the chest. All 12 conventional leads are connected on the ECG. The six precardiac leads identify bio-potentials that run down the body's horizontal plane, while the six limb leads, each at 30 degrees, disperse the bio-potential across the frontal plane. The 12 leads offer 3D information on the heart's electrical activity, allowing any aberrant rhythm in the heartbeat to be detected. Tseng et al. (2010) introduced a remote computer to take an ECG for 15 s with a total of 12 leads.

3.3 ECG ARRHYTHMIAS

Several heart rhythms can be detected using ECG data. The human body is extremely vulnerable to certain ECG rhythms, which can increase the risk of death. There are a variety of serious heart arrhythmias and dangers linked with AF, as depicted in Figure 3.8.

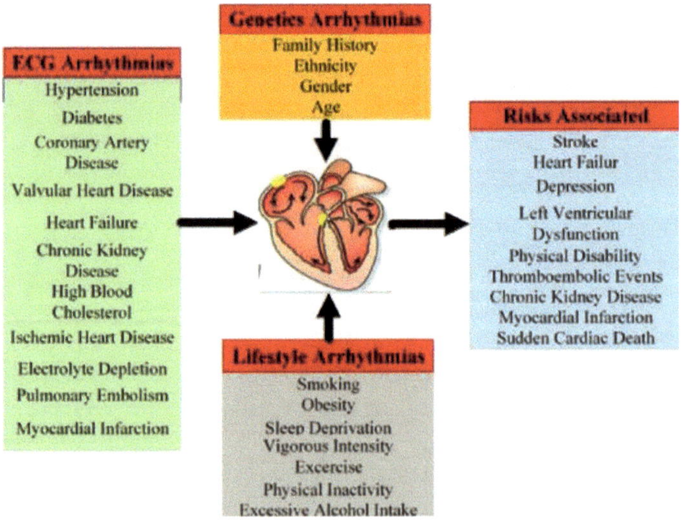

FIGURE 3.8 ECG arrhythmia's and risks associated with atrial fibrillation.

3.4 ATRIAL FIBRILLATION AND ITS TYPES

AF is a heart rhythm that is irregular and often rapid, which can raise the risk of strokes, heart failure, and other complications. The upper chambers of the heart (atria) beat in time with the lower chambers. There may be no symptoms at all, but when they do appear, they include palpitations. Some persons may have chest pain, weakness, or a rapid heart rate as a function of depression and fatigue. Symptoms, etiology, electrophysiology, and other factors can all be used to classify AF (Lubitz et al., 2010). The American Heart Association (AHA), the American College of Cardiology, and the European Society of Cardiology (ACC&ESC) proposed this temporal rhythm-based categorization scheme (Fuster et al., 2007). Because of its simplicity and clinical relevance, they suggest this classification approach. It is the most widely used and approved categorization method for AF.

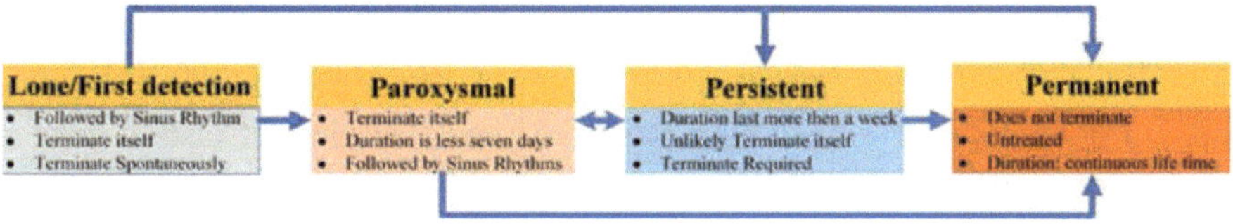

FIGURE 3.9 Types of atrial fibrillation.

Figure 3.9 depicts the four main classifications identified in this methodology, which are addressed further down. In essence, a single episode of each kind of AF has the identical pattern or electrical signature. The frequency with which those episodes occur and the length of time they continue are used to classify them. The main four types of AF:

1. Paroxysmal of AF (PAF)
2. Persistent of AF (PeAF)
3. Long term PeAF
4. Permanent of AF

3.4.1 PAROXYSMAL AF

In paroxysmal, what happens is that the irregular and rapid heartbeat starts abruptly and stops by itself within seven days. It is quite difficult to keep a check on the AF when it is in action. The identity of this disease is also very significant, as medication has high efficacy in the treatment.

3.4.2 PERSISTENT AF

It is also a heart disorder characterized by irregular and rapid heartbeats. If the symptoms persist for more than seven days but resolve on their own, they are still treatable, and effective observation can assist in the early diagnosis of therapy.

3.4.3 LONG-TERM PEAF

When this happens, the arrhythmic episodes last up to seven days. The current cardioversion lasts between 48 and 7 days. It has been an occurrence of AF regularly for more than a year.

3.4.4 PERMANENT AF

It is not possible to correct the abnormal heart rhythm. It lasts a year or more and is not going away. To undergo long-term medication and electroshock treatment, there are more variations such as *Lone AF*, *Valvular AF,* and *Non-Volvular AF*. Lonely AF, which means that there is no underlying heart disease, can lead to poor blood circulation and blood clots are more likely to occur as a result of this and heart abnormalities.

The direction of arrows in Figure 3.9 highlights the evolution of AF from one stage to the next. For PAF patients, the chronic phase can be reached depending on another severity and prevalence of their AF incident or how well their medications work. It is quite unlikely to reverse AF once it has become permanent. It is difficult to recognize AF promptly might raise the likelihood of AF progressing to an advanced stage. It can also lead to other common disorders. As a result, the earlier AF is recognized, the better the odds of taking preventative or corrective actions to avert serious illnesses such as stroke or heart failure. ML is frequently used to evaluate AF (Pourbabaee et al., 2018), forecast AF episodes (Zong et al., 2001), and distinguish between different forms of AF (Akbilgic et al., 2016).

3.5 AF DETECTION APPROACHES

AF detection methods are discussed in this section. AF may be detected using a collection of machine and deep learning methods, but the data must first be transformed into a format that classifiers can utilize to find the most relevant classifications.

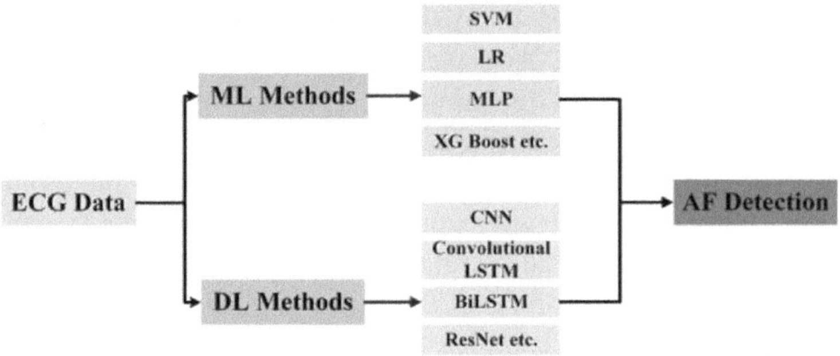

FIGURE 3.10 AF detection methods.

Source: Reprinted with permission from Liaqat et al., 2020. Copyright © 2020 by the authors. Licensee MDPI, Basel, Switzerland. http://creativecommons.org/licenses/by/4.0/

As a result, DL approaches challenge these principles and surpass efficiency methods in several applications, including text classification and picture classification (Kwon et al., 2020). The abstract characteristics of raw data are extracted and classified using DL techniques (Grégoire et al., 2020). This section discusses some significant approach approaches for detecting AF. Figure 3.10 depicts the suggested conceptual framework, which is addressed in depth in the following sections.

3.5.1 AF DETECTION USING MACHINE LEARNING TECHNIQUES

Bruser et al. (2012) used bed-mounted sensors to develop a method for detecting AF using heart vibration signals. Patients are observed remotely, and the effectiveness of the strategy is evaluated using a variety of machine learning classifiers (Bruser et al., 2012). Furthermore, Xiong et al. (2018) suggested a k-means-based technique for finding the AF. The methodology's efficiency is assessed using the PubMed dataset; empirical findings show that maximal entropy outperforms alternative approaches (Xiong et al., 2018). However, an algorithm based on spectral entropy and linear categorization of ECG signals has been presented. Thirteen patients were used to evaluate the procedure's effectiveness. Instead of looking for cardiac peaks in the ECG data, this method can function with any frequency of ECG signal (Hurnanen et al., 2016). Asgari et al. (2015) recommended using stationary wavelet transforms and machine learning approaches like support vector machines to evaluate AF. The technique does not rely on evaluating P and R peaks. This technique had good outcomes when compared to other algorithms, according to the results. Furthermore, Andersen et al. (2019) described a machine learning algorithm-based technique for predicting AF from long-term ECG records. With the use of the information, traits might be extracted and incorporated into the strategy. Classifiers produce a huge number of false positives while analyzing improperly classified data, which affects the approach's output. The technique's efficiency can be improved by manually locating and removing the noise exposure in the ECG signal, but it is computationally complexity (Andersen et al., 2019). In order to improve the performance, Wu et al. (2019) has proposed and investigated many DL based algorithms such as CNN and LSTM, with the conclusion that neural networks generate best and high achieved the performance measures without processes the extraction of the features. A hybrid CNN/LSTM approach was used to improve AF detection performance (Wu et al., 2019). However, Nemati et al. (2016) used machine learning techniques to develop a system for detecting various diseases. The approach detects AF based on wrist-based noise. The movement's duration and ambulatory pulsatile rate are also measured. The proposed approach had good experimental results after a 10-fold cross-validation exercise (Nemati et al., 2016). The novel approach to detecting AF in the general population is first and foremost proven to be exceptionally accurate in monitoring AF. Following feature extraction, several ML classifiers (e.g., including SVM, logistic regression, MLP, XGBoost, CNN, and LSTM) were used to test the mechanism's performance. SVM was the most effective, followed by logistic regression, MLP, and LSTM for testing.

3.5.1.1 SUPPORT VECTOR MACHINE (SVM)

To find the hyperplane in the n-dimensional input space, we use the well-known machine learning technique SVM. Nonlinear classifier problems can be solved using the SVM by utilizing a variety of kernel functions (Suykens et al., 1999). The SVM's fundamental premise is to use a decision boundary to divide the space between data points.

3.5.1.2 MULTILAYER PERCEPTIONS (MLP)

The MLP is made up of neurons, which are interconnected processing components that are connected to distinct weighted inputs. The sum of all connected inputs is a neuron's output, and a nonlinear processing unit known as a transfer function is then applied. MLP's goal is to understand the connection between input and output to translate inputs into understandable outputs and to provide a solution to problems that are not yet known (Naraei et al., 2016). MLP's architecture can be shown in Figure 3.11. An MLP classifier is trained by extracting characteristics from the fully connected layer and using them to identify the AF automatically. A hidden layer is found in the MLP classifier, according to the findings of the experiments. In terms of MLP performance, the 0.09 learning rate is the best. To train the MLP classifier, there are 100 epochs used in the process.

3.5.1.3 LOGISTIC REGRESSION (LR)

A statistic uses logistic regression, also known as logit regression, to estimate the probability of an event based on previous data (Dashtipour et al., 2019). Regression using logit can be used to analyze both binary and multi-class data.

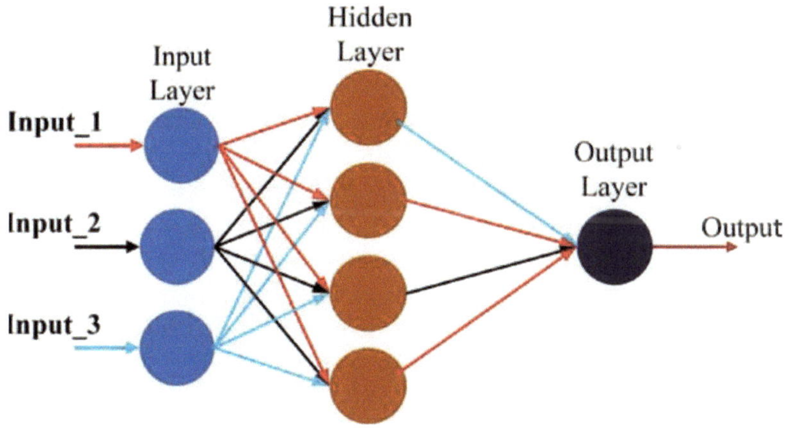

FIGURE 3.11 AF detection methods.

3.5.1.4 XGBOOST

XGBoost is widely used and known as a classifier to identify AF due to its outstanding performance on large datasets. Because it is so versatile, it can solve many regression and taxonomy problems. To train the classifier with XGBoost, we utilized the skicit learn package.

3.5.2 AF DETECTION USING DEEP LEARNING TECHNIQUES

CNN is a classification algorithm that may be used to pictures, text, and a variety of other domains. CNN, on the other hand, is known as shift invariant since it can share weights and other properties. Sentiment analysis, recommendation systems, picture classification, healthcare, and other applications can all benefit from CNN (Jiang et al., 2021). CNN is simply an upgraded version of the multi-layer perceptron, in which each neuron is linked to every other neuron in the network. Some properties may lose their functionality if regularization is applied to them. Using more complicated techniques to find a modest and basic pattern to regularize a CNN's regularization has numerous advantages. Biological processes, such as the neuron-to-visual brain connection pattern, inspired CNN. While feature extraction is not essential in deep learning, it is in machine learning techniques, and the extracted features might degrade performance if the framework does not pick the right ones (Gogate et al., 2020). In comparison to other implementations, the CNN model employed in the technique has a unique architecture. Because of its parameter sharing and sparse connectivity, the CNN classifier has recently become one of the most widely used supervised learning algorithms in computer vision (Gogate et al., 2017). The key benefit of utilizing a CNN classifier for this task is that it can locate relevant attributes without the need for human participation. CNN can learn the exact characteristics of each class using a significant amount of data. The CNN also saves so much time in terms of calculation. To be clear, most DL classifiers do not need hand- crafted features or choice, which could save work during the training or modeling, which is essential step in basic traditional machine learning modeling methods. Table 3.3 displays some notable AF detection approaches employing ML and DL from recent and previous years.

The *Long Short-Term Memory* (LSTM) architecture is made up of an input layer, an LSTM layer, and a linking layer on top of that. To make an LSTM, you will need two layers of 128 cells each, then 0.2 probability dropouts on top of that, then a dense layer with two unique neurons below that. For the main recommended design, we chose adam optimizer as a starting point. For image processing applications, r*esidual networks* (ResNet) separate input into several groups. In 2015, the model was a big winner in the ImageNet competition. Deep neural networks are taught to utilize the ResNet fundamentals, which include two-layer res netblocks,

TABLE 3.3 Previous and Recent Techniques for the Detection of AF Using ML and DL.

Reference	Proposed technique	Database	Features used	Features used	Remarks
Luo et al. (2017)	Deep learning classifier with stacked denoising auto-encoder and a softmax layer	Arrhythmia dataset: 44 non-pacemaker records- MIT-BIH	MFSWT-modified frequency slice wavelet transform with time-frequency features	ACC = 97.5%	Feature extraction and classifier in 1 unit to classify 4 heartbeats to ANSI-AAMI
Isin and Ozdalili (2017)	Backpropagation neural network (BPNN)	MIT-BIH arrhythmia database	QRS features using transferred DCNN (AlexNet) feature extractor	ACC = 98.5%	Classify the 3 groups of heartbeats
Pourbabaee et al. (2018)	CNN with SVM, KNN, and MLP	PAF prediction challenge database PAF prediction challenge database	5-layer CNN. The o/p from the CNN is used as i/p features for the classified	Recall = 87.58%	Detection of PAF
Manogaran et al. (2018)	An adaptive neuro-fuzzy model with multiple kernel learning	KEGG metabolic reaction network database	Blood pressure, heart rate, body temperature, cholesterol, etc.	Sen = 98%, Spe = 99%	Classify heart disease and healthy patients
Satija et al. (2018)	CEEMD + NCC	MIT-BIH arrhythmia data	Signal quality assessment base temporal features	Sen = 99.67%, Ppv = 98.88%	Classify 4 classes of heartbeats
Hasan and Bhattacharjee (2019)	DCNN with softmax regressor	St. Petersburg (SP), MIT-BIH, and PTB datasets	Modified ECG signal using empirical mode decomposition (EMD)	ACC = 99.71%	Heartbeats classify according to the datasets
Chen et al. (2020)	Deep learning model (CNN 5 Blocks)	China Physiological signal challenge (CPSC)	ECG recordings	F1 = 84%	8 Heartbeats classification

TABLE 3.3 *(Continued)*

Reference	Proposed technique	Database	Features used	Features used	Remarks
Dokur and Ölmez (2020)	CNN (Walsh function)	MIT-BIH arrhythmia data	2-D ECG images	ACC = 99%	Small-size NN for classifying 11 heartbeats
Chen et al. (2021)	CNN	MIT-BIH AF database	Automated AF detection	ACC = 98.92%, Spe = 97.04%, Sen = 9.19%	Detection atrial fibrillation
Shi et al. (2021)	Discriminant canonical correlation analysis (DCCA)	Cardiology challenge 2017AF database	Automated AF detection	ACC = 91.7%, Spe =93.2%, Sen = 90.4%, F1= 88%	Automated AF detection

two common residual blocks, and a two-layer R-R block for deep neural networks.

3.6 FUTURE SCOPE

In collaboration with the present study we will highlight the following difficulties that need to be addressed in future ECG signal analysis research. Since real-time ECG measurements from a group of individuals can produce very different classification results, much of the research is based on MIT-BIH data sets. It is also necessary to create a new, more accurate database of ECG data from a wide range of patients to account for inter-patient differences in ECG. The majority of researchers have utilized the AAMI classification criteria for ECG heartbeats (in five different rhythm classes), while others have used classifications given in a public database. Comparing the relative performance of several heartbeat categorization algorithms that have been described is challenging as a result. Researchers have created ways to remotely monitor and analyze ECG data utilizing wireless sensor networks and the internet-of-things (IoT) for the detection of cardiac illness. Although simulink ML techniques for quick and reliable ECG beat classification on distant networks have been suggested and tested by researchers, their use in genuine hospital environments remains a study area owing to the complexity and execution time needed by the various methods. ECG signals are a concern for academics because low-power nodes and lightweight measurement equipment are required, and modern healthcare systems require a simple and rapid classification approach for long-term continuous recording of ECG data.

3.7 CONCLUSION

To improve smart healthcare and AF management, noninvasive ML, DL-based solutions for automatic detection and prediction of low-cost and high-precision AF and its variants are especially significant. On the other hand, with the feature extraction strategies in this paper as well as the use of various artificial intelligent algorithms, we have identified issues related to ECG data processing of noise mitigation methods. A comparative test of various advanced AF detection technologies is also provided. The gaps that must be filled to create a smart wearable solution for AF recognition are also discussed. However, we plan to develop a real-time AF detection method that does not require labeled data to detect AF.

KEYWORDS

- **atrial fibrillation**
- **ECG signals**
- **machine learning**
- **deep learning**
- **electrocardiogram**
- **cardiovascular**
- **cardiac arrhythmia**

REFERENCES

Akbilgic, O.; Howe, J. A.; Davis, R. L. Categorizing Atrial Fibrillation via Symbolic Pattern Recognition. *J. Med. Stat. Inform.* **2016,** *4* (8), 1–9.

Andersen, R. S.; Peimankar, A.; Puthusserypady, S. A Deep Learning Approach for Real-Time Detection of Atrial Fibrillation. *Expert Syst. Appl.* **2019,** *115*, 465–473.

Andrysiak, T. Machine Learning Techniques Applied to Data Analysis and Anomaly Detection in Ecg Signals. *Appl. Artif. Intell.* **2016,** *30* (6), 610–634.

Asgari, S.; Mehrnia, A.; Moussavi, M. Automatic Detection of Atrial Fibrillation Using Stationary Wavelet Transform and Support Vector Machine. *Comput. Biol. Med.* **2015,** *60*, 132–142.

Athanasiou, L. S.; Fotiadis, D. I.; Michalis, L. K. In *Atherosclerotic Plaque Characterization Methods Based on Coronary Imaging*; Academic Press, 2017.

Bruser, C.; Diesel, J.; Zink, M. D.; Winter, S.; Schauerte, P.; Leonhardt, S. Automatic Detection of Atrial Fibrillation in Cardiac Vibration Signals. *IEEE J. Bomed. Health Inf.* **2012,** *17* (1), 162–171.

Calvert, J. W.; Lefer, D. J. Overview of Cardiac Muscle Physiology. In *Muscle*; Elsevier, 2012; pp 57–66.

Cervigón, R.; McGinley, B.; Craven, D.; Glavin, M.; Jones, E. The Effects of Compression on the Detection of Atrial Fibrillation in Ecg Signals. *Appl. Sci.* **2021,** *11* (13), 5908.

Chen, X.; Cheng, Z.; Wang, S.; Lu, G.; Xv, G.; Liu, Q.; Zhu, X. Atrial FibrillationDetection Based on Multi-Feature Extraction and Convolutional Neural Network for Processing ECG Signals. *Comput. Methods Programs Biomed.* **2021,** *202*, 106009.

Chen, T. M.; Huang, C. H.; Shih, E. S.; Hu, Y. F.; Hwang, M. J. Detection and Classification of Cardiac Arrhythmias by a Challenge-Best Deep Learning Neural Network Model. *Iscience* **2020,** *23* (3), 100886.

Chinchkhede, K.; Yadav, G. S.; Hirekhan, S.; Solanke, D. On the Implementation of Fir Filter with Various Windows for Enhancement of ECG Signal. *Int. J. Eng. Sci. Technol.* **2011,** *3* (3), 2031–2040.

Dashtipour, K.; Raza, A.; Gelbukh, A.; Zhang, R.; Cambria, E.; Hussain, A. In *Present 2.0: Persian Sentiment Lexicon Enriched with Domain-Specific Words*, International Conference on Brain Inspired Cognitive Systems; Springer, 2019; pp 497–509.

Dokur, Z.; Olmez, T. Heartbeat Classification by Using a Convolutional Neural Network Trained with Walsh Functions. *Neural Comput. Appl.* **2020,** 1–20.

Dua, M.; Gupta, R.; Khari, M.; Crespo, R. G. Biometric Iris Recognition Using Radial Basis Function Neural Network. *Soft Comput.* **2019,** *23* (22), 11801–11815.

El Attaoui, A.; Hazmi, M.; Jilbab, A.; Bourouhou, A. Wearable Wireless SensorsNetwork for Ecg Telemonitoring Using Neural Network for Features Extraction, *Wirel. Pers. Commun.* **2020,** *111* (3), 1955–1976.

Fuster, V.; Rydén, L. E.; Cannom, D. S.; Crijns, H. J.; Curtis, A. B.; Ellenbogen, K. A.; Halperin, J. L.; Le Heuzey, J. Y.; Kay, G. N.; Lowe, J. E. Acc/aha/ESC 2006 Guidelines for the Management of Patients with Atrial Fibrillation–Executive Summary. *Revista Portuguesa de cardiologia: organ Oficial da Sociedade Portuguesa de Cardiologia= Portuguese J. Cardiol* **2007,** *26* (4), 383–446.

Gogate, M.; Adeel, A.; Hussain, A. In *Deep Learning Driven Multimodal Fusionfor Automated Deception Detection*, IEEE Symposium Series on Computational Intelligence (SSCI), 2017; pp 1–6.

Gogate, M.; Dashtipour, K.; Adeel, A.; Hussain, A. Cochleanet: A Robust Language-Independent Audio-Visual Model for Real-Time Speech Enhancement. *Inf. Fusion* **2020,** *63*, 273–285.

Goldberger, A. L.; Goldberger, Z. D.; Shvilkin, A. In *Clinical Electrocardiography: A Simplified Approach e-book*; Elsevier Health Sciences, 2017.

Grégoire, J.; Gilon, C.; Subramanian, N.; Bersini, H. Forecasting Episodes of Atrial Fibrillation Using a New Machine-Learning Algorithm. *Arch. Cardiovasc. Dis. Suppl.* **2020,** *12* (1), 103.

Hasan, N. I.; Bhattacharjee, A. Deep Learning Approach to Cardiovascular Disease Classification Employing Modified ECG Signal from Empirical Mode Decomposition. *Biomed. Signal Process. Control* **2019**, *52*, 128–140.

Hornick, J.; Costantini, O. The Electrocardiogram: Still a Useful Tool in the Primary Care Office. *Med. Clin.* **2019,** *103* (5), 775–784.

Hurnanen, T.; Lehtonen, E.; Tadi, M. J.; Kuusela, T.; Kiviniemi, T.; Saraste, A.; Vasankari, T.; Airaksinen, J.; Koivisto, T.; Pankaala, M. Automated Detection of AtrialFibrillation Based on Time-Frequency Analysis of Seismo-Cardiograms. *IEEE J. Biomed. Health Inf.* **2016,** *21*(5), 1233–1241.

Isin, A.; Ozdalili, S. Cardiac Arrhythmia Detection Using Deep Learning. *Procedia Comput. Sci.* **2017,** *120*, 268–275.

Jiang, F.; Kong, B.; Li, J.; Dashtipour, K.; Gogate, M. Robust Visual Saliency Optimization Based on Bidirectional Markov Chains. *Cogn. Comput.* 2021**,** *13*, 69–80.

Kalra, A.; Lowe, A.; Al-Jumaily, A. Critical Review of Electrocardiography Measurement Systems and Technology. *Meas. Sci. Technol.* **2018,** *30* (1), 012001.

Klabunde, R. In *Cardiovascular Physiology Concepts*; Lippincott Williams & Wilkins, 2011.

Kwon, S.; Hong, J.; Choi, E. K.; Lee, B.; Baik, C.; Lee, E.; Jeong, E. R.; Koo, B. K.; Oh, S.; Yi, Y. Detection of Atrial Fibrillation Using a Ring-Type Wearable Device (Cardio Tracker) and Deep Learning Analysis of Photoplethysmography Signals: A Prospective Observational Proof-of-Concept Study. *J. Med. Int. Res.* **2020,** *22* (5), e16443.

Lee, S. H. Development of Ventricular Fibrillation Diagnosis Method Based on Neuro-Fuzzy Systems for Automated External Defibrillators. *Int. J. Fuzzy Syst.* **2017,** *19* (2).

Longoni, M.; Carrera, D.; Rossi, B.; Fragneto, P.; Pessione, M.; Boracchi, G. A Wearable Device for Online and Long-Term Ecg Monitoring. *IJCAI* **2018,** 5838–5840.

Lubitz, S. A.; Benjamin, E. J.; Ruskin, J. N.; Fuster, V.; Ellinor, P. T. Challenges in the Classification of Atrial Fibrillation. *Nat. Rev. Cardiol.* **2010,** *7* (8), 451–460.

Luo, K.; Li, J.; Wang, Z.; Cuschieri, A. Patient-Specific Deep Architectural Modelfor Ecg Classification, *J. Healthcare Eng.* **2017,** 1–13.

Luz, E. J. D. S.; Schwartz, W. R.; Cámara Chávez, G.; Menotti, D. ECG-Based Heartbeat Classification for Arrhythmia Detection: A Survey. *Comput. Methods Programs Biomed.* **2016,** *127*, 144–164.

Mahmoud, S. S.; Hussain, Z. M.; Cosic, I.; Fang, Q. Time-Frequency Analysis ofNormal and Abnormal Biological Signals. *Biomed. Signal Process. Control* **2006,** *1* (1), 33–43.

Manogaran, G.; Varatharajan, R.; Priyan, M. Hybrid Recommendation System for Heart Disease Diagnosis Based on Multiple Kernel Learning with Adaptive Neuro-Fuzzy Inference System. *Multimed. Tools Appl.* **2018,** *77* (4), 4379–4399.

Naraei, P.; Abhari, A.; Sadeghian, A. In *Application of Multilayer Perceptron Neural Networks and Support Vector Machines in the Classification of Healthcare Data*, 2016 Future Technologies Conference (FTC), 2016; pp 848–852.

Narasimhan, C.; Verma, J. S.; Kishore, A. R.; Singh, B.; Dani, S.; Chawala, K.; Haque, A.; Khan, A.; Nair, M.; Vora, A. Cardiovascular Risk Profile and Management of Atrial Fibrillation in India: Real-World Data from Realiseaf Survey. *Indian Heart J.* **2016,** *68* (5), 663–670.

Nemati, S.; Ghassemi, M. M.; Ambai, V.; Isakadze, N.; Levantsevych, O.; Shah, A.; Clifford, G. D. In *Monitoring and Detecting Atrial Fibrillation Using Wearable Technology*, 38th Annual International Conference of the IEEE Engineering inMedicine and Biology Society (EMBC), 2016; pp 3394–3397.

Pourbabaee, B.; Roshtkhari, M. J.; Khorasani, K. Deep Convolutional Neural Networks and Learning Ecg Features for Screening Paroxysmal Atrial Fibrillation Patients. *IEEE Trans. Syst. Man Cybern. Syst.* **2018,** *48* (12), 2095–2104.

Prabhakaran, D.; Jeemon, P.; Roy, A. Cardiovascular Diseases in India: Current Epidemiology and Future Directions. *Circulation* **2016,** *133* (16), 1605–1620.

Satija, U.; Ramkumar, B.; Manikandan, M. S. A New Automated Signal Quality-Aware ECG Beat Classification Method for Unsupervised ECG Diagnosis Environments. *IEEE Sens. J.* **2018,** *19* (1), 277–286.

Shi, J.; Chen, C.; Liu, H.; Wang, Y.; Shu, M.; Zhu, Q. Automated Atrial Fibrillation Detection Based on Feature Fusion Using Discriminant Canonical Correlation Analysis. *Comput. Math. Methods Med.* **2021,** 1–10.

Silva, H. P.; Carreiras, C.; Lourenço, A.; Fred, A.; das Neves, R. C.; Ferreira, R. Off-the-Person Electrocardiography: Performance Assessment and Clinical Correlation. *Health Technol.* **2015,** *4* (4), 309–318.

Subramanian, B. ECG Signal Classification and Parameter Estimation Using Multi-Wavelet Transform. *Biomed. Res.* **2017,** *28* (7), 3187–3193.

Suykens, J. A.; Vandewalle, J. Least Squares Support Vector Machine Classifiers. *Neural Process. Lett.* **1999,** *9* (3), 293–300.

Thomas, H.; Diamond, J.; Vieco, A.; Chaudhuri, S.; Shinnar, E.; Cromer, S.; Perel, P.; Mensah, G. A.; Narula, J.; Johnson, C. O.; et al. Global Atlas of CardiovascularDisease 2000–2016: The Path to Prevention and Control. *Global Heart* **2018,** *13* (3), 143–163.

Trahanias, P.; Skordalakis, E. Syntactic Pattern Recognition of the ECG. *IEEE Trans. Pattern Anal. Mach. Intell.* **1990,** *12* (7), 648–657.

Tseng, Y. L.; Shi, Y. Z; Jaw, F. S. Portable, Real-Time, 12-Lead ECG Monitoring System. *Instrum. Sci. Technol.* **2010,** *38* (4), 305–312.

Vora, A.; Naik, A.; Lokhandwala, Y.; Chopra, A.; Varma, J.; Wander, G.; Jaswal, A.; Srikanthan, V.; Singh, B.; Kahali, D. Profiling Cardiac Arrhythmia, and Heart Failure Patients in India: The Pan-arrhythmia and Heart Failure Observational Study. *Indian Heart J.* **2017,** *69* (2), 226–239.

Wu, X.; Sui, Z.; Chu, C.H.; Huang, G. Detection of Atrial Fibrillation from Short ECG Signals Using a Hybrid Deep Learning Model. In *International Conference on Smart Health*; Springer, 2019; pp 269–282.

Xiong, Z.; Liu, T.; Tse, G.; Gong, M.; Gladding, P. A.; Smaill, B. H.; Stiles, M. K.; Gillis, A. M.; Zhao, J. A Machine Learning Aided Systematic Eeview and Meta-Analysis of the Relative Risk of Atrial Fibrillation in Patients with Diabetes Mellitus. *Front. Physiol.* **2018,** *9*, 835.

Yang, X.; Fan, D.; Ren, A.; Zhao, N.; Alam, M. 5g-Based User-Centric Sensing atc Band. *IEEE Trans. Ind. Inf.* **2019,** *15* (5), 3040–3047.

Zong, W.; Mukkamala, R.; Mark, R. A Methodology for Predicting Paroxysmal Atrial Fibrillation Based on ECG Arrhythmia Feature Analysis. *Comput. Cardiol.* **2001,** *28*, 125–128.

CHAPTER 4

Predicting Resilience of Blood Groups Against COVID-19 Delta Variant Using Machine Learning

ASHUTOSH SINGH[1], ROHIT SRIVASTAVA[1], DIWAKAR YAGYASEN[2], and UPENDRA KUMAR[3]

[1]*Department of CSE, BBDITM, Lucknow, Uttar Pradesh, India*

[2]*Department of CSE, BBDITM, Lucknow, Uttar Pradesh, India*

[3]*Department of CSE, IET, Lucknow, Uttar Pradesh, India*

ABSTRACT

It has been observed that COVID-19 has totally broken down the life style and survival of people in various aspects basically in terms of health issues, wealth issues, and mental level problems. In this chapter, the author is trying to diagnose and predict the resistivity of people against Delta variant of COVID-19 on the basis of their blood groups. Here, we have used some biomedical analysis and applied classification and machine learning techniques in order to predict the human body resistance against Delta variant on the basis of their blood group samples. We have also described a machine learning-based model for the prediction of human body resistance against Delta variant. In general, it was observed that blood groups A, B, and O were connected to vulnerability to get infected with definite microbes, including Delta variant. Here, the author has inspected the association between different types of blood group and clinical results of human beings to be diseased with simple and critical respiratory condition

Advanced Research in Electronic Devices for Biomedical and mHealth.
Rajesh K. Kesharwani, Upendra Kumar, Raj K. Keservani (Eds)

because of Delta variant and equated their blood group scattering with the general population.

4.1 INTRODUCTION

Corona Virus: A challenging problem for the entire world introduced on December 2019 and was declared as situation of pandemic by international organization of medical and healthcare commonly known as world health organization. The second variant of this virus was first detected in almost the end of 2020 in India while the nomenclature as Delta variant was done by WHO on May 31, 2021. This was responsible for the death of human being by affecting their lung severely causing infection, blockage of respiratory system, and cardiac arrest. It may be categorized as an artificial bacteria virus mutated by alpha variant of COVID-19 (Gangwar et al., 2020).

The mutation of alpha variant caused a new wave of corona virus basically called as DELTA variant of the severe acute respiratory syndrome (SARS-CoV-2). It was denoted as B.1.617.2 as delta variation of previous COVID-19 virus normally called as alpha version by the World Health Organization (WHO).

It was detected as a carrier of second wave of infections of this virus usually called as COVID-19. This Delta variant further moved on one higher step of danger called as Delta plus Version (AY 1 version). The most infected areas where the cases of this virus were spread rapidly were Kerala, Madhya Pradesh, Karnataka, and Maharashtra. It was earlier stated by Union health ministry that the latest version of corona virus (Delta Plus) should not be considered as a concern of worry as it may produce adverse effects on human beings because of upsurge in transmissibility.

India has previously acknowledged that it was a variation of worry, along with the rinsing cases found in almost 50 samples from almost 12 states in India. One of our states Maharashtra has testified the maximum number of patients of this variant as Delta Plus variant. This version associates the angiotensin transforming enzymes receiver of human being with the protein of spikes and then affects the cells. Later, there was done an unsatisfactory prediction which was generally related with the diabetic patients, patients with hypertension, and disease of coronary artery and patients having poor immune system (Gangwar et al., 2020). It was mentioned in previous research that there is a relation between blood groups and affecting entities (Laguipo et al., 2020). It was also designated that there is established an interaction between antigens of blood groups found inside erythrocytes and some more tissues communicate with some microorganisms, such as viruses, bacteria, and parasites. It was also observed that there is a variation of infection level susceptibility for different blood groups of human beings. This observation may play a very important act in infections by working like a receiver and co-receiver for different blood groups and various infectious entities, such as viruses, parasites, microorganisms, and blood group antigens (Wang et al., 2020).

There is also done an analysis on A, B, and O antibodies to obtain the immunity of these blood groups against bacterial infections and enclosed virus transporting active antigens of A, B, and O blood groups (McPherson et al., 2007). There are many different viruses mentioned here, such as vibrio cholerae, hepatitis C Virus, virus for human immune deficiency, SARS-CoV-2, and *Helicobacter pylori* are some of the active infectable entities that are found to get associated with blood groups of human bodies (Cheng et al., 2005).

An analysis has also been done based on clinical study to examine the connection between different blood groups of human beings and Delta plus version of COVID-19 (SARS-Cov-2) (Chung et al., 2020). It was also observed from previous analysis and studies that there is a huge gap between populations of different zones and their respective blood groups. Frequency of blood groups varies between groups of populations (Zhou et al., 2014).

There is also done an analysis in order to compare the distribution of blood groups of patients infected with Delta plus version on the basis of some attributes like hospitalized patients, recovered patients at their home and dead patients of a specific area. So it is considered very important that the relation between patients infected with Delta version of COVID-19 and their respective blood groups (Zhou et al., 2020).

Because of high transmissibility ratio and sharp increment in spread of Delta plus version of COVID-19 among whole world have created a strained position for the currently present healthcare and research and testing resources. It was also observed that effect of COVID-19 varies among people to people (Zheng et al., 2020). It was analyzed that some of the peoples are affected with slightly mild symptoms while some of the peoples needed to get hospitalized and rather than this situation some of the patients could not survive due to the effect of SARS-Cov-2. It was totally impossible to observe and analyze any individual's situation based on some symptoms or level of effectiveness of infection. Based on some pathogenesis of suspected SARS-CoV-2 and their respective failure of respiratory are doubtful till date, but we can say that the death ratio is bonded with the counts of patients with higher age male people. This is not enough to understand the seriousness of SARS-CoV-2 on the basis of biologically examined factors and this has been observed by many studies that the patients having blood group of A, B, and O type, then there is involved some risk factor for various diseases, such as myocardial infraction, cancer, kidney issues etc. with such type of blood groups. The blood group of A, B, and O may affect the vulnerability of COVID-19 and the sternness of the infection (Cheng et al., 2005). The goal of the analysis is to read if there is an association amid the A, B, and O blood groups and SARS-Cov-2 (accountability and sternness).

The delta plus version of corona virus (SARS-CoV-2) has spread very fast across the whole world as well as in India. As per the scenario of August 2020, almost 7.5 lakh cases of death and 22 lac infected cases were found in all over world. Various risk factors associated with SARS-Cov-2 are in existence in the case of infected patients and their death ratio. These factors of risk are associated with some specific parameters, such as age, gender, diabetes, smoking habitual, cardiac vascular, and respiratory issues and hypertension. It was observed from previously done analysis that patients already having mentioned above issues may get affected widely with this virus.

It was analyzed from the latest work that there exists a relational factor of infection level of Delta plus version on different A, B, and O type blood groups. It was found that patients having "A" type blood group are affected with high risk while patients having "O" type blood group are associated with mild risk factor. Rather than this, it was also observed that the requirement of ventilators is mainly raised by the patients having any blood group besides "O." So, the computed odd ratio is not compatible with this analysis and providing the low level of satisfaction. The ABO blood category peculiarity reproduces polymorphisms inside the *ABO* genetic factor. This genetic factor is related with huge amount of additional qualities, as well as dangerous features for COVID-19 disease and death.

An association called genome-wide analyzed and correlated the variants inside A, B, and O type of blood groups with the ACE (angiotensin-converting enzyme), RBC, and concentration of hemoglobin, hematocrit, coronary artery disease, and diabetes. It was observed from a meta-analysis done in 2012, the people having Non-O blood group are having very significant risk factors by their gene for venous thromboembolism (Ellinghaus et al., 2020).

These circumstances are also related with SARS-CoV-2, as coagulopathy is considered as a normal problem for COVID-19 patients and the risk factor of venous thromboembolism must be treated and managed with a lot of care. There are various relations between situation and type of blood group of a patient of COVID-19 which gives out a validated reason to adapt the truth regarding death and infected community based on their blood groups (Latz et al., 2020).

In earlier work, it has recognized relations between ABO blood groups and an amount of diverse toxicities or sickness sternness ensuing infections containing SARS-CoV-1 (Liu et al., 2020). Rh (D) phenotypes (positive and negative Rh blood types) are related with precisely few illnesses equaled to ABO (28). Similarly, ABO, Rh type is significant factor for type compatibility and response of immunity. For instance, hemolytic sickness of the newly born is an apprehension when there is mismatching between Rh (D) of mother and children (Rossez et al., 2012). Various analysis done by different other studies have originated the proof that Rh-positive individuals are endangered from the effects of hidden toxoplasmosis (Aspholm-Hurtig et al., 2004); however, *Toxoplasma gondii* is treated like a eukaryotic organism (Hari et al., 2020), not a virus like SARS-CoV-2.

4.2 RELATED WORK

4.2.1 ANALYSIS BASED ON COMPARISON OF BLOOD TYPE USING DESCRIPTIVE APPROACH

In a research, it was described that COVID-19 virus produces an angiotensin-converting enzyme which works as receptor along with the spike protein and then causes to communicate a disease to the cells of human body. It is having a direct involvement to produce infection by working as receptor for antigens of blood groups. The basic objective of the research was to make a comparison between clusters of patients on behalf of their blood groups who are infected with SARS-CoV-2. A survey of almost 850 patients was taken with their positive test result of COVID-19 infections. Their positive test results and clinical symptoms and situations are also the part of this research. Finally, this result was compared with the human beings having normal conditions without infections. It was observed from the study that the effect of SARS-CoV-2 in higher in a, B, and AB type of blood groups. Rather than this, people having "O" type of blood group is having lower risk of infections. This analysis also agrees with the previous studies resultant as lower risk factor for the people with 'O' type of blood group. Though, this approach was not sufficiently established to allow special prophylaxis recommendations for non-O individuals. (Zhou et al., 2020)

According to another analysis done in King Fahd Hospital of Almadina Almonoura where total 507 were analyzed who was completely declared with infected by COVID-19, and it was derived that almost 70% of patients required to admit in isolation and almost 21% in ICU. This analysis varies with a standard deviation of ± 9 along with a factor of age of 54 years and a male to female ratio of 303 male (approx. 59.67%) and 204 females (approx. 40.23%) till 15th April 2020.

It has been observed from that patients having smoking habit, diabetes, and indulge with hypertension are affected higher than a normally infected patient. The confirmation of COVID-19 was done based on positive result of RT-PCR (real-time reverse transcriptase polymerase chain reaction test) which was performed through nasal and pharyngeal swab of suspicious patients. Further the infection level of COVID-19 was categorized into different levels of effectiveness as mild infected, very low infected, moderate level, severe infected and critically infected (Hoffmann et al., 2019).

A statistical analysis of using version 12 of SPSS was done for the patients less than 18 years followed based on means and standered deviation for the variables of continuous type and numeric, and percentage for the variable of categorical type with accepted level of significance at $P \leq (1/20)$ (Yang et al., 2020).

Analysis of the results of the study was found appropriate with the above-mentioned value as 59.7% for male infected people and 40.20% for female infected people (Hosseini et al., 2012).

4.2.2 ANALYSIS USING CHI-SQUARE TEST, REGRESSION ANALYSIS, AND FINE GRAY MODEL

In this study, the sample of blood group from NYP (New York Presbyterian) hospital was considered for the analysis of prevention of SARS-CoV-2 among A, B, and O types of blood group. This study basically involves three techniques as mentioned above. This analysis has taken the sample of almost 14,112 patients who are declared positive for at least one time through performing swab test. A test was done using Chi-square method for the analysis of individuals but resulting unsatisfactory to conclude with the statement that it becomes variation in frequency of blood group between tested and non-–tested peoples of SARS-Cov-2. If someone is declared positive after test, then the relation between individual's blood type and outcome of SARS-CoV-2 was documented in terms of prevalence of infection, analysis regarding survival and death ratio among infected patients which were declared positive after swab test.

Initially it was observed that resilience against infection was greater in A and B blood type while it was lower in O blood type (Laguipo et al., 2020).

Frequencies of different blood types may vary based on previous and inherited diseases. Because of this, an analysis using confounding effect was done for inherited and ancestry issues by adjusting their inheritance or ancestry. A comparison was done toward infection resilience using linear regression where blood type O is reference group for blood type A, B, O, and Rh (D) factor. Further making use of bootstrap almost 95% confidence intervals were computed for every estimate.

After making modification in patient's race and ancestry, the resilience level among different types of blood is computed as A, AB, and B types of blood groups are having higher resilience and O type of blood group is associated with higher risk of infection and severity (Chung et al., 2020).

After analyzing the rapid growth in count of patients, it was considered that blood type associating with A, AB, and B was having higher resilience than O type of group. Patients with Rh (+ve) and Rh (–ve) are having almost 2.7% reduced factor of risk of primary level of infection after making arrangement for ancestry, having consistency with a reduced risk factor before arrangement. Further, an examination was done about intubation and mortality applying survival outline to get understood that how the blood group affects growth in disease output as a growth in time. To estimate and compute the above-mentioned scenario, a fine gray model which is capable to estimate the function for growth in incidents during computing the challenging risk and managing covariates. Generally, the mortality and recovery of patients were the comprising issues for intubation while recovery was just an opposite incidence for mortality or death.

An estimation was done since the cohort entry which defines the time of entry in hospital after getting infected positively at very first test or within 4 days of being positive. A criterion was also defined for a patient having recovered from the infection after at least 10 days of cohort entry that the patient can resume his working according to the guidelines provided by the CDC (Zhaohai et al., 2020).

4.2.3 *RELATION BETWEEN INFECTION AND BLOOD TYPE*

HBGAs are concerned in the pathogenesis of several contagions. In precise, the ABO blood category has been related with, for instance, we have analyzed some diseases, such as tuberculosis, malaria, cholera, norovirus, retrovirus, Chikungunya virus, *Helicobacter pylori* (*H. pylori*) and *Escherichia coli* (27). The essential mechanisms vary from general (e.g., receptor ligand communications) to multifaceted and may be partial to a précised pathogenic creation, straining, or sickness level. For ABO, possible clarifications comprise ABH antigens by way of receptors for pathogens, natural antibodies, and lectins by way of inhibitors, and molecular mimicry by blood group antigens among pathogens and patients. A precise example is mentioned which deals with p antigen in the blood group of globoside. This is a very important antigen but not so much sufficient to protect RBC from the entry of parvovirus. It requires some co-receptors for infection (p5–39, 40). The allotment of p antigen in addition to comparatively great expression by RBC along with their antecedents, is reliable with parvovirus B19 clinical conditions containing aplastic anemia (Hari et al., 2020).

Additionally, the patients having deficiency in P antigen are having resistivity for such type of infection (Zhao et al., 2020). In case of some other infections HGBAs are preferred as toxin receptor. Furthermore, HGBA can also show their involvement to pathogens by excretions, body fluids, or non-erythyroid tissues.

In brief, it can be assumed that association between HGBAs and some special infections must preferably satisfy the hypothesis of Koch. Nevertheless, this is generally very hard to record the study of human as document, so an individual can only represent that special types of blood or HGBA are having much susceptibility for infection and any individual without HGBA are fully resistant from such infections as well as from severe decease. Various examplesare shown regarding this in order to show that HGBAs can communicate with pathogens at the primary stage of infection or it can increase the effect or severity of decease.

Many observations were performed during the severe condition of SARS-CoV-2 on different blood types, and it was found that there is less susceptibility in blood group O of various patients (Latz et al., 2020). The same was also analyzed for SARS-CoV-2. Several studies have been done to find the resultant with accurate computation that which blood group is having higher resilience among ABO blood type.

Further, most studies recognized a great number of group A, and lesser number of patients of group O, among a lot of COVID-19 patients, as equated to healthy controls (Hari et al., 2020). These studies comprised patients with SARS-CoV-2 pneumonia reaching in harshness from slight to censoriously ill and needful for motorized ventilation or intensive care unit (ICU) admission. For instance, in one analysis, the number of group A infected patients was suggestively greater than that in healthy controls (38% vs. 32_2%, P < 0_001), whereas group O was suggestively lesser (25_7% vs. 33_8%, P < 0_001); however, the patients of group A had greater occurrences of fundamental comorbidities. Additional reflective analysis had almost similar conclusions but did not designate the comorbidities (Chung et al., 2020).

Alternatively, some study explained more infection inside group AB patients and a lesser degree in group O patients (Latz et al., 2020). In gap, a supplementary study did not treasure any association between blood group A position and COVID-19; nevertheless, group O persons had a poorer threat of COVID-19 and group B and AB persons had a greater threat (Zhou et al., 2014). One possible motive for these changing outcomes is that numerous such analyses did not have justification for many confounders (e.g., age, diabetics), comprising comorbidities. Additional possible confounder for few selected studies could be the use of arbitrarily designated as helper blood donors as controls, due to the risk of group O epidemiological prevalence because of blood collectors selectively employing group O contributors or donors. Significantly, volunteer blood donors are not essentially demonstrative of universal inhabitants; though suitable, their consumption as a control group is not best (Chung et al., 2020).

4.2.4 SEVERITY OF COVID-19 AND ABO BLOOD TYPES

Various analyses have been done to evaluate the effect of COVID-19 over ABO blood types; inn the description of one study, it was described that the patients having blood group of A were having more threat to get hospitalized due to infection of SARS-CoV-2 while the patients belonging to O type of blood group were at below the rate of risk to get hospitalized (Zaho et al., 2020).

Though, the type A patients had more comorbid risk causes for unembellished sickness, which were not accustomed for using a multivariate examination. Another group achieved a GWAS of COVID-19 patients with the failure of respiratory system (Liu et al., 2020), perceiving a consistently important cross-replicating association at 9q34. The 9q34 signal was situated at the ABO blood type locus and a blood type centric examination displayed a greater risk of Spartan COVID-19 with the failure of respiratory for group A individuals and a defensive effect for group O.

With the help of one more example in which an analysis based on nested prospective observational approach of medically sick patients due to COVID-19 in Canada, applying a multivariable adjustment of several risk causes, the patients having blood group of A and AB also were having a greater risk factor involving the requirement of mechanically operated ventilators.

Some additional studies are required to find the severity of COVID-19 infection in association with ABO blood types. Though, gathering evidence proposes that at biochemical and physiological stages, there might be an influence of ABO blood groups to disease biology. It needs to be predictable that host factors previously recognized as subsidizing to COVID-19 severity, a dominant role is being played, paired with well-timed admittance to suitable medical care.

4.2.5 ANALYSIS USING FISCHER'S EXACT TESTS AND ODDS RATIO (OR) TESTS

There were numerous trainings indicating a link between ABO blood group and the risk of COVID-19 infection. We used retrospective observational data from Bahrain to look at the link between ABO blood group and infection risk, as well as susceptibility to severe ICU-requiring infections.

Blood group B was linked to a higher risk, while blood group AB was linked to a lower risk. There was no link found between blood group and the chance of a serious ICU-required infection. Anti-a (blood groups B and O) and anti-b (blood groups B and O) antibodies were used to investigate the connection (blood groups A and O). There is no link between antibodies and infection risk.

The current study, together with the wide range of blood group associations, suggests that blood group may not be the best biomarker for predicting COVID-19 infection risk. In the design of the research, we looked at the link between blood group and the risk of COVID-19 infection and the severity of clinical consequences in this cross-sectional observational investigation. ABO blood group and blood antibody class were used to examine the relationship. The distribution of blood types within a sample of confirmed COVID-19 people in Bahrain was compared with the distribution of blood types among the general population of Bahrain to explore the effect of blood group on susceptibility to a SARS-CoV-2 infection.

The distribution of blood types among a sample of confirmed COVID-19 patients in Bahrain was compared with the distribution of blood types among Bahrain's general population in order to investigate the effect. The distribution of blood types was examined between COVID-19 individuals admitted to an intensive care unit (ICU) and those of the general COVID-19 patients' sample to study the effect of blood type on the severity of clinical outcomes. This was mirrored in the antibody class analysis, with blood groups divided into anti-A (blood groups B and O) and anti-B (blood groups B and O) (blood groups A and O).

The gathering of information, any person who tested positive for SARS-CoV-2 via a nasopharyngeal (NP) swab was considered a confirmed COVID-19 case. Polymerase chain reaction (PCR) analysis employing the E gene as a target was used to check for the presence of SARS-CoV-2 in the NP sample. A PCR assay targeting RdRp was used to validate the presence of the E gene. Using real-time PCR kits from Roche and Invitrogen, all confirmed cases tested positive for the E gene and RdRp. Cases were discovered by community screening targeting close contacts and travellers, as well as random testing in outbreak locations, depending on their clinical presentation to medical care.

To reflect the COVID-19 infected community, a random sample of 3000 COVID-19 positive individuals was picked at random from the

National COVID-19 Database. Of those, 2138 had blood group information documented or available, and were thus included in the study. There were 196 COVID-19 instances with ICU admissions as of July 19, 2020, all of which were included in this analysis. Medical records were used to gather blood group information for all COVID-19 afflicted people. The blood types of 4985 persons who donated whole blood or platelets at King Hamad University Hospital Blood Bank during the past 2 years were obtained to represent the blood type distribution of Bahrain's general population.

The distributions of blood groups and antibodies between samples were compared using Chi-squared (χ^2) and Fischer's exact tests. The likelihood of a blood type or antibody category testing positive were studied using odds ratio (OR) tests in a one-vs-all method. The ORs are given with a 95% confidence interval.

At $p = 0.05$, statistical values were considered significant. STATA statistical software was used for the statistical analysis (version 15.1). The National COVID-19 Research Committee has given their approval (Research Approval Code: CRT-COVID2020-084).

4.3 MATERIALS AND METHODS

This retrospective analysis used the data from 250 patients admitted to the hospital between March and June 2021 (Name cannot be disclosed due to government orders). The study enrolled 250 confirmed COVID-19 cases with available blood group (ABO and Rh), demographic, and clinical data. All COVID-19 patients had been confirmed using a reverse transcriptase real-time polymerase chain reaction (RT-PCR) assay specific for the SARS-CoV-2 nucleoprotein (N). Patients' case report forms were used to collect data on their blood group, gender, age, hospitalized ward, and disease outcome. Since the frequency of participants in different age groups varied, the patients were categorized according to their age in the literature. Additionally, patients were classified into various hospitalized wards. This study revealed two outcomes: recovered and deceased (because of COVID-19).

Blood group and antibody distributions were compared between samples using Chi-squared (^{2}) and Fisher's exact tests. The probabilities of a blood type or antibody class testing positive in a one-to-all way were studied using odds ratio (OR) tests. ORs are presented with a 95% confidence interval for the sake of completeness. At a p-value of 0.05, statistical results were deemed significant. To determine the probability of death, researchers used multiple logistic regressions (dependent variable). Blood types, age, gender, and hospitalization wards were all considered independent factors. Also, we established logistic regression-based machine learning based on factors, such as age, gender, blood group, severity level of the patient, respiratory problems and finally person was suffering from diabetes. These all factors were used to determine the mortality rate. For this prediction, we have employed the machine learning model of random forest classifier (Zhao et al., 2020).

Using ensemble-based learning methods, random forest classifiers are a subset of machine learning. They're easy to set up, quick to use, and have had great results across a wide range of industries. The random forest approach builds several "basic" decision trees during the training step and then uses a majority vote (mode) to classify the results. This voting technique has the added benefit of correcting decision trees' tendency to over fit training data, among other things. Random forests use a technique known as bagging to train separate set of information using individual trees during training stage (Chung et al, 2020).

4.4 RESULTS

A total of 231 patients had a positive outcome, whereas 19 patients had a negative outcome (died). There were 135 male cases and 115 female cases out of all the cases. The average patient age was 55.21 years with a standard deviation of 15.17 years (median 54 years with a range of 1–90 years). Patients were divided into five age ranges: 16–30 years old, 31–40 years old, 41–50 years old, 51–60 years old, and older than 60 years old. The hospital had ICUs, CCUs, emergency rooms, infectious disease wards, post-ICUs, isolated rooms, and others. A breakdown of the demographics (gender/age/hospital ward/blood group) of all patients, living or dead. We used confidence interval (CI) and p-value for the exploratory studies. The use of p-values makes it possible to identify any statistically significant findings. As well as the strength and direction of an effect, confidence intervals reveal the range within which the correct value is most likely to be found.

4.4.1 CONFIDENCE INTERVAL (CI)

Estimates of the intensity of an effect can be estimated using confidence ranges. Convention dictates that 95% confidence intervals are used when reporting results. These ranges show the 95% confidence intervals in which the treatment effect can be assumed to fall. There is a 95% probability that the difference between the two study labels is between 6 and 10 deaths if the mean difference in visual acuity is 8 (95% confidence interval: 6–10 mortality rate).

4.4.2 P-VALUE

A p-value determines the likelihood that the observed result—or one that is more extreme—occurs by chance, given that no differences exist among the target blood type labels. A p-value of 0.05, for example, indicates that the difference between labels of blood types being compared has a 5% probability of occurring by chance. When this probability is modest, it becomes less likely that the null hypothesis is correct—or that the chance of a group difference is high.

Gender had no significant impact on the results of COVID-19 in this investigation. Data revealed a strong link between patient age and prognosis for the condition. Over 60-year-olds had a higher risk of dying from COVID-19-associated causes than younger adults. We discovered a strong link between the patient's hospitalization ward and the disease's final result. Those admitted to intensive care units, critical care units, or emergency rooms had a greater death rate than those with infectious diseases. The most common blood type among those who died from COVID-19 was O+, while the least common was AB-, and the majority of those who died had O+. According to a logistic regression study, the odds of dying were 1.81 times higher in group A- than in group A+, but the difference was not statistically significant. Type B+ had a lower mortality rate than type A+. The risk of death from COVID-19 is 3.8 times higher for those with blood type B– than for people with the A+ blood type. Death rates were lower in the AB+ group than in the A+ group. Finally, the risk of death was lower for blood groups O+ and O- than for A+.

TABLE 4.1 CI and p-Value for the Dataset.

Blood Group	Population	CI: 95%	p-value
A+	70	0.946 (0.667–1.294)	0.874
A–	8	1.821 (0.931–3.662)	0.091
B+	65	0.617 (0.393–0.793)	0.004
B–	6	3.9 (1.881–7.719)	0.002
AB+	18	0.879 (0.492–1.611)	0.698
AB–	3	-	-
O+	75	0.969 (0.692–1.374)	0.896
O–	5	0.884 (0.498–1.646)	0.882

A- patients had 1.79-times higher death rates than A+ patients, while patients with type B- blood had 3.6 -times higher COVID-19 mortality rates than A+ patients, according to our research. While A+ was associated with a higher death rate, other blood types like B+, AB+, O+, and O- were less likely to perish. COVID-19 has not yet been linked to a specific blood type. People with blood type A are more likely than those with blood type O to get the condition, according to some research. There were a

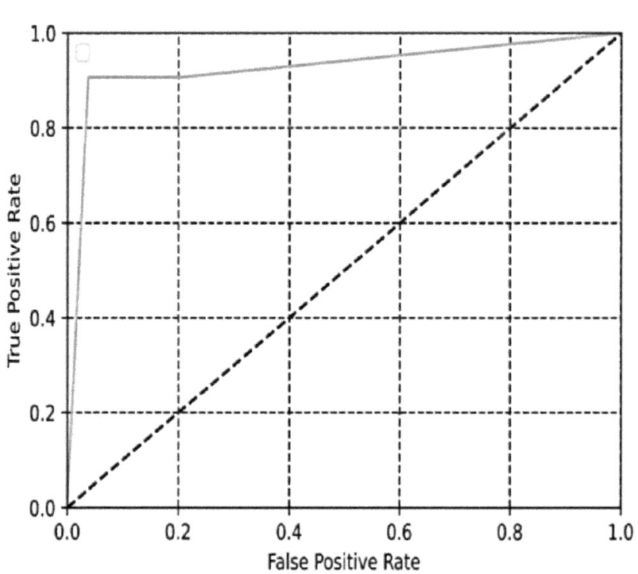

FIGURE 4.1 ROC curve for the dataset.

few researches that found a link between blood type and COVID-19, but the results were mixed. People with Rh- blood type had decreased infection, intubation, and death rates, while people with Rh+ blood type were more susceptible to COVID-19. In contrast, an Iranian study found no link between COVID-19 and Rh blood type. There was also no connection between Rh blood types and hospitalizations, ICU stay artificial ventilator assistance and case fatality rates.

We also conducted study on the susceptibility of the patient suffering from COVID-19 along various other factors, such as blood group, age, gender, and diabetic. There were three outcomes, the person suffering from COVID-19 survives just through quarantine (class 0), person is admitted to the hospital then survives (class 1) and finally person succumbs to COVID (class 2). We recorded an accuracy of 95% that how accurately we identify the above scenario.

It is possible to see the accuracy of a classification by looking at the receiver operating characteristic (ROC) curve. Analysis of ROC curves shows how a predictive model's accuracy is affected by varying likelihood thresholds. When looking at the ROC curve, the false-positive rate (FPR) is shown on the x-axis, while the true-positive rate (TPR) is shown on the y-axis. TPR metric measures how well a classifier can identify individuals of the positive group while FPR the rate at which the classifier misclassifies a negative class as a positive one. Because of this, a connection is made between FPR and TPR that can be utilized to derive an FPR threshold for optimal TPR. We recorded a TPR of 91% at 20% and 96% at 50% false acceptance rate (FAR) as shown in Fig. 4.2. Due to small dataset, the reported ROC curve cannot be better plotted, and with the increase in collection of more individuals, it might increase to desired values.

To efficiently illustrate the performance of deep learning models, a confusion matrix can be built utilizing true-positives (TP), true negatives (TN), false positives (FP), and false-negatives (FN). TP is the number of instances that are accurately classified as positive while FP represents any observations that the model incorrectly classifies as positive but are, in fact, negative. Similarly, TN represents incorrectly assigned instances to a negative classification and FN represents instances that were assigned to the negative class by the model but are actually positive. The confusion matrix makes it easy to see how many correct and wrong predictions there are in each class. It demonstrates the categorization model's ambiguity

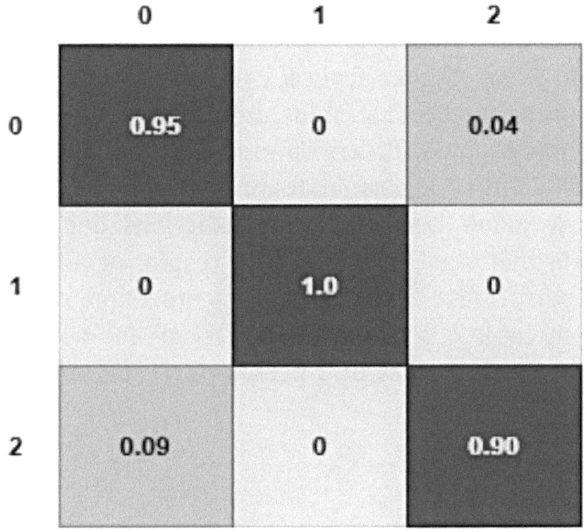

FIGURE 4.2 Confusion matrix for the dataset.

while making predict ions. The x-axis and y-axis, respectively, show the actual and expected class designations. Each square in the confusion matrix represents the likelihood of the projected class matching the actual class. Although there is no positive or negative class in multiclass problems, the number of TP, TN, FP, and FN cannot be computed immediately. These figures can be calculated separately for each class. The TP for class "0," for example, will be the number of right predictions for that class. The number of TN for class "1" is the sum of probabilities in all squares of the confusion matrix that does not belong to class "1" in either predicted or actual label. In Fig. 4.2, for class '0,' the model misclassified only 0.04% of the whole samples while for class "1," none of the samples were misclassified. Finally, for class "2," 0.09% of the samples were misclassified as class "0."

TABLE 4.2 Precision Recall and F1-Score for the Dataset.

	Precision	Recall	F1-Score
0	0.91489	0.95556	0.93478
1	1.0000	1.0000	1.0000
2	0.95122	0.90698	0.92857

For symmetric databases, where false-positives (FP) and false-negatives (FN) have the same cost, accuracy is a helpful performance parameter. However, higher accuracy models are not always preferable. As a result, other performance indicators including as precision, recall, and F1-score are studied. Precision measures the number of predictions that correctly identify a particular class while Recall is a metric that measures how many correct class predictions could be made given all of the data that was available. The results of all machine learning methods for performance criteria, such as precision, recall, and F1-score are reported in Table 4.2. The precision recall and F1- Score is reported highest for the second class of a person surviving after admitted to the hospital.

4.5 CONCLUSIONS

Following are the massive outbreak of the COVID-19 since last year. Many factors were into consideration for finding out situations and distribution of virus among population. The impact of the virus ranged from normal quarantine to severe case of pneumonia type symptoms including susceptibility. The purpose of the research was to find a correlation between the resilience of blood group types against the virus. This would help the population to better prepare for the pandemic.

Regarding the link between blood type and the risk of COVID-19 infection, we found that people with blood group A had a higher frequency of infection and a higher risk, whereas people with blood group O had a lower frequency and a lower risk. In line with findings by Latz et al., we found no connection between blood group A and COVID-19 infection susceptibility in our study. The risk linked with blood group B was also found to be significant. People with blood group AB had a lower chance of COVID-19 infection, which is consistent with a small number of publications. However, in all of these studies, including this one, the sample size for this group was very small. No link was found between having blood group O and a lower risk of infection, according to previous research. Finally, our results add further evidence to the previously discovered associations between blood types and COVID-19.

KEYWORDS

- **COVID-19**
- **machine learning**
- **receiver operating characteristic**
- **reverse transcription**
- **polymerase chain reaction (RT-PCR)**
- **SARS-CoV-2**
- **confidence Interval**
- **p-value**

REFERENCES

American College of Emergency Physicians (ACEP). COVID19 Severity Classification. 2020.

Boren, T.; Falk, P.; Roth, K. A.; et al. Attachment of Helicobacter Pylori to Human Gastric Epithelium Mediated by Blood Group Antigens. *Science (New York, NY)* **1993,** *262,* 1892–1895.

Branch, D. R. Blood Groups and Susceptibility to Virus Infection: New Developments. *Curr. Opin. Hematol.* **2010,** *17* (6), 558–564.

Brown, K. E.; Hibbs, J. R.; Gallinella, G.; et al. Resistance to Parvovirus B19 Infection Due to Lack of Virus Receptor (Erythrocyte P Antigen). *N. Engl. J. Med.* **1994,** *330,* 1192–1196.

Cheng, Y.; Cheng, G.; Chui, C. H.; Lau, F. Y.; Chan, P. K.; Ng, M. H.; Sung, J. J.; Wong, R. S. ABO Blood Group and Susceptibility to Severe Acute Respiratory Syndrome. *JAMA* **2005,** *293* (12), 1450–1451.

Chung, C. M.; Wang, R. Y.; Chen, J. W.; et al A Genome-Wide Association Study Identifies New Loci for ACE Activity: Potential Implications for Response to ACE Inhibitor. *Pharmacogenom. J.* **2020,** *10,* 537–544.

Chung, C.-M.; Wang, R.-Y.; Chen, J.-W.; Fann, C. S. J.; Leu, H.-B.; Ho, H.-Y.; Ting, C.-T.; Lin, T.-H.; Sheu, S.-H.; Gérard, C.; Maggipinto, G.; Minon, J. M.; A Genome-Wide Association Study Identifies New Loci for ACE Activity: Potential Implications for Response to ACE Inhibitor COVID-19 and ABO Blood Group: Another Viewpoint. *Br. J. Haematol. 190,* e93–e94.

Cooling, L.; Blood Groups in Infection and Host Susceptibility. *Clin. Microbiol. Rev.* **2015,** *28* (3). 801–870.

Cooling, L. L.; Koerner, T. A.; Naides, S. J. Multiple Glycosphingolipids Determine the Tissue Tropism of Parvovirus B19. *J. Infect. Dis.* **1995,** *172,* 1198–1205.

Coronavirus Disease 2019 (COVID-19) Weekly Epidemiological Update World Health Organization WHO Coronavirus Disease 2019 Weekly Epidemiological Updates, 2020.

Ellinghaus, D.; Degenhardt, F.; Bujanda, L.; Buti, M.; Albillos, A.; Invernizzi, P.; Fernández, J.; Prati, D.; Baselli, G.; Asselta, R.; et al. Genomewide Association Study of Severe Covid-19 with Respiratory Failure Karlsen *N. Engl. J. Med.* **2020**. DOI:10.1056/nejmoa2020283.

Gangwar, M.; Ojha, B. K.; Shukla, H. K.; Singh, A. P.; Srivastava, R.; Singh, S. Covid 19: A Challenging Situation for the World. *Int. J. Adv. Sci. Technol.* **2020,** *29* (05), 12373–12382.

Hari. Blood Type and COVID-19 Risk: O may Help, A May Hurt. *N. Engl. J. Med.* **2020,** *11,* 325–329.

Hoffmann, M.; Kleine-Weber. H.; Krüger, N.; Müller, M.; Drosten, C.; Pöhlmann, S. The Novel Coronavirus 2019 (2019-nCoV) Uses the SARS-Coronavirus Receptor ACE2 and the Cellular Protease TMPRSS2 for Entry into Target Cells. bioRxiv. 2020. DOI: 10.1101/2020.01.31.929042v1

Hosseini, S. M.; Feng, J. J. How Malaria Parasites Reduce the Deformability of Infected Red Blood Cells. *Biophys. J.* **2012,** *103* (1), 1–10.

https://www.who.int/docs/default source/coronaviruse/situation-reports/20200817-weekly-epi-up date-1.pdf

Laguipo, A. B. B. Blood Types and COVID-19 Risk Confirmed. *N. Engl. J. Med.* **2020**.

Latz, C. A..; et al. Blood Type and Outcomes in Patients with COVID-19. *Ann. Hematol.* **2020,** *99,* 2113–2118.

Li, J.; Wang, X.; Chen, J.; Cai, Y.; Deng, A.; Yang, M. Association Between ABO Blood Groups and Risk of SARS-CoV-2 Pneumonia. *Br. J. Haematol.* **2020,** *190* (1), 24–27.

Liu, N.; et al. The Impact of ABO Blood Group on COVID-19 Infection Risk and Mortality: A Systematic Review and Meta-Analysis. *Blood Rev. 1,* 100785.

McPherson, R.; Pincus, M.; eds. *Henry's Clinical Diagnosis and Management by Laboratory Methods*, 21st ed.; Philadelphia: Saunders Elsevier, 2007.

Rossez, Y.; Maes, E.; Lefebvre Darroman, T.; et al. Almost All Human Gastric Mucin O-Glycans Harbor Blood Group A, B or H Antigens and are Potential Binding Sites for Helicobacter Pylori. *Glycobiology* **2012,** *22,* 1193–1206.

Wang, P. G. Relationship Between the ABO Blood Group and the COVID-19 Susceptibility *medRxiv* 2020, DOI: 10.1101/2020.03.11.20031096

Weigel-Kelley, K. A.; Yoder, M. C.; Srivastava, A. Alpha5beta1 Integrin as a Cellular Co Receptor for Human Parvovirus B19: Requirement of Functional Activation of Beta1 Integrin for Viral Entry. *Blood* **2003,** *102,* 3927–3933.

World Health Organization (WHO). Coronavirus Disease 2019 Situation Reports. 2020. https://www.who.int/docs/default-source/coronaviruse/situation-reports/20200405-sitrep-76-covid-19.pdf?sfvrsn=6ecf0977_2

Yang, X.; Yu, Y.; Xu, J.; Shu, H.; Xia, J.; Liu, H; et al. Clinical Course and Outcomes of Critically Ill Patients with SARS-CoV-2 Pneumonia in Wuhan, China: A Single-Centered, Retrospective, Observational Study. *Lancet. Respir Med.* **2020,** *8* (5), 475–481.

Zhao, J.; Yang, Y.; Huang. H.; et al. Relationship Between the ABO Blood Group and the COVID-19 Suspectibility. 2020. https://doi.org/10.1101/2020.03.11.20031096.8

Zheng, Z.; Peng, F.; Xu, B.; Zhao, J.; Liu, H.; Peng, J.; Li, Q.; Jiang, C.; Zhou, Y.; Liu, S.; … Tang, W. Risk Factors of Critical & Mortal COVID-19 Cases: A Systematic Literature Review and Meta-Analysis. *J. Infect.* **2020**. DOI: 10.1016/j.jinf.2020.04.021

Zhou, F.; Yu, T.; Du, R.; et al. Clinical Course and Risk Factors for Mortality of Adult Inpatients with COVID-19 in Wuhan, China: A Retrospective Cohort Study. *Lancet* **2020,** *395*(10229), 1054–1062.

Zhou, F.; Yu, T.; Du, R.; Fan, G.; Liu, Y.; Liu, Z.; Xiang, J.; Wang, Y.; Song, B.; Gu, X.; … Cao, B. Clinical Course and Risk Factors for Mortality of Adult Inpatients with COVID-19 in Wuhan, China: A Retrospective Cohort Study. *Lancet* **2020**. DOI: 10.1016/s0140-6736(20)30566-3

Zhou, S.;Welsby, I. Is ABO Blood Group Truly a Risk Factor for Thrombosis and Adverse Outcomes. *World J. Cardiol.* **2014,** *6* (9):985.

CHAPTER 5

Key Role of Convolutional Neural Networks in Biomedical Imaging Applications

MANJU DEVI[1], SUKHDIP SINGH[1], and SHAILENDRA TIWARI[2]

[1]*Deenbandhu ChhotuRam University of Science and Technology, Murthal, Haryana, India*

[2]*Thapar Institute of Engineering and Technology (TIET), Patiala, Punjab, India*

ABSTRACT

Artificial intelligence (AI) has revolutionized the world and increasing human abilities in significant ways. There are numerous AI-based techniques such as machine learning and deep learning, each with its own set of benefits and applications. Convolutional neural networks (CNN) is a model of artificial neural network (ANN) that is gaining popularity in a variety of applications, particularly in computer vision and medical science. This chapter presents the comprehensive details of CNN model with their detailed architecture, such as building elements, convolution, pooling, and fully connected layers to automatically acquire temporal orders of knowledge and adapt via backpropagation. Also, presents key role of CNNs in the field of Biomedical Imaging. The chapter ends with the discussion of current challenges (limitations) of CNN, some benchmark datasets and a conclusion.

Advanced Research in Electronic Devices for Biomedical and mHealth.
Rajesh K. Kesharwani, Upendra Kumar, Raj K. Keservani (Eds)

5.1 INTRODUCTION

Deep learning techniques are built around neural networks, which are a subset of machine learning. Node layers are made up of input, one or more hidden, and an output layer. Every node has weight and a threshold that it links to. When a single node outcome reaches a specific level, it is activated, and information is transferred to the network's next layer. Instead, no data are transferred. Our focus was on convolutional neural networks (CNNs) in this article. It is a sort of multilayer neural network for spatial analysis which is unique among other deep learning (Tachibana, 2014) architectures. CNN's design is based on how living creatures perceive the world. However, it was not until the ImageNet competition in 2012 that their true worth was realized, resulting in a revolution thanks to the reliable utilization of Graphics Processing Units (GPU's), corrected linear units, innovative dropout regularization, and appropriate data augmentation (Lecun et al., 2015). CNNs, which were named one of the top 10 breakthroughs of 2013, has resurfaced as a widely known learning machine, not just in the computer vision field, but also in a variety of applications spanning from natural language processing (NLP) to remote sensing processing and computer-aided diagnosis.

CNNs' incredibly huge achievement can be categorized into two major groups: (I) their modular features extraction structure, which adjusts architecture benchmark parameters for a specific job which needs less prior knowledge, and (II) their end-to-end framework training approach, that enables for the optimal design of all elements of an image-processing piping system. CNNs have lately gained popularity in the computer vision area because of their benefits over classical learning-based techniques. There's a significant amount of work demonstrating the excellent properties of CNNs in medical imaging challenges over the previous 3 years. Many classic technologies relying on hand-engineered analytic methods and image characteristics have been found to outperform CNN-based methods in most of these domains. Segmentation in optics (Shelhamer et al., 2017) cardiology imaging (Tran, 2016), morphological point localization (Ghesu et al., 2016; Štern et al., 2016), spatially imaging alignments (Miao et al., 2016), and anomaly identification (Jamaludin et al., 2016) are few excellent techniques.

5.1.1 BACKGROUNDS OF CONVOLUTIONAL NEURAL NETWORK

David Hubel and Torsten Wiesel, two neurophysiologists, examined and eventually wrote the article "Receptive fields of single neurons in cat's striate cortex" (Hubel and Wiesel, 1968) in 1959, describing how the neurons within a cat's brain are formed in numbers of a layer. Such layer learns to detect data features by retrieving local information first, afterward merging them for higher-level representation. Eventually, this concept became a key premise of deep learning. Kunihiko Fukushima created the neocognitron model (Fukushima, 1980) in 1980, and that's a self-organizing neural network with numerous layers smart enough to learn to recognize visual patterns spatially, so this structure became the first theoretical framework of CNN as depicted in Figure 5.1. In 1998, LeCun et al. made a significant upgrade to neocognitron's architecture by producing LeNet-5, a recent CNN framework that effectively understood the MNIST hand-written integer dataset. LeNet-5 is also prepared with the error back-propagation technique or could identify data features immediately from unprocessed input data without the use of some external feature selection method. CNN did not perform well in numerous complicated tasks after the discovery of LeNet-5 due to several limitations, such as a lot of significant training data, an absence of method creativity, and insufficient computer power. However, in the information technology era, the researchers got a huge labeled dataset, quite inventive techniques, as well as particularly impactful GPU's workstation. In 2012, Krizhevsky et al. built AlexNet, which obtained excellent efficiency within "ImageNet Large Scale Visual Recognition Competition" (ILSVRC) (Russakovsky et al., 2015) using these kinds of improvements. AlexNet's success opened the door for the development of other CNN models (Sultana et al., 2018) while also their use in several fields of machine learning and computer vision.

The chapter will help readers gain a better knowledge of CNN and will create opportunities for new research and application advances in the field. The rest of the chapter is divided into sections: Describe working principles of CNN in Section 5.2, CNN models are defined in Section 5.3, applications in radiology are defined in Section 5.4; the article will come to a close with Section 5.5, which is the final section.

5.2 WORKING PRINCIPLES OF CONVOLUTIONAL NEURAL NETWORK

The main significant approach in DL (Devi, Singh, Tiwari, et al., 2021) is CNN. LeCun (Lecun et al., 2015) has implemented CNNs as templates for functionality in extraction activities so that the data are spatially configured preserved, and the property of invariance of translation is assured. It is a kind of multi-layer neural network that is an expert at the processing of high data volumes with greater accuracy, and less computational cost. Why are CNNs more important in computer vision than other types of neural networks?

The classification layer and the feature extraction layers train simultaneously in CNN, which improves the model's output better ordered and depends on the extracted features.

The weight share function of CNN's, which reduces the number of trainable parameters inside networks and helps the architecture avoiding over fitting as well as improve generalizations, is one of the key reasons for adopting CNN in this circumstance.

When the alternative form of a neural network is used instead of CNN's, the implementation of a big network becomes more complicated.

Within radiology specialists, CNN also has published a variety of studies in fields, such as segmentation (Christ et al., 2016), image reconstruction (Zhang and Dong, 2020), and other fields. CNN's fundamental structure involves convolution, pooling, flattening, and fully connected layers (Kim et al., 2020). Convolution layers are accountable for feature extraction. CNN obtains characteristics by itself, unlike machine learning. The dimension of the inputs is reduced in the pooling layer. To flatten the entire network, use a flattening layer. The flattening layer converts the whole feature map matrix pooled into a single column. Two main parameters in CNN are the dropout layer and the activation function described below.

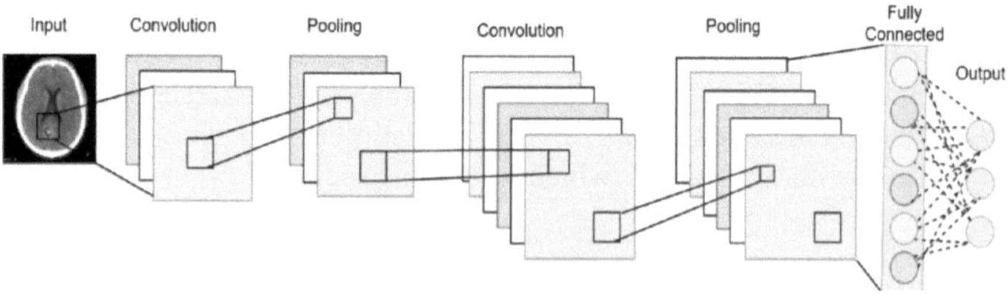

FIGURE 5.1 Convolution neural network architecture.

5.2.1 CONVOLUTION LAYER

This layer is an integral portion of the CNN model that extracts features, usually consisting of a blend of linear and nonlinear processes, which means convolution and activation function.

5.2.1.1 CONVOLUTION

This is a linear feature extraction process in which a limited set of numbers, known as the kernel, is inserted throughout the input that is a number of a set known as a tensor. At every position of the tensor, every aspect of the kernel and input tensor is determined and the output value is computed at the respective location of the output tensor, named the feature map. The process repeats by analyzing different kernels to construct an undefined number of a parameter representing multiple input tensor attributes; multiple kernels may therefore be regarded as different feature extractors. The type and shape of the kernel seem to be the main hyperparameter that describes the process of convolution. Usually, the initial is 3×3, but often 5×5 or 7×7. The above is conditional and defines the depth of the maps of output functions.

The gap among the two consecutive positions of the kernel is considered as a stride that determines the operation of convolution as well. The typical value of the step is 1; interestingly, a step greater than one is often used to downsample the feature maps. Down sampling is performed by pooling operation which is defined below. A parameter is a variable that throughout the training period is automatically optimized, and a hyperparameter is a variable that needs to be set accordingly.

For example: Take the following 5×5 with a 3×3 image input and filter matrix: The dimension of a visual area is also determined by the filter size or kernel. The filter is deployed toward a portion of the image, as well as the quantitative assessment between both the input pixels and the filter is computed. Thereafter, the weighted sum is loaded inside an output vector. The filter after this move through the stride, as well as the process is performed till its kernel has traversed the entire image. The ultimate output of a series of dot products out from input as well as the filter is a feature vector or activation function.

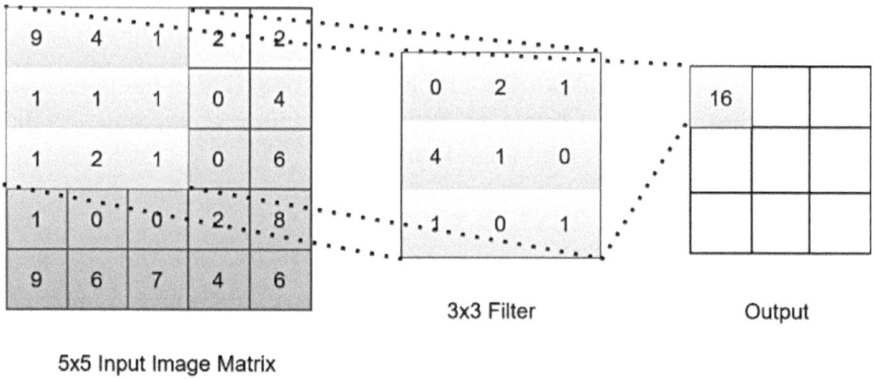

FIGURE 5.2 Convolution layer.

5.2.1.2 NONLINEAR ACTIVATION FUNCTION

The convolution output is moved through an activation function. There are several nonlinear functions like sigmoid or hyperbolic tangent () tanh, swish, but still, the Rectified Linear Unit (ReLU) is a popular nonlinear activation function, allowing the system to convergence very rapidly.

a) Sigmoid

The sigmoid function has an 'S' shaped curve. The sigmoid function accepts true values as input and outputs in between [0, 1] range. The sigmoid is represented mathematically as:

$$f(x)_{sigm} = \qquad (5.1)$$

b) Tanh

Visually, it approximates to sigmoid function and seems to have a similar S-shape. The function uses a true number as input and outputs a number within [−1, 1]. The Tanh (also known as "tanh" and "TanH") function is a hyperbolic tangent activation function. The tanh is represented mathematically as:

$$f(x)_{tanh} = \frac{e^{x} - e^{-x}}{e^{x} + e^{-x}} \qquad (5.2)$$

c) ReLU

In CNNs, the Rectifier Linear activation function is the most popular one. ReLU (Agarap, 2018) is a piece-wise linear function, it outputs instantly if the inputs are positive; otherwise, it returns zero. As a result, a structure which utilizes this is easier to train and gives superior outcomes, because it is considered the usual activation function for a variety of methods. ReLU's mathematical description is:

$$f(x)_{ReLU} = \max(0, x) \tag{5.3}$$

Because of the vanishing gradient issue, the sigmoid and hyperbolic tangent activation functions cannot be employed in networks with numerous layers. The vanishing gradient issue is resolved by using a rectified linear activation function, which allows models to learn quicker and function effectively.

5.2.2 POOLING LAYER

This layer offers a standard down sampling process. This layer effectively decreases the number of network parameters and computations, restricting over fitting by gradually decreasing the network spatial scale. There are two kinds of pooling: max and average pooling. Max-Pooling produces the highest value from the image area represented by a Kernel. Contrarily, Average pooling produces the average of all the values from the image's

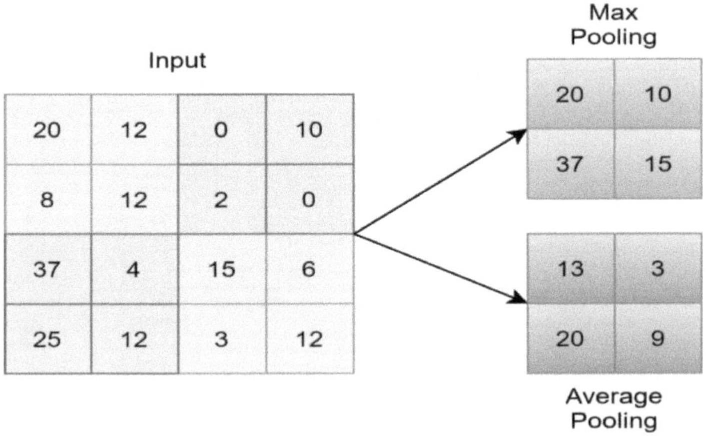

FIGURE 5.3 Pooling layer.

Kernel section. Max-pooling operation is used in this layer. Only the limit is taken from a pool. This is achieved with the use of filters that slide over the input; the maximum variable is extracted out at each step and the rest is removed. The network is simply downsampled. The pooling layer does not change the number. of hidden layers like the convolution, and the depth dimension stands constant.

5.2.3 FULLY CONNECTED LAYER

This layer was the final step of the CCN model. CNN is consisting of hidden layers and fully connected (FC) layers. The neuron has a total relation to all the activation of the previous layers. Therefore, their activations can be calculated with a multiplication of a matrix supported by a bias offset. Usually, the final FC layer has a similar output node as the number of classes. A nonlinear function, such as ReLU, follows every fully connected layer.

5.3 CONVOLUTIONAL NEURAL NETWORK MODELS

5.3.1 LENET-5

LeNet-5 was created to recognize handwritten and machine-printed characters. LeCun et al. (1998) first proposed it in 1998. Three convolutional and two fully connected layers make up the LeNet-5's five weighted (trainable) layers. The first two convolution layers are preceded by a max-pooling layer, and the final layer is then accomplished by two fully linked layers. The classifier that can categorize up to 10 digits is the final layer of such completely connected layers.

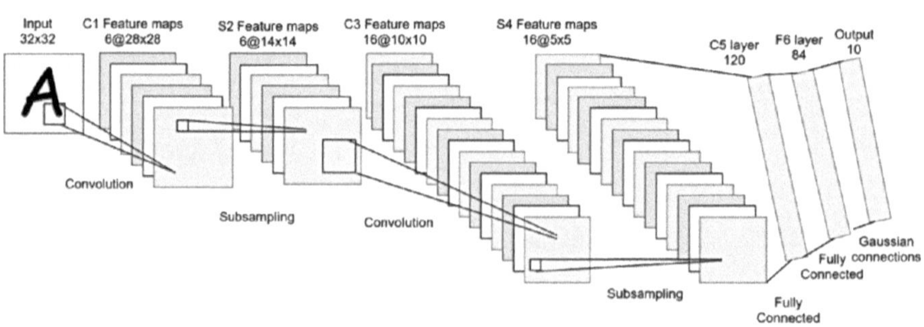

FIGURE 5.4 Structure of LeNet-5.

Source: Adapted from Data Science Central, 2018. https://www.datasciencecentral.com/lenet-5-a-classic-cnn-architecture/

5.3.2 *YOLO*

You Only Look Once (YOLO) (Redmon et al., 2016) is a standard identification method that incorporates end-to-end trained CNN's architecture to instantly detect objects along with their actual location. YOLO splits the data into a set number of grids, and afterward uses a correct label to build a fixed number of bounding box locations from each grid. The object is then selected and located inside the image using a threshold value (where the probability of a given class is far less than a threshold value).

5.3.3 *ALEXNET*

In 2012, Krizhevky et al. created AlexNet (Gonzalez, 2007) that was developed to classify ImageNet data and was motivated by LeNet-5. It is made up of eight trainable layers, the first five of those are convolutional and the final three of these are fully linked layers. The very last output layer, which was created for ImageNet data, uses 1000 units to categorize the source images through each of the 1000 classes in the ImageNet datasets. AlexNet has become a sophisticated model capable of achieving excellent results on some very difficult datasets. AlexNet's performance will suffer significantly if either of these convolutional layers is erased. AlexNet is a premier structure for any particle identification task, and it has a lot of potential in the computer vision AI area. Figure 5.5 depicts the architecture of AlexNet.

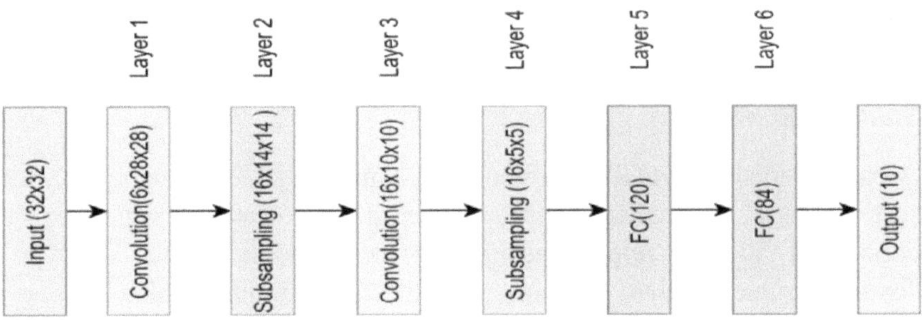

FIGURE 5.5 Structure of AlexNet.

5.3.4 *SEGNET*

For semantic segmentation, the researcher utilized an encoder–decoder structure (Badrinarayanan et al., 2017). The encoder employs 13 levels of the VGG16 network, which are used in opposite directions by the decoder. A pixel-by-pixel classification layer is a final layer. SegNet recalls the "max-pooling variables" at the associated encoder layer during the decoding stage to upsample the layers. Because the network does not have to learn the up-sampling weights again, the training process is simplified.

5.3.5 *GOOGLENET*

All prior CNN designs are substantially highly complicated and deep than the GoogLeNet model described in Szegedy et al. (2015). Also, it includes a new method named "Inception," which combines filters of various shapes and sizes into a single module. GoogLeNet has nine "Inception," 2 convolution, and 2 pooling layers. 6 convolutions and 1 pooling layer make up every "Inception" layer. GoogLeNet is the most up-to-date CNN structure for the ILSVRC task, with a top-five classification error of 5 x 5% on the ImageNet challenge, comparing to 15.3% for AlexNet.

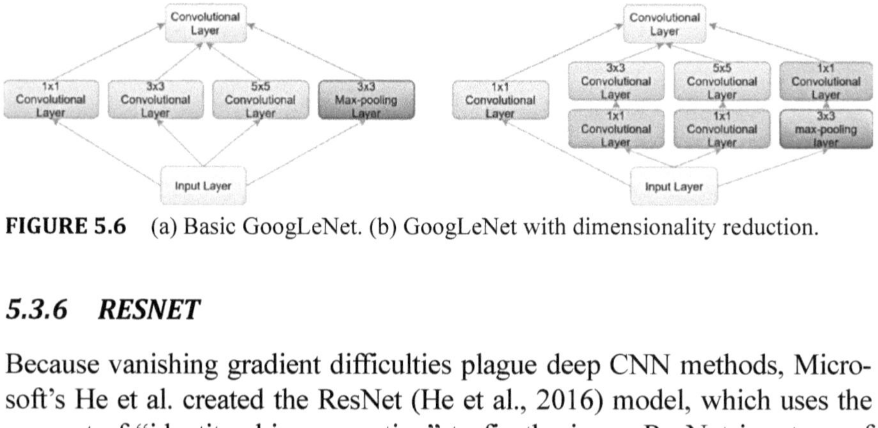

FIGURE 5.6 (a) Basic GoogLeNet. (b) GoogLeNet with dimensionality reduction.

5.3.6 *RESNET*

Because vanishing gradient difficulties plague deep CNN methods, Microsoft's He et al. created the ResNet (He et al., 2016) model, which uses the concept of "identity skip connection" to fix the issue. ResNet is a type of "exotic structure" that uses microarchitecture modules (also known as "network-in-network structures") rather than standard sequential CNN models like AlexNet, Over Feat, and VGG. Rather than learning a straight mapping $(x) = F(x)$, the ResNet technique provides residual mapping $(x) = f(x) - x$, and all those blocks are known as residual blocks. Numerous residual blocks with 3×3 convolution layers make up the entire ResNet structure. The contrast between direct and residual mapping is depicted in Figure 5.7.

ResNet is significantly smaller than VGG16 and VGG19, owing to the use of world average pooling despite fully connected layers, which decreases the model size to 102 MB for ResNet50.

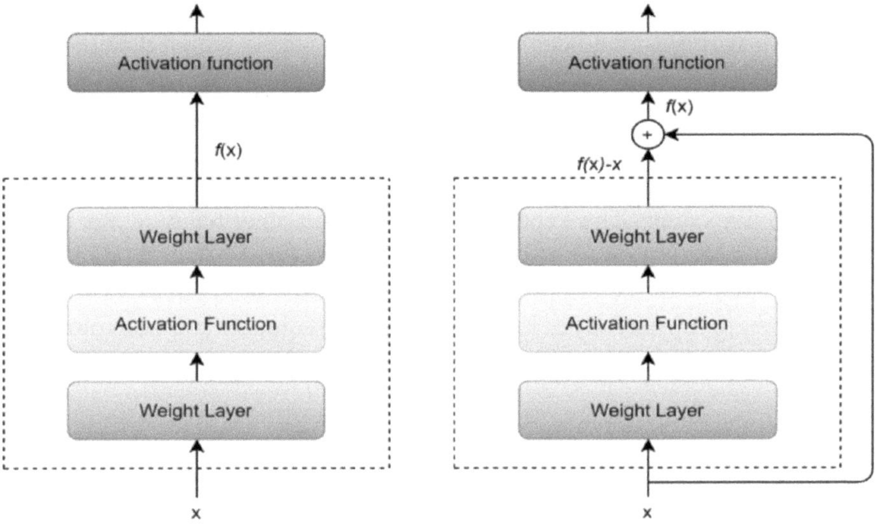

FIGURE 5.7 (a) Straight mapping block. (b) Residual block.

5.3.7 DENSENET

As demonstrated in Figure 5.8 DenseNet (Huang et al., 2017) expanded the concept of residual mapping by distributing the output of every block to everyone subsequent block within every dense block in the network. It enhances feature propagation abilities and solves the vanishing gradient issue by concept is to create in both forward and backward directions throughout the training stage. Huang et al. presented DenseNet in 2016, and that was awarded the champion of the ILSVRC-2016.

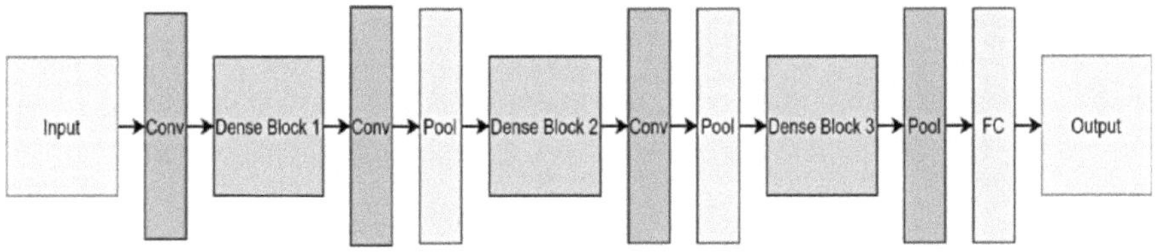

FIGURE 5.8 DenseNet architecture.

5.3.8 U-NET

Olaf Ronneberger et al. presented U-Net, a type of CNN technique, in 2015 to improve segmentation on biomedical imaging. U-Net is a CNN architecture that has grown in size despite very minor changes to the CNN model. It was created to deal with medical images in which the goal is not just to classify whether or not there is an infection, but also to pinpoint the infection's location. A u-shaped contraction and expanded passage make up this architecture (Olaf Ronneberger and Computer, 2015). The contraction route is made up of two 3 × 3 convolutions, ReLU, and 2 × 2 max-pooling steps. The expanded route, on the other hand, is made up of 2 × 2 up convolution, 3 × 3 convolution, and ReLU. The feature vector is combined with the clipped feature vector from the convolutional layer from the appropriate layer in between up convolution and convolution in expanding path.

5.3.9 VGG NET

VGG Net (Simonyan and Zisserman, 2015), created by Simonyan and Zisserman in 2014, is among the most prominent CNN architectures. The developers provided six distinct CNN setups, the far more popular of which are VGGNet-16 (setup D) and VGGNet-19 (setup E). VGGNet-16's structure is depicted in Figure 5.9 the success of VGG Net can be attributed to its structural clarity and use of small-sized filters for convolutional operations. VGG Net, regrettably, has two significant flaws:

Training is excruciatingly slow.

The weights of the network design are quite large (in terms of disk/bandwidth).

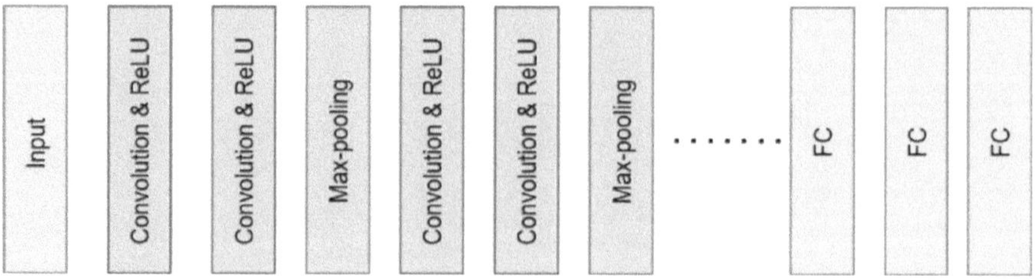

FIGURE 5.9 Structure of VGG net.

5.3.10 DEEPLAB

Deep CNN has two problems when it comes to semantic segmentation: downsampling as well as spatially invariance. The researchers employed the holes technique for solving the first problem. The author employed conditional random fields (CRF) to get information to solve the second difficulty. In the PASCAL VOC 2012 semantic segmentation challenge, DeepLab (L. C. Chen et al., 2018) obtained 71.6% Intersection over Union (IoU) accuracy in this challenge. The major point between DeepLabv1 and DeepLabv2 is an advanced technique known as Atrous Spatial Pyramid Pooling (ASPP).

5.4 APPLICATIONS IN RADIOLOGY

5.4.1 CLASSIFICATION

Because of its great accuracy, CNNs are employed for image classification and recognition. In the task of medical classification, the CNN-based deep neural system is commonly utilized. Because CNN is such a good feature extractor, using it to identify medical images can save time and money on feature selection. To categorize image patches of lung illness, Q. Le et al. (2014) proposed a modified CNN with a relatively small ConvLayer. The technique would be used on different medical image databases, according to the researchers. Furthermore, it was discovered in other research, CNN-based systems are trained using a large Chest X-ray (CXR) film dataset and state-of-the-art with good accuracy and sensitivity results on their dataset, such as the Stanford Normal Radiology Diagnostic Dataset, that also contains over 400,000 CXR, and the latest CXR database (ChestX-ray8) that contains 108,948 front-view CXR (Wang et al., 2017). Furthermore, training an acceptable model with insufficient data are difficult. The invention of AlexNet in 2012, which won the ILSVRC (Kermany et al., 2018) contest the same year, was the first achievement in image classification. Following that, researchers have made significant enhancements to the CNN architecture over time, making CNN the first choice for image classification problems.

5.4.2 SEGMENTATION

By heavily employing CNNs to solve classification challenges, that is time to go deeper into CNN's capabilities. Besides classification, CNN is being utilized for more complex tasks, such as image segmentation, object identification, and so forth. Image segmentation is a computer vision procedure that divides an image into segments that represent each of the image's multiple classes. In an image, segmentation aids in identifying where objects of various classes are present. Kim et al. used deep learning-based approaches, particularly the U-Net structure, to create a web-based application for segmenting spine imaging data from CT scans (Kim et al., 2020). Vania et al. (2017) developed a technique for automatically segmenting the spine from CT scans using CNN and redundant class labels. Two and three Convolutional fully connected layers made up the implementation framework. Using a generative adversarial network, Izadi et al. (2018) introduced a novel approach for segmenting skin lesions. The input image is split into two categories: lesion and backdrop Osadebey et al.'s (2021) work takes advantage of deep learning methods by presenting a three-step segmentation in which each stage is executed using a deep learning methodology. During the preprocessing phase, a CNN classifies the input into lung and none lung areas. The preprocessing step used a CNN-based U-net, whereas the post-processing phase used another U-net and CNN for contour refinement and high false filtration, etc. Pathak et al. (2019) proposed an efficient low-dose computed tomography reconstruction algorithms using a novel dictionary learning techniques modified with differential equations and have done a remarkable work in the field of medical imaging.

5.4.3 DETECTION

Object detection in computer vision was an earlier and essential topic (Li et al., 2015; Pedersoli et al., 2015; Qiang et al., 2020). The problems frequently stem from determining how to precisely and effectively pinpoint an object in images or video. CNN's have been used for detecting and locating since the 1990s (Nowlan and Platt, 1995). In contrast to image classification, source images potentially come with many objects. With CNN models, we attempt to recognize those items in the source image by properly identifying each object as well as correcting placement within the image. Region-Based Convolutional Neural Networks (R-CNNs) are a class of algorithms for solving object recognition and localization tasks that are optimized for models efficiency. YOLO is the second group of object identification systems that are designed for speed and real-time use.

5.4.4 OTHERS

Low-dose CT is becoming more used for healthcare situations (Devi et al., 2021). Low-dose CT, for example, was shown to be successful in diagnosing lung cancer (Aberle et al., 2011). While noisy low-dose CT images made it difficult to evaluate CT images accurately, numerous image processing methods were employed to de-noise low-dose CT images. Past research has shown that deep learning can efficiently de-noise low dose and ultra low-dose CT images (Chen et al., 2017; Nishio et al., 2017). U-net was previously employed to tackle the inverse problem in images for creating a de-noising CT image reconstructed from projection data in a previous study (Jin et al., 2017). U-net is trained to reconstruct a noise-less CT image from raw data using (a) noisy CT images generated from raw data using Filtered Back projection (FBP), (b) de-noising the images derived from the raw data. While it was easy to train U-net to reconstruct CT images immediately from the phantom, the researchers reported that doing the FBP first substantially simplified the training.

5.5 SOME BENCHMARK DATASETS

1. **MNIST Dataset:** Handwritten digits are represented in grayscale in the MNIST dataset, which comprises photographs in gray-scale. Random selection of 100 photos from MNIST. In all, it is divided into 10 different categories, one for each number from 0 to 9. There is a fixed size of 28 × 28 pixels for each grayscale image. Digits are normalized in size, centered within the image, and centered within the image itself. MNIST has a total of 70,000 images, divided into 60,000 training and 10,000 test images.
2. **BraTS:** There is a collection of brain tumor MRI scans with expert annotations in the brain tumor segmentation challenge (BraTS). Multiple MRI scans of patients with confirmed GBM/HGG and low-grade glioma (LGG) are included. A native T1 scan, post-contrast T1 scan, T2-weighted scan, and a T2-FLAIR scan are among the modalities used in these studies. Enhanced tumor, peritumoral edema and necrotic, and non-enhancing tumor core are all annotated.

3. **MICCAI 2015 Multi-Atlas Abdomen Labeling Challenge:** Fifty abdominal CT scans were randomly selected from an ongoing colorectal cancer chemotherapy trial and a retrospective ventral hernia investigation under the supervision of the Institutional Review Board (IRB). In the portal venous contrast phase, 50 images were taken in different volumes (512 × 512, 85-198) and fields of view (approx. 280 × 280 × 280 mm^3 − 500 × 500 × 650 mm^3). When it comes to the in-plane resolution, it goes from 0.54 mm^2 to 0.98 mm^2, while the slice thickness spans from 2.5 to 5.0 millimeters. NiftyReg generated the normal registration information.
4. **LUNA:** In 2017, the Kaggle Data Science Bowl featured a lung segmentation dataset in the Lung Nodule Analysis (LUNA) competition. For lung segmentation, this dataset contains 2D and 3D CT images with corresponding label pictures. About 70% of the data is used as the train set, while the remaining 30% is used as the test set. Each image is 512 by 512 pixels in size. Because the lung region in CT scans has nearly the same Hausdorff value as non-objects of interest like bone and air, learning the lung region through learning its soft tissue is worthwhile. Data from the LIDC-IDRI chest CT scan reference database is used in LUNA competitions for automatic nodule identification systems.
5. **ChestX-ray8:** It consists of 108,948 frontal X-ray images taken from 32,717 individual patients between 1992 and 2015, with eight common disease labels extracted from radiological reports using NLP techniques.
6. **Medical segmentation decathlon (MSD):** Simpson et al. (2019) developed a huge, open-source, hand-annotated medical images data set comprising numerous anatomical segments. This data collection can be used to objectively assess generic segmentation technique using extensive standards, as well as provide medical image data accessible to the public. Anatomical components, models, and data sources from numerous resources are all included in the data set, which includes 2633 three-dimensional medical images. And 10 subcategories are included in the study.

a. **Brain Tumor:** There are 750 labels in total, separated into two sections: glioma (necrotic/active cancer), and edema. An MRI scan performed as part of standard clinical care.

b. **Heart:** One cardiac phase (free breathing with respiratory and electrocardiogram (ECG) gated) yielded 30 mono-modal MRI scans of the complete heart. The left atrium was chosen as the ROI for this study. There was a limited training data set combined with considerable anatomical diversity that made this data set ideal.

c. **Liver:** Patients with colorectal, breast, and lung original malignancies had 201 contrast-enhanced CT scans taken from patients with primary cancer and metastatic liver illness. Those ROIs corresponded to liver segmentation and malignancies within the liver. An important reason for choosing this data set was the fact that it had a major label imbalance between large and tiny target areas (liver and tumor) (ROIs).

d. **Hippocampus:** A total of 394 are present, and the labels are hippocampus (the brain), head, and body. In this case, it is MRI. There were 90 healthy people in the study and 105 people with a non-affective psychotic condition.

e. **Prostate:** There are 48 prostate multiparametric MRI scans in the data collection. These include T2-weighted, diffusion-weighted, and T1-weighted contrast-enhanced series. It was decided to use a subset of two series, transverse T2-weighted and apparent diffusion coefficient (ADC). Both of these ROIs corresponded to areas of interest in prostate tissue (TZ). This data set was chosen because of the difficulty in segmenting two adjacent regions with a substantial inter-subject variability. In Nijmegen, The Netherlands, the data were collected at the Radboud University Medical Center and Nijmegen Medical Center.

f. **Lung:** Lung tumor is the name given to 96 of them. CT is a method of imaging that uses X-rays. Stanford University patients with non-small-cell lung cancer were included in the lung data set. An expert thoracic radiologist used OsiriX to mark the tumor location on a typical CT cross-section.

g. **Pancreas:** There are 421 portal venous phases CT scans of patients who had pancreatic tumors removed, and the data set is comprised of these scans. The pancreatic parenchyma and pancreatic bulk were the two ROIs that were analyzed in this study (cyst or tumor). An unbalanced labeling system between large (background) and small-structured tumors led to the selection of this batch of data. The data were collected at the Memorial Sloan Kettering Cancer Center in New York, United States of America.

h. **Hepatic Vessel:** Each of the 443 hepatic vessels has a unique label: liver vessels. CT is the imaging method used.

i. **Spleen:** There are 61 in total, and the spleen is the label. CT is the imaging method used. Memorial Sloan Kettering Cancer Center collected spleen data from individuals having chemotherapy for liver metastases.

j. **Colon:** In the data set, 190 individuals with primary colon cancer had portal venous phase CT scans. Colon cancer primary tumors were the ROI goal. This data collection was chosen because of its heterogeneous look and the difficulty of annotating it. The data were collected at the Memorial Sloan Kettering Cancer Center in New York, United States of America.

In Table 5.1, we summarize the some of the benchmark dataset in medical images.

5.6 CURRENTHE CHALLENGES (LIMITATIONS) OF CNN

On data that are either time series or has a grid-like architecture, CNNs have shown to be effective. Furthermore, deep CNN systems have been used to solve several additional problems. The following are some of the major issues that come with various convolutional networks:

Because of the numerous layers, millions of parameters and sophisticated nonlinear data structures, it is difficult to interpret CNNs. Without assessing uncertainty in the findings gained, CNN researchers focused on building accurate models. It is necessary to make successful use of

TABLE 5.1 Benchmark Dataset in Medical Imaging.

Dataset	Object	Modality	Tasks	Images	Size of images	URL
Medical MNIST	Abdomen, Brest	CT,MRI	Classification	58954	64×64	https://www.kaggle.com/andrewmvd/medical-mnist
Breast Ultrasound Images	Breast	US	Classification, Detection and Segmentation	780	512×512	https://www.kaggle.com/aryashah2k/breast-ultrasound-images-dataset
Data Science bowl 2018	Cell nuclei	Microscopy	Segmentation	670	96×96	https://www.kaggle.com/c/data-science-bowl-2018/data
NIH Chest X-ray	Chest	X-ray	Reconstruction	112,120	1024×1024	https://www.kaggle.com/nih-chest-xrays/data
LiTS	Liver	CT	Segmentation	331	512×512	https://competitions.codalab.org/competitions/17094
BRATS	Brain	MRI	Segmentation	-	255×255	https://www.med.upenn.edu/sbia/brats2018/data.html
DRIVE	Eye	Funduscopy	Segmentation	400	-	https://drive.grand-challenge.org/
LIDC-IDRI	Lung	CT	Segmentation	1012	$64 \times 64 \times 64$	https://wiki.cancerimagingarchive.net/display/Public/LIDC-IDRI
Brain CT Images with Intracranial Hemorrhage Masks	Brain	CT	Detection and Segmentation	2500	624×624	https://www.kaggle.com/vbookshelf/computed-tomography-ct-images
3 DIRCADB	Liver	CT, MRI	Segmentation	-	-	https://www.ircad.fr/research/3d-ircadb-01/
MSD	Various	MRI, CT	Segmentation	2633	-	http://medicaldecathlon.com/
MICCAI 2017	The whole heart	CT	Segmentation	50	512×512	https://wiki.cancerimagingarchive.net/display/Public/Challenge+competitions
JSRT	Chest	CXR	Segmentation	247	-	http://db.jsrt.or.jp/eng.php

the CNN in medical diagnostics and this confidence needs to be able to determine the model's uncertainty or certainty or to describe the outcome achieved. This field requires more investigated. While heat maps, class activation (CAM), grade CAM, grade CAM++ were suggested by the researchers for viewing CNN outputs, the visualization area remains a challenge.

In the existence of prior information or knowledge about the image to be interpreted, understanding of medically based images would be more effective. CNNs would be more efficient in this scenario if the data were made not just by images but also by patient history. The next difficult issue would be to develop models to make decisions, which might be the next research trend, as well as to provide input for both photos and patient history.

Low level type of information could also be collected by using small kernels to improve speed. However, greater computational complexity during training comes at a cost. In addition, CNN can be improved using many paths design. The efficiency of the processors and the memory can be increased due to the collective learning of global textual characteristics and local detailed characteristics.

The choice of hyperparameters has a significant impact on CNN performance. A small modification in the hyper-parameter values can have a big impact on a CNN's entire functionality. As a result, careful selection of hyper-parameters is a critical design flaw that must be handled using an appropriate optimization technique.

In addition, because of their significant depth and scale, CNNs require a great deal of memory and computer power to train. The deeper CNNs include millions of train input parameters that could lead to a widespread and ineffective model, particularly with limited datasets. It requires models that are lightweight and that can also draw key characteristics such as dense models. Also examine the lightweight CNNs.

Deep learning has its own set of issues. It concentrates on three topics in particular: network structure design, 3D data segmentation model design, and loss function. It is worth looking into the network structure's architecture. Modifying the network structure has a major impact that can be easily transferred to other jobs. When 3D medical data are cut slice by slice, it can more effectively capture the geometric information of the target, which can be lost. As a result, designing 3D convolution models to process 3D medical picture data is a researchable direction. Loss function design has long been a challenge in deep learning research.

CNN models are similar to black boxes in that they are difficult to analyze and explain. As a result, verifying them can be challenging at times.

The imbalanced class issue where the positive class is underrepresented, and the majority of the images belong to the ordinary class, is one of the challenges in medical data. CNNs are a challenge in developing unbalanced data. However, by integrating additional underrepresented data, researchers tried to address this difficulty. Denser CNNs could also cause the problem of the disappearing gradient to be addressed by using skip connections such as the inceptionNet architecture.

Since CNNs are invariant in translation, rotation, and size invariance without explicitly increasing, the data are often terrible for handling.

The following are a summary of the many obstacles and ways to overcome particular medical image interpretation challenges as shown below in Table 5.2.

TABLE 5.2 Number of Challenges and Their Solutions.

Number of Challenges in medical images	Solutions for overcome difficulties
Sparsity of labeled data	Semi-supervised deep CNN
Extract local and global features	Multipath way CNN
Less training samples	Augmentation
Reduce classification errors	Train on misclassified image patches
Imbalanced label distributions	Two phase training
Noise in images	Gaussian filtering
Heart classification	Two path CNN, for spatial and temporal features
Thicker CT images of brain	Geometric normalization

AI-assisted diagnosis of various diseases realizes the concept of long-term medical treatment. For medics, it becomes a useful tool. However, because it is still an open subject, we can expect a slew of new technologies and study findings in the next years.

5.7 CONCLUSION

In image, video, and text processing, deep CNNs have made substantial progress. In this article, we explored CNNs and examined how they might be improved in terms of layer design, activation function, and loss function, among other things. We've also covered how CNN may be used for image classification, object recognition, and image segmentation, among other things. Discuss the some benchmark dataset and challenges of CNN. We believe that even this work not only aids future research and applications advances in the field of CNNs but also gives a better knowledge of CNNs.

KEYWORDS

- **deep learning**
- **convolutional neural networks**
- **image classification**
- **segmentation**
- **computer vision**

REFERENCES

Aberle, D. R.; Adams, A. M.; Berg. C. D.; Black, W. C.; Clapp, J. D.; Fagerstrom, R. M.; Gareen, I. F.; Gatsonis, C.; Marcus, P. M.; Sicks. J. D. Reduced Lung-Cancer Mortality with Low-Dose Computed Tomographic Screening—The National Lung Screening Trial Research Team. *N. Engl. J. Med.* **2011,** *365* (5), 395–409.

Agarap, A. F. Deep Learning using Rectified Linear Units (ReLU). **2018,** *1,* 2–8.

Badrinarayanan, V., Kendall, A., Cipolla, R. SegNet: A Deep Convolutional Encoder-Decoder Architecture for Image Segmentation. *IEEE Trans. Pattern Anal. Mach. Intell.* **2017,** *39* (12), 2481–2495.

Chen, H.; Zhang, Y.; Zhang, W.; Liao, P.; Li, K.; Zhou, J.; Wang, G. Low-Dose CT Denoising with Convolutional Neural Network. In *Proceedings—International Symposium on Biomedical Imaging*, 2017; pp 143–146. https://doi.org/10.1109/ISBI.2017.7950488

Chen, L. C.; Papandreou, G.; Kokkinos, I.; Murphy, K.; Yuille, A. L. DeepLab: Semantic Image Segmentation with Deep Convolutional Nets, Atrous Convolution, and Fully Connected CRFs. *IEEE Trans. Pattern Anal. Mach. Intell.* **2018,** *40* (4), 834–848.

Christ, P. F.; Elshaer, M. E. A.; Ettlinger, F.; Tatavarty, S.; Bickel, M.; Bilic, P.; Rempfler, M.; Armbruster, M.; Hofmann, F.; D'Anastasi, M.; Sommer, W. H.; Ahmadi, S. A.; Menze, B. H. Automatic Liver and Lesion Segmentation in CT Using Cascaded Fully Convolutional Neural Networks and 3D Conditional Random Fields. In *Lecture Notes in Computer Science (Including Subseries Lecture Notes in Artificial Intelligence and Lecture Notes in Bioinformatics), 9901 LNCS*, 2016, pp 415–423. https://doi.org/10.1007/978-3-319-46723-8_48

Devi, M.; Singh, S.; Tiwari, S. CT Image Reconstruction using NLMfuzzyCD Regularization Method. *Curr. Med. Imag. Form. Curr. Med. Imag. Rev.* **2021,** *17,* 1–11. DOI: 10.2174/1573405617999210112195819

Devi, M.; Singh, S.; Tiwari, S.; Chandra Patel, S.; Ayana, M. T. A Survey of Soft Computing Approaches in Biomedical Imaging. *J. Healthc. Eng.* **2021,** *2021.* DOI: 10.1155/2021/1563844

Fukushima, K. Neocognitron: A Self-Organizing Neural Network Model for a Mechanism of Pattern Recognition Unaffected by Shift in Position. *Biol. Cybernet.* **1980,** *36* (4), 193–202.

Ghesu, F. C.; Georgescu, B.; Mansi, T.; Neumann, D.; Hornegger, J.; Comaniciu, D. An Artificial Agent for Anatomical Landmark Detection in Medical Images BT—Medical Image Computing and Computer-Assisted Intervention. *Miccai* **2016,** *2016*, 229–237.

Gonzalez, T. F. Handbook of Approximation Algorithms and Metaheuristics. In *Handbook of Approximation Algorithms and Metaheuristics*, 2007, pp 1–1432. DOI: 10.1201/9781420010749

He, K.; Zhang, X.; Ren, S.; Sun, J. In *Deep Residual Learning for Image Recognition*, Proceedings of the IEEE Computer Society Conference on Computer Vision and Pattern Recognition, 2016-Decem, 2016; pp 770–778.

Huang, G.; Liu, Z.; Van Der Maaten, L.; Weinberger, K. Q. In *Densely connected convolutional networks*, Proceedings—30th IEEE Conference on Computer Vision and Pattern Recognition, CVPR 2017, 2017 Janua, 2017, pp 2261–2269.

Hubel, D.; Wiesel, T. <Jphysiol01104-0228.Pdf>. *J. Physiol.* **1968,** 215–243. DOI: 10.1113/jphysiol.1968.sp008455/abstract?rss=1

Jamaludin, A.; Kadir, T.; Zisserman, A. SpineNet: Automatically Pinpointing Classification Evidence in Spinal MRIs. In *Lecture Notes in Computer Science (Including Subseries Lecture Notes in Artificial Intelligence and Lecture Notes in Bioinformatics), 9901 LNCS*, 2016, pp 166–175. DOI: 10.1007/978-3-319-46723-8_20

Jin, K. H.; McCann, M. T.; Froustey, E.; Unser, M. Deep Convolutional Neural Network for Inverse Problems in Imaging. *IEEE Transac. Image Proc.* **2017,** *26* (9), 4509–4522.

Kermany, D. S.; Goldbaum, M.; Cai, W.; Valentim, C. C. S.; Liang, H.; Baxter, S. L.; McKeown, A.; Yang, G.; Wu, X.; Yan, F.; Dong, J.; Prasadha, M. K.; Pei, J.; Ting, M.; Zhu, J.; Li, C.; Hewett, S.; Dong, J.; Ziyar, I.; … Zhang, K. Identifying Medical Diagnoses and Treatable Diseases by Image-Based Deep Learning. *Cell* **2018,** *172* (5), 1122–1131.e9.

Pathak, Y.; Arya, K. V. Tiwari, S. An Efficient Low-Dose CT Reconstruction Technique Using Partial Derivatives based Guided Image Filter. *Multimed. Tools Appl.* **2019,** *78,* 14733–14752.

Kim, Y. J.; Ganbold, B.; Kim, K. G. Web-based Spine Segmentation Using Deep Learning in Computed Tomography Images. *Healthc. Inform. Res.* **2020,** *26* (1), 61–67.

Lecun, Y.; Bengio, Y.; Hinton, G. Deep Learning. *Nature* **2015,** *521* (7553), 436–444.

Lecun, Y.; Bottou, L.; Bengio, Y.; Ha, P. In *LeNet, Proceedings of the IEEE, November*, 1998; pp 1–46.

Li, Q.; Cai, W.; Wang, X.; Zhou, Y.; Feng, D. D.; Chen, M. In *Medical Image Classification with Convolutional Neural Network*, 2014 13th International Conference on Control Automation Robotics and Vision, ICARCV 2014, 2014 December; pp 844–848.

Li, Y.; Wang, S.; Tian, Q.; Ding, X. Feature Representation for Statistical-Learning-based Object Detection: A Review. *Pattern Recognition*. **2015,** *48* (11), 3542–3559.

Miao, S.; Wang, Z. J.; Liao, R. A CNN Regression Approach for Real-Time 2D/3D Registration. *IEEE Transac. Med. Imag.* **2016,** *35* (5), 1352–1363.

Nishio, M.; Nagashima, C.; Hirabayashi, S.; Ohnishi, A.; Sasaki, K.; Sagawa, T.; Hamada, M.; Yamashita, T. Convolutional Auto-Encoders for Image Denoising of Ultra-Low-Dose CT. *Heliyon* **2017,** *3* (8), e00393.

Nowlan, S.; Platt, J. A Convolutional Neural Network Hand Tracker. *Adv. Neural Inf. Process. Syst.* **1995,** 8–10. DOI: 10.1.1.40.9668&rep=rep1&type=pdf

Olaf Ronneberger, P. F., Computer, T. B. U-Net: Convolutional Networks for Biomedical Image Segmentation. *IEEE Access*. **2015,** *9* (may), 16591–16603.

Osadebey, M.; Andersen, H. K.; Waaler, D.; Fossaa, K.; Martinsen, A. C. T.; Pedersen, M. Three-Stage Segmentation of Lung Region from CT Images Using Deep Neural Networks. *BMC Med. Imag.* **2021,** *21* (1), 1–19.

Pedersoli, M.; Vedaldi, A.; Gonzàlez, J.; Roca, X. A Coarse-to-Fine Approach for Fast Deformable Object Detection. *Pattern Recogn.* **2015,** *48* (5), 1844–1853.

Qiang, B.; Chen, R.; Zhou, M.; Pang, Y.; Zhai, Y.; Yang, M. Convolutional Neural Networks-based Object Detection Algorithm by Jointing Semantic Segmentation for Images. *Sensors (Switzerland)* **2020,** *20* (18), 1–14.

Redmon, J.; Divvala, S.; Girshick, R.; Farhadi, A. In *You only Look Once: Unified, Real-Time Object Detection*, Proceedings of the IEEE Computer Society Conference on Computer Vision and Pattern Recognition, 2016 December, 2016; pp 779–788. DOI: 10.1109/CVPR.2016.91

Russakovsky, O.; Deng, J.; Su, H.; Krause, J.; Satheesh, S.; Ma, S.; Huang, Z.; Karpathy, A.; Khosla, A.; Bernstein, M.; Berg, A. C.; Fei-Fei, L. ImageNet Large Scale Visual Recognition Challenge. *Int. J. Comp. Vision* **2015,** *115* (3), 211–252.

Izadi, S.; Mirikharaji, Z.; Kawahara, J.; Hamarneh, G. In *Generative Adversarial Networks to Segment Skin Lesions, Proceedings of the IEEE 15th International Symposium on Biomedical Imaging*, Washington, DC, USA, 2018; pp 881–884.

Shelhamer, E.; Long, J.; Darrell, T. Fully Convolutional Networks for Semantic Segmentation. *IEEE Transac. Pattern Anal. Mach. Intell.* **2017,** *39* (4), 640–651.

Simonyan, K.; Zisserman, A. In *Very Deep Convolutional Networks for Large-Scale Image Recognition, 3rd International Conference on Learning Representations, ICLR 2015 - Conference Track Proceedings*, 2015; pp 1–14.

Simpson, A. L.; Antonelli, M.; Bakas, S.; Bilello, M.; Farahani, K.; van Ginneken, B.; Kopp-Schneider, A.; Landman, B. A.; Litjens, G.; Menze, B.; Ronneberger, O.; Summers, R. M.; Bilic, P.; Christ, P. F.; Do, R. K. G.; Gollub, M.; Golia-Pernicka, J.; Heckers, S. H.; Jarnagin, W. R.; … Cardoso, M. J. A Large Annotated Medical Image Dataset for the Development and Evaluation of Segmentation Algorithms. 2019, http://arxiv.org/abs/1902.09063

Štern, D.; Bischof, H.; Urschler, M.; Payer, C.; Darkoˇdarkoštern, D. Regressing Heatmaps for Multiple Landmark Localization using CNNs Automatic Age Estimation from Skeletal and Dental MRI Data Using Machine Learning View Project SEE PROFILE

Regressing Heatmaps for Multiple Landmark Localization using CNNs. *Miccai, June*. 2016, https://www.researchgate.net/publication/304024957

Sultana, F.; Sufian, A.; Dutta, P. In *Advancements in Image Classification Using Convolutional Neural Network*, Proceedings - 2018 4th IEEE International Conference on Research in Computational Intelligence and Communication Networks, ICRCICN 2018, 2018; pp 122–129. DOI: 10.1109/ICRCICN.2018.8718718

Szegedy, C.; Liu, W.; Jia, Y.; Sermanet, P.; Reed, S.; Anguelov, D.; Erhan, D.; Vanhoucke, V.; Rabinovich, A. In *Going Deeper with Convolutions*, Proceedings of the IEEE Computer Society Conference on Computer Vision and Pattern Recognition, 07-12 June, 2015; pp 1–9. DOI: 10.1109/CVPR.2015.7298594

Tachibana, H. 葉月ちゃんでもできる Deep Learning. *Sig2D'14*, 2014, 1. http://files.sig2d.org/sig2d14.pdf#page=5

Tran, P. V. A Fully Convolutional Neural Network for Cardiac Segmentation in Short-Axis MRI. 2016; 1–21. http://arxiv.org/abs/1604.00494

Vania, M.; Mureja, D.; Lee, D. Automatic Spine Segmentation using Convolutional Neural Network via Redundant Generation of Class Labels for 3D Spine Modeling. 2017; pp 1–18. http://arxiv.org/abs/1712.01640

Wang, X.; Peng, Y.; Lu, L.; Lu, Z.; Bagheri, M.; Summers, R. M. In *ChestX-ray8: Hospital-Scale Chest X-Ray Database and Benchmarks on Weakly-Supervised Classification and Localization of Common Thorax Diseases*, Proceedings - 30th IEEE Conference on Computer Vision and Pattern Recognition, CVPR 2017, 2017 Janua, 2017; pp 3462–3471. https://doi.org/10.1109/CVPR.2017.369

Zhang, H. M.; Dong, B. A Review on Deep Learning in Medical Image Reconstruction. *J. Operat. Res. Soc. China*. **2020,** DOI: 10.1007/s40305-019-00287-4

CHAPTER 6

The Most Recent Developments and Applications of Smartphone-based Devices in Biomedical and mHealth

UPENDRA KUMAR[1], RAJESH KUMAR KESHARWANI[2], and MANOJ KUMAR PAL[3]

[1]*Department of Computer Science and Engineering, IET Lucknow, Uttar Pradesh, India*

[2]*Nehru Gram Bharati (Deemed to be University), Prayagraj, Uttar Pradesh, India*

[3]*Indian Institute of Information Technology, Allahabad, Prayagraj, Uttar Pradesh, India*

ABSTRACT

Smartphone-based applications revolutionize biomedical practice with artificial intelligence. Due to all time need of presence of experts in cloud and continuous data connectivity to the device, rising demand for high-quality medical services, telemedicine suffers from its inherent limitations. These limitations can be overcome by using computer-aided diagnosis (CAD) in which abnormalities can be detected without manual intervention. Commercially available traditional medical equipment restricts the installation of new software and, therefore, the integration of CAD-based intelligent algorithms cannot be done along with the existing equipment. Therefore, an external computing device is essentially required to capture image data from traditional medical equipment, perform CAD operations and finally result is generated. Smartphones are now playing important

Advanced Research in Electronic Devices for Biomedical and mHealth.
Rajesh K. Kesharwani, Upendra Kumar, Raj K. Keservani (Eds)

roles in personalized healthcare due to its universal known computing capability. Smartphones have shown to be versatile with embedded CAD technology which can be utilized as a smart computing device for automated diagnosis and other biomedical applications. It can be used remotely and even in resource-less conditions and have highly influential to handle both quantity and quality of medical care. Additionally, smartphone-based embedded devices have shown their application interest in the field of tele-imaging, food quality control, education, etc. In this chapter, the most recent applications and development of smartphone devices are discussed toward histopathological-based examination, bacteria and virus detection, food technology, and routine diagnosis. Incorporation of machine and deep-learning methods with smartphone-based biomedical devices has shown their capability to significantly enhance the efficiency of detection and analysis of biological samples in biomedical and mHealth applications.

6.1 INTRODUCTION

With rising healthcare costs throughout the world, a need arises for reducing its cost and resolving the complexity of biomedical devices (Thekkek et al., 2008). Additionally, with rapidly growing demand for high-quality healthcare services in the demographic area in the world which have below low level of medical infrastructure especially found in developed countries, portable devices such as smartphones can transmit relevant medical-related data to remote medical experts which in turn may have a high impact on quantity and quality of medical care. Hospital-centralized-based healthcare system suffers from its inherent limitations that patients have to visit the hospitals regularly even for routine check-ups like monitoring of blood pressure, diabetes, electrocardiography, etc. As a result, this increases the cost of healthcare and also acts as an add-on difficulty for old-person and remote patients, who are incapable to reach the hospitals due to mobility problems. In developing countries, heavy pressure is experienced by healthcare infrastructure due to high population growth. Mobile health (mHealth) system can address these issues by providing out of smartphone-based hospital healthcare (Vaidya et al., 2013). Demand for mHealth arises due to the tremendous needs of emergency healthcare, point of care (POC) diagnostics, remote monitoring, and rural healthcare, etc. Smartphones are no-doubt widely used handheld devices in mHealth applications due to its well-known computing capability, Wi-Fi, 3G, 4G, inbuilt communication modules like Bluetooth, flexibility of environment running multiple healthcare applications, sufficient storage memory to store patients' data in huge amount, etc. Significance and importance of smartphone devices in mHealth and its contribution in improving one's well-being with low cost and effort are reported in (English et al., 2013). A variety of applications like fall detection to assist the senior without press the call button, heart rate monitoring, diabetes monitoring, ECG monitoring, etc., using smartphone devices have been reported in (Rodrigues et al., 2014; Quero et al., 2007). Tele-diagnosis system is utilized by the patient to transmit data from smartphones to the healthcare expert side for getting diagnosis and treatment. The medical expert who is sitting away remotely can guide the patient based on the above-said transmitted data received from the smartphone devices. In tele-diagnosis system, still intervention of medical experts is essentially required to monitor and guide the patient; as a result it will add to the cost of healthcare. Additionally, this architecture is also not suitable and applicable for remote areas where there is no facility of data connectivity. In these situations, the computer-aided diagnosis (CAD) embedded with smartphone devices will be very beneficial. This reduces the cost of healthcare by minimizing the intervention of medical expert and also eliminating the need of availability of data connectivity to the smartphone devices.

Microscopes are imaging devices, whose growth has been observed gradually in terms of the resolution and they produce high sensitivity for detection of pathogen and diagnosis of diseases. The availability of such high-end microscopes is often not easily possible in masses in remote areas due to its high cost and lack of technical facilities. Therefore, it causes delay in-time diagnosis resulting fatalities in almost all resource-less areas (Panagariya, 2014). To overcome from this problem, smartphone-based imaging devices (SIDs) can be used alternatively. These devices can be used as a platform to utilize the imaging capability of smartphone and are utilized for variety of imaging applications other than conventional photography. A strong capability has been shown by them to be used as microscopic devices, sensing and analytical detection devices, pollution and contaminants monitoring devices, as well as devices dedicated for educational purposes also. SIDs have more advantages in comparison to conventional optical microscope in such areas which have limited human resource and where there is tremendous need of rapid diagnosis. SIDs are portable devices with either add-on attachment components or built-in camera setup-based modifications are required for advanced imaging applications. Additionally, other benefits could be getting diagnosis confirmation, sharing of medical experts' knowledge, and rapid and in-time data sharing for faster medical analysis. This enhancement makes the whole diagnostic system more affordable and helps in easily reaching out to a larger portion of the society due to low cost and flexible nature (Zimic et al., 2009). The current age smartphone in integration with improved high-end hardware and software can be utilized as a stand-alone application platform in terms of built-in source of information, detector, and the computational procedure. It has been also continuously exploited in order to develop autonomous mobile sensing devices highly applicable for various analytical applications as discussed in (McCracken et al., 2016; Yang et al., 2016; Vashist et al., 2015). The smartphone devices have become a foremost affordable choice especially in the area of biomedical and mHealth services due to their fast growing development.

Many researchers have incorporated different optical improvements and techniques to convert the smartphone devices into a laboratory-grade microscopic device dedicated to carry out various bio-analytical analyses with improved accuracy. Zhu et al. have shown in their work the usability of the smartphone device as a cost-effective imaging-based analytical tool using a combination of single 1-mm ball lens along with light-emitting diode (LED) configuration for cost-effective rapid blood analysis (Zhu et al., 2013). The study done by Roy et al. includes the incorporation of shadow imaging technique without using lens in a smartphone-based platform to perform the counting of blood cells (Roy et al., 2014), whereas Ozcan has proposed the application of a fluorescent optofluidic-based imaging platform with smartphone to find the density of white blood cells present in the sample (Zhu et al., 2011). Many scientific articles have been proposed by researchers on the development of different SIDs as well as explaining their applications in variety of domains. However, it is often difficult for new researchers to find a comprehensive review based on smartphone in order to understand the basic principles and working of such embedded devices and biomedical systems with wide range of multidiscipline in context to their applicability. In this chapter, various applications of SIDs have been discussed in histopathology, food quality control, pathogen detection, diagnosis, integration of machine learning with smartphone devices, and 3D-printed optomechanical attachments containing sensors-based specialized device for particular examinations and other related area. A variety of different possible biomedical applications of SIDs as well as their advantages is discussed in Table 7.1.

6.2 SMARTPHONE-BASED AUTOMATED SYSTEMS FOR DISEASE DIAGNOSIS

Routine diagnosis process plays a key role in the initial and pre-screening of patients based on disease at any healthcare unit. High specific, accurate, and rapid detection are desirable at a faster rate. However, with the current traditional benchtop methods, detection and pre-screening are attained at a higher diagnosis cost. Also, these highly cost devices are not always available in limited resource remote areas. With the rapid and advanced development of smartphone imaging technology-based capabilities, SIDs can be utilized for various routine diagnosis-based applications. Microscope-based histopathological examination in current healthcare unit is considered to be a gold standard method for laboratory-based diagnostic examination of variety of diseases. This approach requires the preparation of laboratory-based thin stained sections and its examination needs pathologists to understand and examine the underlying tissue architecture (Rubin et al., 2018). This whole process consumes more time and often it is not easy to perform their examination especially in resource-limited remote regions. Thus, a portable, flexible, and automated analytical system for the diagnosis process would be beneficial. It will help in saving time especially during critical and fatal situations like a rapid surgery or a case of emergency (Gurcan et al., 2009). With the rapid development and current age smartphone-based imaging capabilities, SIDs have shown efficient to be used for histopathological laboratory-based examination of various diseases. Along with the great potential and capabilities in fast diagnosis, SIDs have also shown their capability for easier transmission of medical data to medical expert analyst for further validation (Carusi et al., 2016).

6.3 SMARTPHONE-BASED RETINAL IMAGING SYSTEMS (SRIS) FOR DETECTION OF DIABETIC RETINOPATHY

As per estimation done by World Health Organization (WHO), around 347 million people are suffered from diabetes worldwide and this number may increase up to 552 million expected by the year 2030. In the United States, the number of American people suffered from diabetes is more

TABLE 6.1 List of Application Area and Uses of Smartphone-based Imaging Devices (SIDs).

S.No.	Application area of SIDs	Uses	Advantages
1	Routine diagnosis	-Hematological and histopathological examinations used for diagnosis and study of diseases of the tissues -Rapid and in-time examination of metabolites such as intermediates and end products of cellular regulatory processes in blood and body fluids -Fast and in-time monitoring for vital health parameters such as pulse rate, temperature measurement of body, respiration rate, and blood pressure	-Portable and easy to use devices with improved sensitivity in comparison to traditional diagnostic methods -Fast and in-time detection, portable devices act as POC for detection in nature -Cost-effective and time-saving methods
2	Bacterial detection	-Fluorescence- and autofluorescence-based technology having capability to monitor bacterial loads a factor which delays healing -Immunoassays a biochemical test for real-time detection of bacterial species in a biological sample in which the presence or concentration of a macromolecule is measured using an antibody or an antigen -Combining microfluidic devices as analytical platform along with SIDs for analysis of bacterial load with high performance	-Reduces time required for bacterial culture test which can help to find harmful bacteria in our body and easier compared to traditional analytical tests -Real-time detection of bacterial species with high sensitivity and specificity
3	Virus detection	-Colorimetric and fluorescence immunoassay, a biochemical method that identifies and quantifies unknown analytes (protein, lipid, and nucleic acid, etc.) present in biological solution incorporation with smartphone for detection of viral strains -Loop-mediated isothermal amplification (LAMP) assays and RT-LAMP assays to detect viruses accurately -Nucleic acid molecules-based imaging technology to understand and analyze the pathology of viruses	-Easily quantifiable and visible output directly on the smartphone devices -Less time-consuming, i.e., in-time solution than traditional benchtop methods -Enabling on-time detection of virus in resource-less remote location

TABLE 6.1 *(Continued)*

S.No.	Application area of SIDs	Uses	Advantages
4	Food quality control	- Cytometric methods based on digital image processing can be used for detection and analysis of food contaminants which are usually spoiled or tainted foods as they comprise microorganisms like bacteria or parasites that make them unfit for consumption -Can be used as spectroscopic methods as a device for detection of contamination of bacteria and viruses in food -Colorimetric assays such as reactions that lead to a change of color due to an enzymatic interaction between spotted reagents and the analyte for faster and accurate detection of allergens and toxins in food	-Faster and rapid detection and observation of food contaminants -Pre-screening of fresh and hygienic live stocks and meat products to monitor and maintain their quality -Can be utilized for regular monitoring of the food products by quality control authorities
5	Deep learning (DL) methods used for smartphone based imaging devices	-Rapid detection and laboratory observations of cancers and blood anomalies -Studying recent development and behavior in model organisms that are non-human species and used in the laboratory to help medical scientists to have better understanding of biological processes -Widely useful in non-biological applications such as study and analysis of air quality, road quality, detection of the efflorescence deposit, and spalling in old historical buildings.	-DL may help in rising capacities of existing SIDs -DL helps in improving the detection efficiency and sensitivity of SIDs to higher and more accurate -Biomedical-based applications can also be trained to be used for non-biological applications -DL helps in saving time, money, and motivates the whole analysis process more accurate and sensitive.

than 9% (around 29 million) and 8 million out of those are undiagnosed (Karakaya and Hacisoftaoglu, 2020). A diabetic person is at very high risk of eye-related disease including diabetic retinopathy, cataract, diabetic macular edema (an accumulation of fluid in the macula part of the retina), and glaucoma. The most common cause of vision loss is due to diabetic retinopathy (DR) because of bleeding of the small blood vessels present in the retina. If anyhow these bloody retinal vessels are untreated, it may high impact, may result in vision loss of varying degrees and even may finally results in blindness. Due to the silent nature of DR disease, it may cause no symptoms of disease or only creates mild vision problems (Aiello et al, 2011). Since early stage detection of DR could suggest for right treatment helps to prevent eye blindness, medical experts suggest the eye check-up for diabetic patients at regular interval. With early stage diagnosis and accurate evaluation of DR disease severity, regular coordination of diabetic eye care is possible and prompt appropriate treatment may be followed for prevention of eye blindness and visual loss (Karakaya and Hacisoftaoglu, 2020). However, current survey shows that access to such traditional medical care systems in developed countries ranges between 60 and 90%, whereas developing countries have significantly very lower rates (Hartnett et al., 2005). Patients without such eye care facility do not takeout benefit from the potential of early disease detection and consequently getting effective and in-time treatment.

Among rural areas and resource-less populations, a significant disparity is observed in pre-screening-based early diagnosis and access to traditional eye care system. In the retinal examination, medical experts use special type of optical devices such as an ophthalmoscope, 20D lens, and fundus camera. Having different salient features like easier storage, better quality image, and faster electronic data transfer, fundus cameras are broadly used in traditional system to detect eye diseases using their digital image processing-based features. However, retinal imaging method with a fundus camera is very time taking and it involves complete manual process. An imaging expert person is required in order to capture retinal image and then another expert is required for the evaluation report obtained from these imaging devices which may take a few days to submit. Also standard fundus cameras are large in size to carry and heavy for transportation and also very costly affair to be purchased by every healthcare center. Thereby, they appear to be inconvenient to be widespread used as a pre-screening tool. The need of such infrastructure for DR disease screening process becomes more tedious as the number of diabetic patient increases. Therefore, huge demand arises for small, portable, light weight, and inexpensive retinal imaging systems which can perform disease pre-screening for DR. Recent technological developments have highly encouraged and enabled use of widespread available smartphones in designing small-sized, low-power, light weight, and under-cost biomedical imaging devices. These systems are capable of incorporating imaging, on-board processing, and wireless communication technology. Therefore, smartphone-based imaging systems are widely applicable from healthcare sector to entertainment because such systems become small, easy to handle and portable. Since fundus camera systems are usually of large-size, heavy-weight, and high-cost imaging devices, they are ready to become good option to be transformed into a small and portable device in order to perform fast DR disease screening.

Developing current age technology-based portable retinal imaging devices using smartphones is an emerging innovation and research area that highly attracts several research universities and industries. Figure 7.1 depicts the smartphone-based retinal imaging system (SRIS) (Karakaya et al., 2020). Figure 7.1(a) shows different types of smartphone based imaging systems utilized in the market. 20D Lens embedded with a smartphone is one of the early retinal imaging device designs to record video on human and rabbit eyes is shown in Figure 7.1(a)(i) This early design generally used the Filmic Pro mobile application in order to adjust focus, exposure, and even light intensity by manual method. Another simple smartphone-based imaging device design is the iExaminer system. It is made by attaching a smartphone device to a PanOptic ophthalmoscope system as shown in Figure 7.1(a)(ii) These systems have requirement of attaching the smartphone device to existing medical equipment. Recently, the advent of new SRISs incorporating with medical devices has been seen in the market including D-Eye, Peek Retina, and iNview. D-Eye system reflects the smartphone flashlight to illuminate the retina of the human eye as shown in Figure 7.7.1(a)(iii) Peek retina imaging device uses its own light in order to illuminate the retina and the smartphone is used to capture the image as shown in Figure 7.7.1(a)(iv) iNview smartphone-based retinal imaging device was developed by Volk Optical in order to capture wide angle retinal images as shown in Figure 7.7.1(a)(v) Figure 7.1(b) shows the optical design and view of the SRISs. Each portable SRIS has variety of degrees in angles and direction of retinal views (AoV)

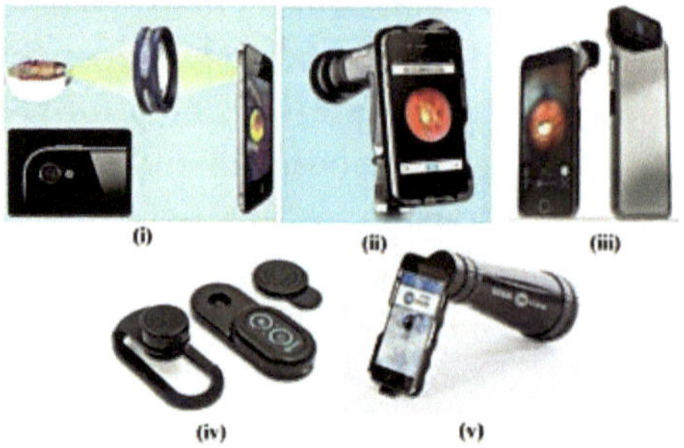

(a) *View of different types of Smartphone-based retinal imaging popular devices available in the market,* **(i)** *Fundus photography method-based system used by Harvard Medical School* **(ii)** *iExaminer system developed by Welch Allyn,* **(iii)** *D-Eye system,* **(iv)** *Peek Retina system, and* **(v)** *iNview system by Volk.*

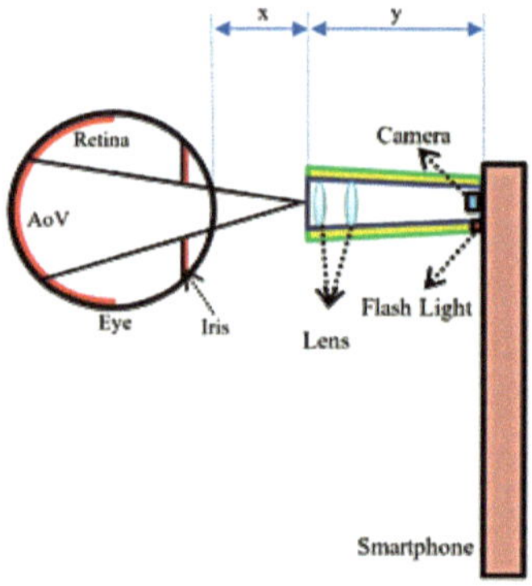

(b) *A view of optical design and functioning of the smartphone-based retinal imaging devices*

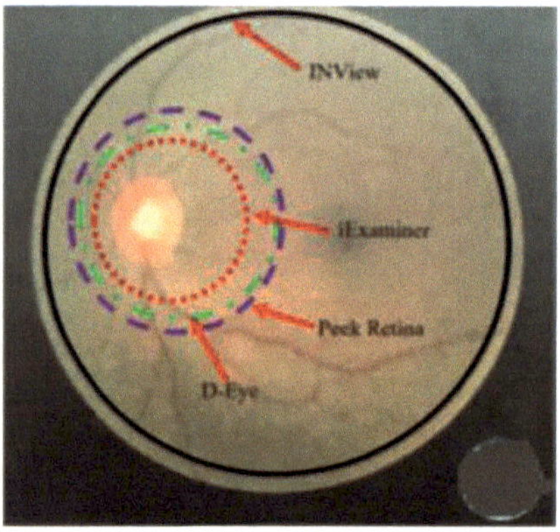

(c) *Comparison in between the different field of view of each smartphone-based retinal imaging system (SRIS) using printed normal retina image. It has various field of view markers where the solid black line is corresponding to iNview, the green dashed-dotted line shows for D-Eye, purple dashed line is representation for Peek Retina, the red dotted line shows for iExaminer*

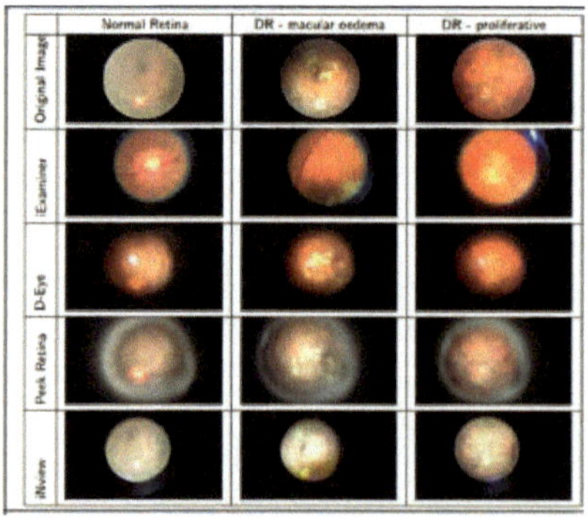

(d) *Variety of retinal images. (1st row) shows original printed real retinal fundus digital images, and their different captured versions using (2nd row) byiExaminer, (3rd row) by D-Eye version, (4th row) by Peek Retina and (5th row) by iNview version*

FIGURE 6.1 Smartphone-based retinal imaging systems. Reproduced from (Karakaya and Hacisoftaoglu, 2020) with their permission.

based on their optical design to capture retinal digital images. Figure 7.1(c) shows the different captured printed retinal digital images using different systems such as iExaminer (inner-most dotted circle), D-Eye (2nd inner-most dotted circle), Peek Retina, and iNview, respectively. It depicts the normal retina-based-printed image from the eye using the field of view-based markers corresponding to each imaging system. Figure 7.1(d) shows the different set of captured printed real-retinal images using variety of systems such as iExaminer, D-Eye, Peek Retina, and iNview. First row shows the original printed real-retinal digital images. The top left corner, retinal image is a normal retinal image which does not have any abnormality. The image present at the middle of the top row categorically belongs to a diabetic retinopathy disease where there is clinically high significant macular edema is visible. On the other hand, the right of the top row, image basically belongs to a proliferative diabetic retinopathy disease where several abnormalities can be observed. The remaining images present on each row are being captured using different SRISs as discussed as above. iExaminer system has been used to capture the retinal images shown at the second row. It appears that quality of these images is good enough and there is clear visibility of presence of optic nerve and few central blood veins. However, the presence of some macula edema can be seen in these images, so they can be used for detection and analysis of diabetic retinopathy. D-Eye system has been used to capture the retinal images present on the third row, where there is no even distribution of illumination present on it. However, the macular edema can be visualized, so they are also helpful for detection and analysis of diabetic retinopathy. Fourth row of Figure 7.1(d) shows the captured retinal images using Peek Retina system. It can be observed from the image that the field of view corresponding to Peek Retina is comparatively larger than iExaminer. Furthermore, these images have clear visibility of the optic nerve and their surrounding vessels, this could help to detect and analyze diabetic retinopathy with better efficiency. The retinal images at the last row are captured using iNview system. It is obvious visible that its field of view appears to be largest in comparison to other SRISs. The quality of its retinal image is very good and illumination is evenly distributed.

In the first set of experiments done by (Karakaya and Hacisoftaoglu, 2020), the printed retina was used to capture the retinal images in the retina box using variety of SRISs. With this set of experiments, the image quality was compared among variety of generated images and field of view of different SRISs. For image classification, they used the CNN-based AlexNet using the transfer learning method because Convolution Neural Network (CNN) is considered usually as one of the highly famous deep-learning frameworks. In the second set of experiments, several experiments were designed for each SRIS to analyze the diabetic retinopathy disease detection performance using deep learning-based framework for smartphone-based systems and were compared with the accuracy of original retinal images. The experimental results obtained in this study show that the SRISs can be used as an alternative solution to the direct ophthalmoscope. However, the variety of different field of view of the SRISs plays a key role in determining the accuracy of automatic diabetic retinopathy disease detection.

6.4 ASSESSMENT OF CARDIOVASCULAR DISEASES BASED ON SMARTPHONE USING ECG AND PPG ANALYSIS

Cardiovascular diseases (CVDs) and other heart-related abnormalities due to coronary artery blockade are some of the leading and responsible causes of severity death around the world. According to survey by WHO, such cardiac abnormalities caused around 31% of total deaths worldwide in 2020 (https://www.who.int/health-topics/cardiovasculardiseases/, accessed on 11 July, 2021). Cardiac arrhythmia is a type of disorder pattern and abnormal heart rhythm, which generally leads to a variety of different heart diseases. The early and faster detection of these cardiac abnormalities is essential in order to minimize the causalities. Electrocardiogram (ECG) is the golden standard method in order to record the electrical activities of the heart and its measurement. The ECG is the most widely used tool for heart disease, adopted in almost all clinic centers, economic, and accurate test viewed by expert to measure the behavior of the activity of the heart.

Further, the study on analysis of ECG is the most effective method in order to project and identify cardiac abnormalities (Ashrafuzzaman et al., 2013). There are a few problems and limitations with the traditional ECG machines. These devices are the only hospital or clinic-based systems and they cannot be moved around easily because of their bulky size. To use these devices for conduction of test need a medical expert. Sometimes, there is possibility that arrhythmias disease may not present at the recording time; therefore, often ECG devices may not be useful and applicable to detect abnormalities, because these tests record are of only 1–2 min. That is why a significant amount of money is being spent regularly every year on the detection and analyzing heart diseases. The hospitals, medical expert of ECG, and healthcare facilities are generally too far away in remote areas of most of the developing countries, so patients need to travel a lot with high cost for the treatment and analysis of cardiac problems. Further, the old age people may not feel it convenient in frequent visit to the hospital. Most of the heart diseases occur suddenly and for proper treatment person reserves only a few minutes. Therefore, the early or in-time detection and start of proper treatment of such heart diseases to be cured is utmost necessary. All such critical issues lead and enforce biomedical researchers to propose new solutions for such healthcare monitoring and treatment to resolve such cardiac problems. Thanks to the developers who developed such technology-enabled Personal Digital Assistants (PDAs) and smart-phone devices; really they made it possible and successful. Nowadays, smartphone devices are easily available equipped with enhanced tiny size but having very powerful sensors, wireless transmission capabilities which is need of hour, high speed processors, extended storage options, and long-lasting batteries. Additionally, smartphone devices are used in variety of domains such as business, entertainment, education, social connectivity, and every other important field of life. In a survey, the smart-phone technology-based society of UK states that around 93% of their population widely uses smartphones (Zhang et al., 2011). Considering, this extensive applications and enhanced wide capabilities to perform analysis by smartphone devices, many researchers have proposed and developed smartphone-based healthcare monitoring systems. The aim of this study is to perform review and have detailed discussion on those cardiac monitoring systems which utilize smartphones directly or indirectly in order to perform ECG-based analysis and Photoplethysmography (PPG) analysis.

PPG technology can be defined as the measurement and signature of changes in blood volume. It can be exploited to measure and estimate many underlying parameters of heart such as blood pressure (BP), toxcity, telemetr, heart rate rhythm, and heart rate (HR), etc. PPG technology is widely used in many cardiac-related current age medical devices such as pulse oximeters and BP-based beat-to-beat measuring devices. A variety of features are provided by smartphone-based devices such as mobile and ambulatory health monitoring, real-time feedback system by patients, ease of usage, portability, wireless-enabled in-time service, and faster transmission of data. They can be classified as invasive or non-invasive.

Additionally, the use of built-in or wearable sensors-based devices made it possible to capture ECG or PPG signals. These cardiac signals are easily transmitted using wireless data transmission-based technologies and further processed using various machine learning techniques and algorithms. With the current age technological advancements like machine learning and computer vision technology, it is even more motivating and encouraging now-a-days to solve this burning topic-based issue.

Automatic medical imaging-based diagnostic system is an emerging branch of study under computer vision which includes in-depth analysis and outcome on patient's status (Thevenot et al., 2017). The first subcategory of ECG recording devices consists of those systems record ECG signals using built-in sensors embedded within smartphone or other wearable devices. Once the recording is done, these data are sent through the smartphone in digital form using wireless transmission methods such as infrared signals, Bluetooth, or other radio-based transmission techniques for analysis and prognosis purpose. These ECG signals are thereafter visualized on PDAs or smartphone devices screens for further analysis and taking appropriate action on-time. Using such devices, the patient can themselves view the signals and forward them to the medical expert/cardiologist for analysis in-time. Unfortunately, these systems has major drawback, i.e., the task of abnormality and disease detection is still a manual process. This procedure is very time-consuming which is not tolerable and acceptable in the case of heart diseases due to its severity. Consequently, to make the abnormalities detection task automatic, some scientists have developed automated systems comes under second subcategory. Such automatic systems are developed and modeled as a client–server architecture where smartphone device acts as a client. This client receives signals (ECG or PPG) from the sensors embedded and is transmitted to a server via different technologies such as Wi-Fi, GSM technology, 3G, or 4G network. Such servers are usually programmed and equipped with algorithms based on ECG analysis in which abnormality is detected and report/alert is send back to patient and medical experts/cardiologist for further treatment. Though these systems are capable of analyzing and detecting abnormality automatic, this process has a significant drawback, i.e., lack of real-time feedback process. Additionally, necessary parameters for the system to work efficiently are the light traffic on the transmission medium, congestion free traffic, high cost, and optimum performance of the wireless network and server. These all issues are clearly mentioned in final and especially third subcategory of the proposed model where acquisition, processing, abnormality detection of ECG signals, and generation of report/alert is performed completely on the smartphones. This type of automated system provides continuous analysis of ECG, in-time detection of ECG abnormalities, real-time feedback system in the form of a report/alert to patient, caretaker, and medical experts for further study.

A general representation of above-mentioned all three subcategories of smartphone-based cardiac monitoring system are presented in Figure 7.2. Additionally, PPG-based non-invasive systems have been discussed by many researchers. These systems can help in real-time patient monitoring and estimation of parameters of cardiac abnormalities by putting the index finger of the relevant subject in front of the camera of a smartphone devices. Traditionally, ECG recording has been used for regular cardiac monitoring, but with experiments, some researchers have proved that there exist strong correlation between PPG signals and ECG waveforms (Zhang et al., 2011). An ECG cycle composed of five feature points/segments such as P, Q, R, S, and T and three important time intervals (PR, QRS, and QT) used for analyzing it. These time intervals and feature points contain important cardiac information and have been used by many researchers for initial diagnosis (pre-screening of disease) and abnormality detection. There exists strong correlation between peak-to-peak intervals of PPG with the RR interval segment of ECG. This following section reviews the non-invasive systems comprised built-in cameras of the smartphone in order to record and capture PPG signals and process them in smartphone devices for estimating cardiac-based parameters using various current age processing techniques. In most of the cases, the subject puts its index finger on the camera embedded with smartphone devices while letting embedded LED flashlight turned on. In the proposed method by Scully et al. (2011), the PPG signals are recorded using Motorola Droid smartphone in which subject places the index finger on camera embedded within it by turning on flashlight and recording was performed in resolution of 720 × 480. In another work, Lamonaca et al. (2013) developed a smartphone-based system in order to estimate blood pressure from PPG signals using machine learning (artificial neural network [ANN]) based model (Lamonaca et al., 2013). Using pixel brightness level, the signals were enhanced, and ANN model categorically extracts systolic BP (SBP) one type of BP and Diastolic BP (DBP) simultaneously. The author developed ANN model in JAVA to achieve and perform easy integration of application and getting independence from hardware software-based architecture.

Another type of smartphone-based system was evolved to perform analysis based on frequency domain to apply on the PPG signal which calculates HR and also extract various relevant informative features. These extracted features corresponding to variety of sections like the valley point, the systolic peak, and the Dicrotic notch of the PPG signal are thereafter used to estimate different classes of BP such as very low point, low, average point, high, and very high point BP using machine learning (ANN) and Support Vector Machine (SVM)-based classifier (Gaurav et al., 2016). The detection of Hypertension disease was performed on the smartphone devices by analysis of PPG and estimation of HR, HRV, and BP. The authors used Pan-Tompkins algorithm to extract and process the peak point of these signals and used ANN classifier for decision making based on extracted linear and non-linear features. PPG signals can be successfully used to estimate and analyze many cardiac and other physiological-based parameters, but they are easily open to be vulnerable. It may suffer from many limitations which can harm the quality of PPG signals such as, low sampling rate (to refresh itself) of mobile phones, variation in pressure, and movement of the finger on sensor or camera. The baseline drift and presence of other outlier content from PPG signals were successfully removed by constructing and using a mathematical model comprising sum of composition two Gaussian functions (Banerjee et al., 2015). The accuracy of the system for diagnosis can be affected because of different types of noises and artifacts which may occur during acquisition of signal (ECG and PPG). Telemedicine system implemented in these smartphone-based models provides facility of health monitoring and essential urgent suggestions for patients residing in remote locations at distance for better treatment. A variety of issues need to be addressed and solved such as the short-range accessibility of wireless communication-based technologies, i.e., Bluetooth, implementation of advanced algorithms to analyze complex ECG incorporating with smartphones, flexible, effective and adaptive wearable sensors (design needs to be changed), detection of present fewer abnormalities/disease, and security of patient data (ECG and PPG). The concept of tele-medicine using client–server-based approach for distance based on the patient care monitoring and generating alarm for detection of abnormality/disease makes possible the in-time detection and faster treatment of disease in order to minimize mortality rate. This study aims to act as a reference for biomedical researchers and developers to provide base knowledge of the working and limitations of existing smartphone-based systems and their future improvements.

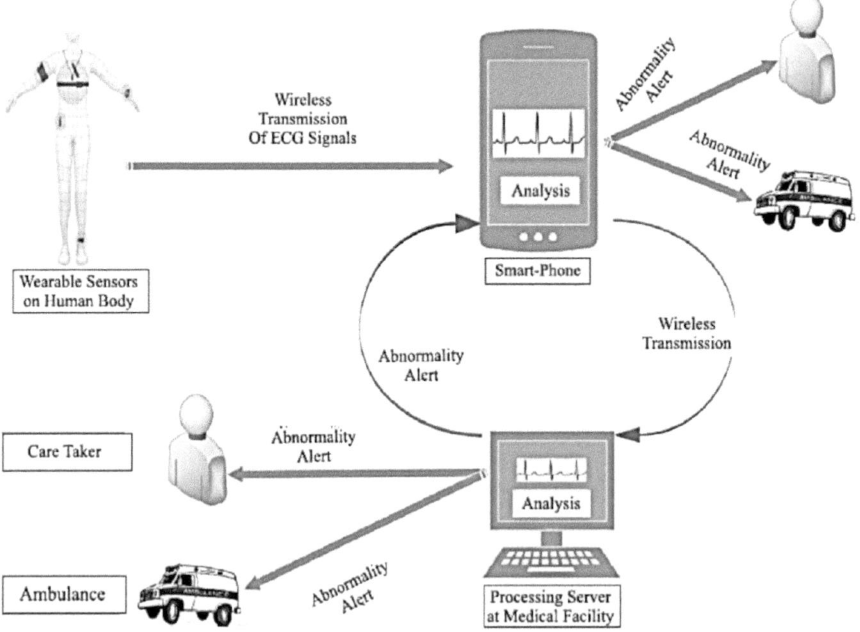

FIGURE 6.2 A typical architecture of smartphone-based monitoring systems for cardiac abnormality. Reproduced from [21] (Shabaan et al., 2020) with their permission.

6.5 AUTOMATIC DETECTION OF ABNORMALITY IN KIDNEY FROM ULTRASOUND IMAGES USING SMARTPHONE

Kidneys are two bean-shaped important body organs which are residing near the middle of the back just below the rib cage which protects the crucial body organs such as the heart, lungs (air-filled organs), and great vessels. It plays regulatory roles for various functional activities in the human body. Kidneys are likely to be affected by different kind of diseases like cysts, stones, infections, etc. It is estimated by a survey done in the United States that around 26 million people have symptoms of chronic kidney disease (CKD) and they are unaware of it may lead to fatality (https://www.kidney.org/news/newsroom/factsheets/FastFacts). Early detection of CKD at initial stage may prevent the kidneys from its permanent failure which may possible by automated diagnosis. Automated abnormality detection system of kidney using ultrasound digital images is a challenging task due to some of the reasons such as acquiring images by ultrasound method have low signal to noise ratio because of the presence of multiplicative noise, i.e., speckles, partially affected with acoustic shadowing which is imaging artifact, kidney in ultrasound image is only partially visible because of occlusions of other present organs like spleen, variation in size and shape of the kidney organ which generally depends on various factors of the patients like their age, weight and height, images with low contrast, and poorly defined edges in digital images of the kidney.

Ultrasound scanning method is the widely used and applicable medical imaging modality for diagnosing the kidney for abnormality detection. Traditionally, ultrasound scanner devices are installed in high-tech city-based established hospitals in resource full area due to its high form factors, cost, and need for an expert professional already trained in sonography for performing scanning. Recent current age technology-based advancements in computing have realized and installed portable ultrasound scanners (PUS), which are now started being used in POC and emergency healthcare (Kim et al., 2012). Additionally, handheld-based ultrasound scanning systems based on system-on-chip (SOC) solution and mobile platforms are presented in (Ahn et al., 2015). Lack of sonographer professionals limits the potentiality and applicability of using ultrasound scanning in POC diagnostics of kidney abnormality. In this work, an android-based application was developed for automatic detection of any abnormality of the kidney in two-dimensional B-mode ultrasound images. In this system, the smartphones can capture ultrasound kidney image using any ultrasound scanner device, process it, and finally produces the diagnostic result of the image for further treatment process as shown in Figure 7.3(a). Additionally, this system doesn't need of data connectivity or any utility software to be installed and it can automatically detect abnormality by directly connecting to any ultrasound scanner. This type of system may be very beneficial in rural healthcare and resource-less area where there is limitation of data connectivity. Authors have also developed an automated algorithm used for classifying cyst and stone abnormalities in captured kidney-based ultrasound images. In the experiment, stones in kidney are hyperechoic and have bright appearance while cysts have dark appearance compared with surrounding region of image of kidney. The appearance of cyst- and stone-related abnormalities of the kidney is clearly shown in Figure 7.3(b). In (Krishna et al., 2014), the authors proposed a hard-threshold-based classification algorithm for automatic detection of abnormality from the kidney images on Field Programmable

Gate Arrays (FPGA) platform. This algorithm is based on computing first- and second-order texture features widely extracted from kidney region to capture existing abnormality. In another work, the authors have proposed fuzzy-neural network-based computer-aided decision support system for the detection of kidney abnormality (Raja et al., 2008).

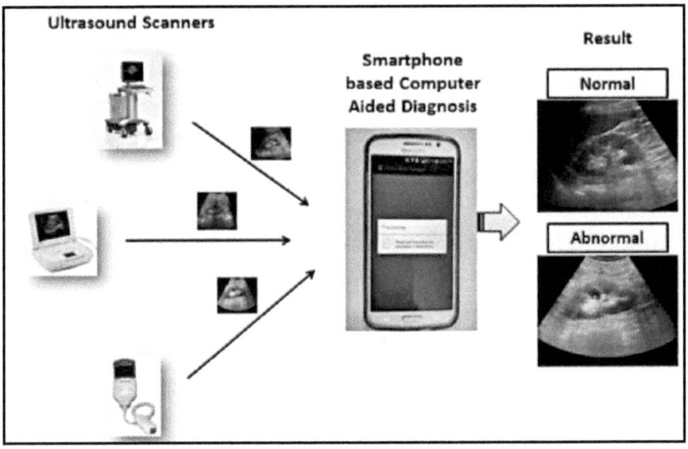

(a) Graphical representation of mobile based CAD.

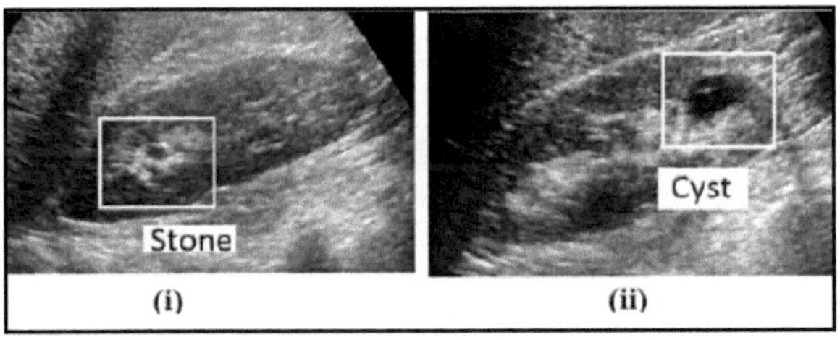

(b) Abnormalities in Kidney (i) Stone (ii) Cyst.

FIGURE 6.3 Smartphone-based abnormality detection of Kidney using Ultrasound Images. Reproduced from (Vaish et al., 2016) with their permission.

6.6 OTHER MEDICAL DIAGNOSIS APPLICATIONS OF SMARTPHONE DEVICES

Optical microscopy (OM) technology since its introduction is well known in medical and has been widely used for various disease diagnostic applications. Identification of pathological changes occurred in subject samples using hematological or histological observations is an important role of OM technology which greatly help in routine diagnosis. Researchers are allowed to evaluate the sample integrity of the subject at anatomical or morphological scales by observing the structural difference among cellular components. Hemocytological disorder examination of blood samples with OM-based hemocytometer equipment or using automatic flowcytometry is common approach for various disease and health conditions detection. Limitations of these techniques are that they consume a lot of time and very costly. Recently, rapid development has been observed using cell phone-based microscopy and presented itself as a global platform for cytological research and studies. A smartphone-based blood analyzer model was developed by Zhu et al. (2013), which can be used as a portable device to examine and measure the concentration of RBCs, WBCs, and hemoglobin from the volume of ~10 μL (very small sample). There are three different optomechanical-based hardware components embedded with the primary camera of the smartphone device in order to measure the concentrations. These attachments comprises of eight LEDs (~470 nm) used to excites the fluorescently labeled WBCs uniformly, whereas the RBC counter attachment comprises of a single white LED used for illuminating the image of unlabeled RBCs. The measurement of hemoglobin concentration is done through absorbance method by using Beer–Lambert law by incorporating a single blue color LED (~430 nm) to illuminate especially the burette comprising samples of lysed blood. The sensitivity of these smartphone-based devices has outperformed in comparison to commercial hemocytometer (Zhu et al., 2013).

Additionally, along with above-mentioned applications of approaches of hemocytological examinations, OM can also be utilized to detect the presence of various parasites in sample of blood. More often, faster screening method is required in order to detect the level and presence of micro-filarial (mf) in blood sample. Existing traditional methods are time-consuming and expensive such as pathological testing of stained blood-smears using a microscope device or using quantitative method such as polymerase chain reaction (qPCR). Alternatively, a smartphone-based video-microscopic device was developed by D'Ambrosio et al. (2015) in order to detect the load/content of mf in blood sample and confirming the presence of parasite in the blood by measuring its wriggling motion. The name of this device is referCellScope Loa in which a reverse camera lens module is connected along with rear camera of smartphone and blood sample is illuminated using a LED array attached to it. A comparison was made between this device with equipment standard microscopy and obtained correlation was 0.99. In the graph between blood smear vs CellScope, no any false-negative results was present, whereas two false-positive cases were observed with certainty of 99.99%. Other applications of such CellScope Loa named device could be observed for rapid screening and quantifying the infectious agents such as filariae, trypanosomes, and other motile blood-borne with high sensitivity (D'Ambrosio et al., 2015). Histological examination using OM device is also used for routine diagnosis. To examine the histological slides, a variety of microscopic-based techniques are usually used for analysis. This process requires extensive setup of microscopy-based system as well as an expert professional to examine the slides visually, may lead to create hindrance to rapid diagnosis of disease in remote resource-less areas (Muehldorfer et al., 2002). Recently, SIDs have been represented as POC systems to be used for a wide variety of application areas along with the incorporation of machine learning algorithms to perform analysis automatically. Histological examination is also used during the process of organ transplantation in order to check their liability.

More often, the basic reason behind liver graft failure is macrovesicular steatosis (MS) because of the accumulation of triglycerides occurred in the cytoplasm of hepatocytes (Olthoff et al., 2010). In a study of Cesaretti et al. (2018), the authors developed an add-on BLIPS lens attached to the rear camera of the smartphone device in order to perform liver-based MS assignment. In this setup, the BLIPS lens was incorporated with camera of smartphone along with sticky pads and the phone was put on a stage made by plexiglass. The components such as smartphone, a light source, i.e., white LED, and slides all three were manually aligned in such a way to obtain the best focus toward the sample plane. The staining of three-micrometer-thick tissue blocks was performed using H&E stain material and used for medical imaging. The empty vacuoles present in the cytoplasm area of the hepatocytes histologically characterized MS and grading of MS is done by using the calculated percentage of such cells. A strong correlation has been observed for the combination of smartphone system with microscopic technology to determine the disease and health conditions (Cesaretti et al., 2018). Histopathological test is the gold standard examination for the detection of suspicious anomalies-based cancer of the cells. This traditional method comprises the model-based performance of biopsy cum OM examination, which is highly painful, time-consuming process, and requires expert professionals (Lingen et al., 2008). The examining oral cancer patients also suffer from these issues. Furthermore, due to generic wounds present in the mouth in large scale, a diagnostic tool with higher sensitivity is required to develop that could be useful in a rural setting. An automated CellScope device was developed by Skandarajah et al. (2017) for screening of oral cancer using a technology based on brush biopsy. In this system, a device comprised of a ×20 objective lens in which white LED light is focused on the sample slide and images are captured using an iPad Mini. Cytobrush Plus GT was used to collect the samples and cells were released out from the brush by titration method. The sample was then spread over in a glass slide and staining was performed using H&E. The application model was developed by acquiring 125 random images from the raster pattern-based slide and images which had greater than 50% cell density were considered for creating the model. 70% sensitivity was obtained by the authors in the examination based on CellScope in comparison to analysis based on standard histological.

In conclusion, SIDs have become better option for variety of medical problems for various routine diagnosis applications, which otherwise need traditional sophisticated equipment and usually consumes more time in processing. These devices are widely helpful in providing low-cost diagnosis to the large populations in even remote resource-less areas with significantly higher specificity and sensitivity in order to help in continuous health monitoring of the patient with ease.

6.7 SMARTPHONE-BASED AUTOMATED SYSTEMS FOR BACTERIA DETECTION

Bacterial pathogens detection and identification from biological samples are the key methods to diagnose a large set of infectious diseases. However, traditional methods of diagnosing include culture-based approach or PCR test, a widely-used, highly sensitive test in which traces of genetic material is found from a specific pathogen, are usually cumbersome, time-consuming, and especially require sufficient resources, i.e., expensive devices and skilled expert professionals (Hameed et al., 2018). The role of SIDs is significantly increased for various bio-analytical applications and widely used as POC detection units for infectious diseases. Bacterial detection process often includes various analytical tools and devices for various clinical- and research-oriented applications. Optical imaging methods have evolved and become essential tools for bacteria screening and detecting process of a wide variety of subjects. However, the conventional microscopic-based devices are heavy, high-cost affair, and require advance level of laboratory setup for proper operation (Ozcan, 2014). In order to fulfill the rising demand for POC devices in healthcare and resolving the existing limitations, an observation of shifting of paradigm is being observed toward the development of low cost, light weight, and portable devices. Consequently, SIDs have shown strong capability of analyzing as compared to conventional devices such as optical microscopes (Hernández-Neuta et al., 2019). The size and shape of bacteria are in microscale, and therefore, need high magnification for imaging. The limitation of smartphone-based devices (SIDs) is that it cannot attain such high magnifications. Therefore, combining and incorporating with techniques based on counter-staining such as fluorescence, SIDs can easily detect and quantify the bacteria content in the sample.

A compact smartphone-based fluorescence microscope-based device was developed by Mullër et al. (2018) for imaging fluorescently labeled bacteria sample for detection and analysis. In this system, in order to illuminate the sample at an angle of 61°, a 488-nm diode-based laser device was used to perform proper diagnosis. An external lens was used to collect the fluorescent signals from the subject sample and a long pass filter was used for removal of noise before it reached the rear camera sensor of smartphone. All the concerned optical components of this system were placed covered inside a 3D-printed optomechanical box. For faster identification and quantification of bacteria pathogen, they were fluorescently labeled with peptide nucleic acid fluorescent-labeled (PNA) probes. This system was able to detect bacteria pathogen to 104 CFU/mL, comparatively larger than traditional microscopic method and also able to capture pathogenic Cronobacter spp. based digital images showing its ability to be used in resource-less areas (Müller et al., 2018). OM-based method is traditionally accepted as standard methodology for examining and analyzing sputum samples for detection of tuberculosis (TB) disease and other widely used procedures involve using PCR test and culture assays. Culture assays-based testing methods are challenging to perform efficiently and require incubation process for a week, whereas the PCR-test technology requires high cost setups, thereby being limitation in applications to high-end resource settings (Boehme et al., 2010). Therefore, sputum smear microscopy-based method is most commonly and widely used in countries having moderate income standard for rapid and reliable identification of patients with tuberculosis (TB). Thus, improving microscope technology-based screening methods by incorporating new technological components could help in diagnosing TB considerably. Fluorescence-based microscopy technology has shown higher performance as compared to the bright-field-based microscopy. With the rising development of different kind of light sources for the method of fluorescence microscopy, the latter approach is becoming cost-effective, ease of use, and usage in different areas is also increased (Ojha et al., 2020).

Cheng et al. (2012) developed a system named CellScope, a fluorescence microscopic system based on smartphone technology for TB detection. Figure 7.4(a) shows the system comprised of 3D printed parts and it is accompanied with inkjet-printed lens attached toward the smartphone camera. In this system, multiple LEDs embedded with fluorescent filters inherently used to excite the bacteria pathogen-based subject samples. There is restriction of focal adjustment of the given sample with the lens because of the non-movability of sample stage. The classification of TB objects is done using the negative ones-based candidates by support vector machines (SVM) classifier and an average precision of 89.2% ± 2.1% was achieved by the authors which in turn enable an easier, faster, and accurate diagnosis of TB from given sputum smear samples (Chang et al., 2012). Due to the presence of bacteria, healing of wounds is usually prohibited by and it is not always easy to detect such bacteria in subject sample due to various issues in identification process and also in-visible symptoms (Bowler et al., 2001). Current traditional methods to monitor infected wounds of the subject require their visual assessment by expert as well as look for clinical-based signs and symptoms for analysis which are less efficient and time-taking process. An automated Portable Real-time based Optical Detection, Identification based, and Guidance for Intervention (PRODIGI) system was developed by Wu et al. (2014), which is a handheld autofluorescence medical imaging-based device used to detect, identify, and quantify the content of bacteria in wounds on subject sample in real-time as shown in Figure 7.4(b). Such a handheld and portable device can be easily carried to the healthcare field or used in home-based setting for easy monitoring of process of wound healing. The PRODIGI system captures both white color light and autofluorescence-enabled signals for higher illumination from tissue components and bacteria. The illumination for bright-field imaging method is provided by broadband white LEDs, whereas excitation of light sources for autofluorescence imaging method is performed using two monochromatic violet-blue LED arrays. In this methodology, a dual-band fluorescence filter is placed in front of the smartphone camera which is used to block the reflected excitation light coming from the skin surface and an emission filter is used to separate the autofluorescence signals emitted from both bacteria and tissue; as a result, a composite RGB digital image is displayed as an output. The device is successfully proved to be useful in the tracking and monitoring of wound healing and associated infections in the subject sample in non-invasive approach and faster method than other conventional methods (Wu et al., 2014).

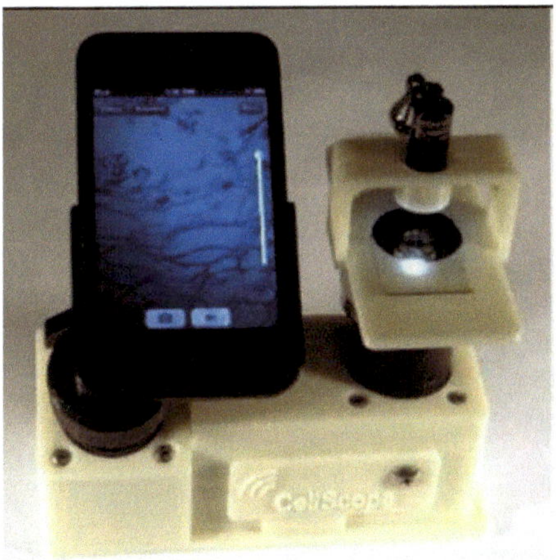

(a) CellScope, a smartphone-based fluorescence microscopic system with 3D printed parts for TB detection developed by Chang et al. (2012).

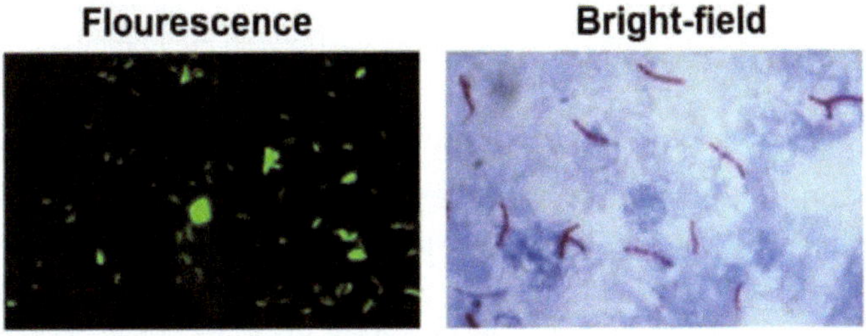

(b) CellScope based fluorescence (green colour) and bright-field (red colur) sample images of TB pathogen, respectively (Chang et al., 2012)

(Figure 6.4 *Continued...*)

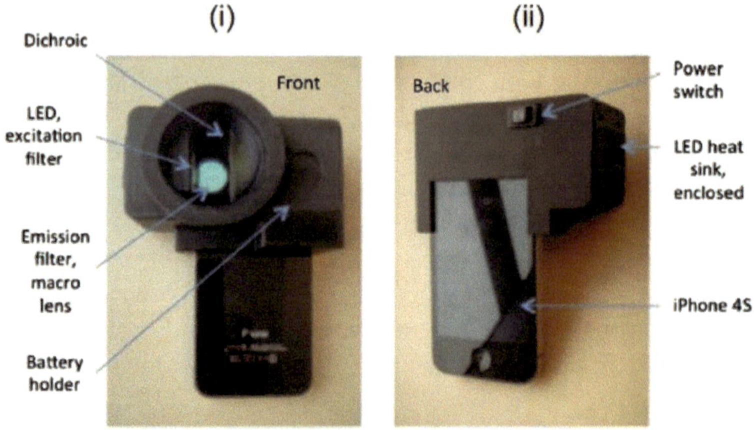

(c) PRODIGI, a smartphone based imaging device developed by Wu et al. (2014)
(i) Front view which is mounted onto a standard iPhone 4S smartphone and shows the optical components and battery holder of the accessory adapter (ii) Back view of the system showing the LCD viewing screen and on/off switch

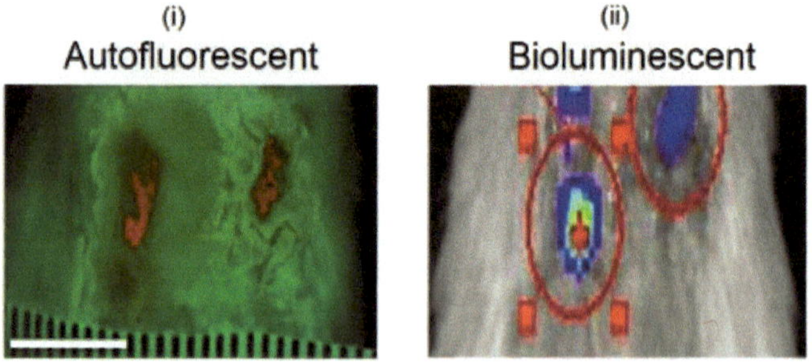

(d) Bioluminescence medical imaging of bacteria in vivo (i) autofluorescent
(ii) bioluminescent when grown in the mouse skin wound model of Wu et al. (2014)

FIGURE 6.4 General view of smartphone-based bacterial pathogen detection system. Reproduced from (Chang et al., 2012; Wu et al., 2014) with their permission.

Fluctuating sensitivity rates are observed for the microscope-based testing/examination and required expert professionals for examinations. On the other way, better sensitivity and accuracy have been observed using analytical assay-based technology in assessment of bacteria using both approaches quantitative and qualitative. A SIDs-based system was developed by Barnes et al. (2018) for diagnosing bacteria pathogen in patients with urinary sepsis infection. In this work, for the generation of fluorescent signal from the sample, the lysed biological sample was mixed with a standardized reaction mixture using loop-mediated isothermal amplification (LAMP) method which regards to amplification. The performance of such smartphone-based system was significantly improved against for analysis of several Gram-positive and Gram-negative bacterial species in comparison to standard assay method using a real-time quantitative testing PCR. The capability of bacteria detection using this approach was within limited range in which positive demonstration is required for detection of urinary tract infection from given clinical culture/samples (Barnes et al., 2018). The sensitivity of the system which is formed by incorporating smartphone devices with LAMP assay increases for the detection of the pattern outputs. Smartphone application is able to recognize a slight change in read out along with capability of reading multiplex analytical results obtained at the same time. However, sometimes sensitivity decreases using LAMP assay-based method with outputs being false-positive. Therefore, for faster detection, nucleic acid-based immunoassay test is preferred with the system. An enzyme-linked aptamer assay in combination with smartphone detection system was developed by Li et al. (2018) for rapid quantification and identification of different strains of mycobacterium. Here, the bacterium was closely bound to the nitrocellulose membrane attached with biotin-labeled aptamers, easily used for detecting mannose-capped lipoarabinomannan present on and over the surface of the bacteria. Then, streptavidin-labeled horse radish peroxidase is mixed with the aptamer and thereby developing a mixture color in the presence of H_2O_2. Thereafter, smartphone was used in order to detect and quantify the bacteria and this approach showed a detection and quantification limit of 104 CFU/mL of given samples. A higher sensitivity and specificity is observed with the experimental results compared to conventional acid-fast staining-based assay (Li et al., 2018).

Similarly, incorporation of smartphone-based detection system with microfluidic methods has significant ability to increase the performance and throughput of the microfluidic device by enabling multiplexing technology and increasing the detection speed. Some of the vivid applications of SIDs have been highlighted by these devices in the field of quantification and detection of bacteria, which is very useful for monitoring and analyzing disease progression. The presence of bacteria can be detected by SIDs in much faster way and with a lower detection limit at very low cost and are often used in place of various conventional techniques to provide read out for the experiments. However, disadvantage with such devices are that differentiation between pair of species of bacteria often comes to a limited result and incorporation of several conventional methods are additionally required by them such as antibody-based detection.

6.8 SMARTPHONE IMAGING-BASED VIRUS DETECTION SYSTEMS

Viruses are sub-microscopic infectious agent, pathogenic particles generally much smaller than bacteria comprised with genetic material, i.e., DNA or RNA. Generally, host cell machinery is used by them to replicate itself inside living cells of an organism and it starts killing the process of the cell. Viruses infect all different kinds of life forms, starting from animals and plants to microorganisms, including even bacteria and archaea also and often their detection and diagnosis process requires specialized experimental tools and high-end processes which are generally not available at resource-less undeveloped remote area-based primary screening health centers (Shors, 2017). The widely used methods of screening of viruses are various traditional analytical approaches such as biochemical assay, immune assay, or PCR-based methods. Although these conventional methods have higher sensitivity and accuracy, due to lack of proper resources, their use is limited in remote resource-less areas. Therefore, researchers have started working toward the design and development of POC devices which may have similar performance and sensitivity. Thereby, the development of SIDs is emerged to support sophisticated laboratory-based technologies to the field, which in turn will help detection and diagnosis to reach to masses (Peruski and Peruski, 2003).

A smartphone-based system was developed by Laksanasopin et al. (2015) by attaching a dongle to it that perform actions similar to traditional benchtop ELISA instrument, which can be used as easily available another POC diagnostic device. It was designed in such a way to perform similar to triplexed immunoassay which can detect three infectious disease markers such as HIV, treponemal syphilis, and non-treponemal syphilis. The smartphone-based devices including microfluidics capability becomes cheap and accessible especially in remote resource-limited areas. The device is portable and easy to carry and it comprises disposable plastic cassettes preloaded with the required reagent to perform the action of immunoassays in which gold nanoparticles and silver ions are used as the substrate for ELISA. In this system, less power is consumed by dongle and the audio jack was used in the smartphone in order to transmit power to it to avoid the use of additional battery. In comparison to standard conventional laboratory detection tests, the results using this device were found to be comparable and sensitivity/accuracy of 92–100% was obtained. This experiment looks advantageous in terms of detection and diagnosis of relevant disease, also makes them easily accessible and affordable to most of the population (Laksanasopin et al., 2015). However, a complex architecture-based device fabrication and arrangement of extensive reagent inside the cassette is required in this system. Furthermore, an additional component such as flow devices are used to make the immunoassay simpler and ease of use in which the membrane has enzymes embedded in. A fluorescent-enabled lateral immunoassay technology in combination with smartphone was developed by Yeo et al. (2016) in order to detect and diagnose avian influenza (AI) named virus strains. These viruses are generally highly susceptible and pathogenic and they become major cause of infections across different species including human also, and in-time detection, diagnosis, and controlling of these pathogenic viruses is important. A smartphone-based system with fluorescence device as mentioned above has already shown its performance and capability in the diagnosis of various viruses. This system comprises a 3D-printed module and LED to excide the fluorescence device with excitation wavelength ~470 nm. The nitrocellulose was used to prepare the strip for the immunoassay and coated and covered using an anti-influenza antibody. Furthermore, dendrimer was used for bioconjugation of the strip before it was introduced with the subject sample. In this experiment, this system was able to detect H5N1 type virus with classification result of 96.55% sensitivity and 98.55% specificity. The advantage of using smartphone-based virus detection and diagnosis method analyze the results within around 15 min, which in turn comparatively faster and rapid than most of the traditional benchtop methods (Yeo et al., 2016). Immunoassays-based technology performed higher sensitivity with better accuracy in order to produce faster analytical results than traditional biochemical tests but very often suffer from lack of specificity. Therefore, PCR-based diagnosis and testing methods are observed to perform comparatively with better sensitivity and specificity. However, PCR technology-based approach is a time-consuming, complex, and highly expensive, thereby generally used for sub-optimal applications (Shukla et al., 2016). Therefore, newly derived reverse-transcription loop-mediated isothermal amplification (RT-LAMP)-based methodology has become emerging technology widely used for such detection and diagnosis of virus pathogen in resource-limited remote area due to its significant features such as sensitivity, portability, accuracy, and majority of all its distinct capabilities despite being very simple and ease of use.

A multiplexed hybrid-based systems incorporating smartphone-based microfluidics with RT-LAMP technique for detection process was developed by Ganguli et al. (2017) to identify and diagnose the Zika virus in combination with Dengue and Chikungunya infectious viruses. This smartphone-based model consists of a polydimethylsiloxane (PDMS) material made microfluidic chip and consists of three inlets to contain three different samples such as lysis buffer, blood sample, and amplification reagent. In this system, amplification reagents are used to lyse and mix with the blood sample and then it is transferred to the microfluidic chip, which comprises pre-loaded RT-LAMP primers for detection of different virus pathogens. Once the setup of smartphone device and microfluidics card was done by placing them in their positions, fluorescence signal was collected from the primers sample related to pathogen in the blood sample by initiating the fluorescence imaging. The detection limit was found in the experiment to be 1.56 × 104 PFU/μL for Zika virus and 1.56 × 104 copies/μL of purified RNA sample for the viruses such as Chikungunya and Dengue from the given complete blood sample (Ganguli et al., 2017). However, amplification process usually involves in RT-LAMP method by using general indicators of the process of total DNA synthesis. In this process, opening the reaction tube is necessary to perform postreaction analysis and, therefore, introduces the risk factor of amplicon contamination and other kinds of complications too (Tian et al., 2016). To overcome the above problems stated herewith, a target-specific and a smartphone in multiplexable format integrated RT-LAMP-based device was developed by Priye et al. (2017) for the detection of virus pathogens such as Zika, Dengue, and Chikungunya involving closed-tube-based experiment. The detection process usually involved the use of technology of quenching of unincorporated-based amplification signal reporters (QUASR). QUASR method has comparatively brighter signals that normal human eye or even a smartphone camera can detect easily and has lower false-positive amplification detections and higher performance. In this, multiplexing targets are also enabled in a single reaction. The device accompanied with three different components such as assay reaction housing module, heating module, and an optical detection module. In this model, the virus pathogen detection rate at 103 PFU/mL was obtained to be 100% specific by using the Zika-specific primers and without preparing any sample (Priye et al., 2017).

The imaging anchored system based on smartphone technology can be used for qualitative detection and it is easier for non-expert people to use it for detection and analysis. The outputs of these devices are easily analyzed using smartphone-based interface which also in turn enables sharing the results with expert professionals in a different location in order to promote and perform cross validation. Furthermore, the importance of imaging technology based on DNA molecules can be highly observed in diagnostic system especially in such diseases caused by viruses and other pathogens in which the structure and form of DNA are changed (Herrick and Bensimon, 1999). Using imaging technology, nucleic acid, important class of macromolecules usually found in almost all cells and viruses also can be used to understand the pathology process and virus life cycle. Although traditional optical imaging-based methods are generally used to study and operate this, but complex and expensive setups are required for its working such as incorporation of confocal fluorescence-based microscopy and super-resolution based microscopy system (Witte et al., 2018). Various optical devices as attachments have played role in making the smartphone-based devices to be advanced in imaging sub-microscopic entities. A model developed by Wei et al. (2013) overcomes these issues and allows smartphone devices to be used for imaging single molecules. This device detects fluorescence signal by integrating a 3D-printed opto-mechanical part with the smartphone camera. In this system, for exciting the source, a laser diode of size 450-nm was used and in-built CMOS sensor attached to the phone was used to record fluorescence signal strength by using attached external lens. In order to block scattered background light, two 500-nm filters were placed in between external lenses and lenses of smartphone camera. An intercalating dye (YOYO-1) was used to label DNA molecules of varying sizes. Thereafter, DNA sample was slightly warmed and then immediately cooled so that sticky ends can be opened and then it was placed between two coverslips result-in linear stretching of the DNA. A specialized MATLAB program was used to measure the length of DNA which provides an accuracy of around <1 kb for 10 kb size or longer DNA molecules.

A cost-effective smartphone-based device integrated with machine learning-based software was proposed by Samacoits et al. (2021) that evaluate the fluorescence signals of the CRISPR (Clustered regularly interspaced-based short palindromic repeats) diagnostic of SARS-CoV-2 virus. The device comprises two different sections such as a three-dimensional (3D)-printed housing container and low-cost optic components which is used for excitation of fluorescent reporters and it performs selective transmission of the fluorescence emission to the smartphone device. The authors have developed custom software integrated with binary classification model in order to quantify the captured fluorescence images and the presence of the virus can also be determined. This detection system has a limitation of detecting (LoD) of 6.25 RNA copies/μL on given laboratory subject samples and in the experiment, a test accuracy of 95% and sensitivity of 97% was obtained on 96 nasopharyngeal swab samples. Figure 7.5(a) depicts a general view of smartphone-based system for virus detection using CRISPR diagnostic (Samacoits et al., 2021). Figure 7.5a. (i) shows a system by combining CRISPR diagnostic and the smartphone-based device and flow chart how to detect SARS-CoV-2 using the proposed system, (ii) shows computer-aided design (CAD)-based system components description, (iii) shows actual image of smartphone-based device used for fluorescence imaging of the CRISPR diagnostic assay, and (iv) shows a step-wise procedure to detect and quantify SARS-CoV-2. Finally, this system has the ability to automatically upload the images and results to a central controlled server which can be used as primary method to keep track of the COVID-19 transmission in real time which is not possible by using traditional methods.

Another smartphone-based POC platform was developed by Xia et al. (2019) for highly sensitive and selective detection and diagnosis of the avian influenza virus using a nanomaterial-enabled colorimetric-based detection method. In this system, to capture the avian influenza virus, the 3D nanostructures were used serving as a support for antibody conjugation and are made on PDMS herringbone structures using a template of ZnO nanorod. Once the image of virus is captured, virus can be detected by naked eyes using on-chip gold nanoparticle-based colorimetric reaction approach with a detection limit of 2.7 × 104 EID50/mL, which is better than that of traditional method fluorescence-based ELISA. This proposed system by incorporating point-of-care microfluidic system with smartphone-based imaging and colorimetric detection devices would provide a fast, ease of use, cheap, sensitive, affordable, and user-friendly platform to detect viruses in remote resource-less field. A general view of smartphone-based system in combination with nanostructured micro-device for virus detection is shown in Figure 7.5 (b). Its part-(i) shows general view of microfluidic device, part-(ii) shows detailed view and process of assay in the system for sandwich virus detection, part-(iii) shows structural view and assembly of the optical system, and part-(iv) shows a general view of the smartphone imaging system design for virus detection.

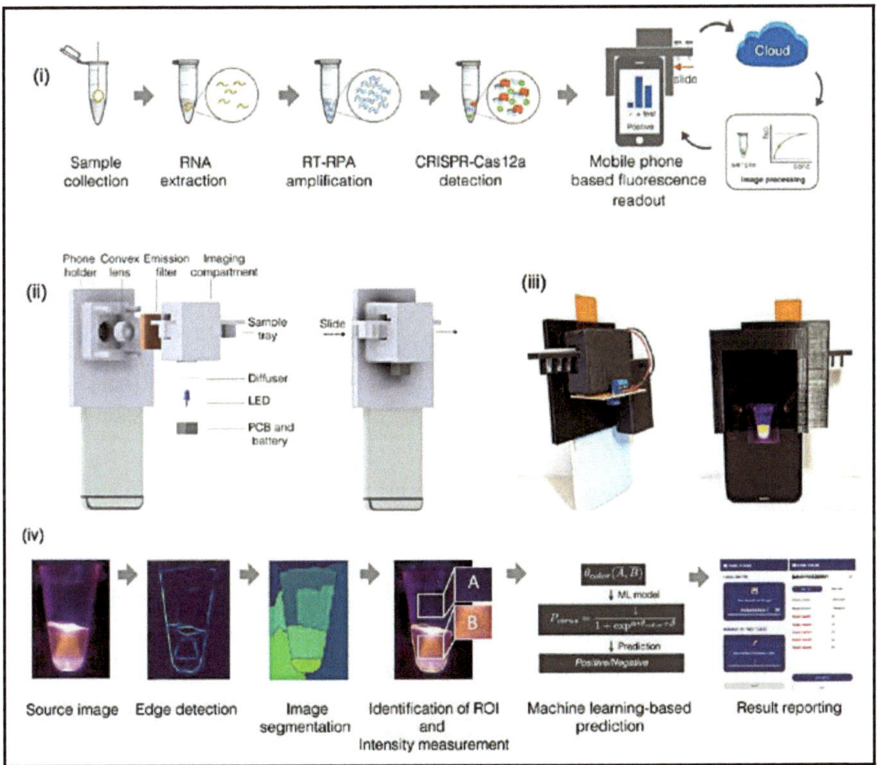

(a) Smartphone based system for virus detection for CRISPR diagnostic (Samacoits et al., 2021) (i) A combination of CRISPR diagnostic and the smartphone-based device and flow chart for detection of SARS-CoV-2. (ii) Computer-aided design (CAD) based system components description (iii) Actual image of smartphone based device used as fluorescence imaging of the CRISPR diagnostic assay (iv) a step-wise procedure for quantification of SARS-CoV-2

(Figure 6.5 *Continued...*)

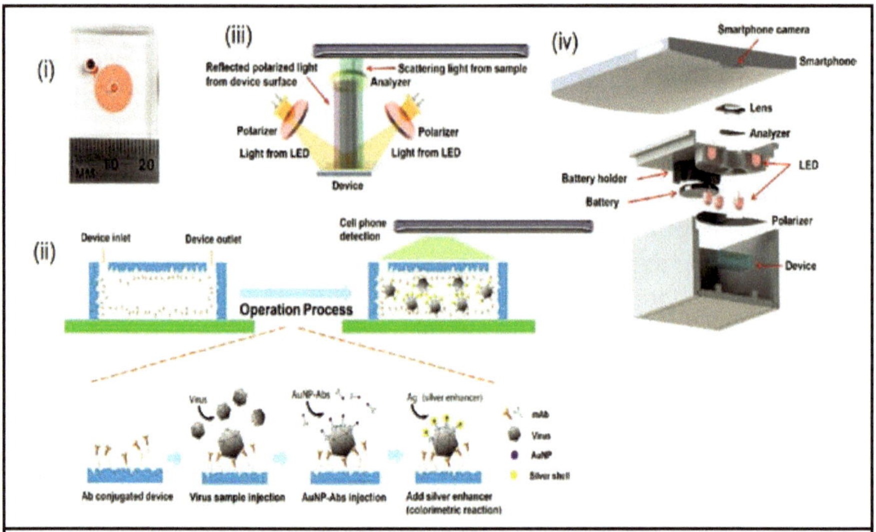

(b) A view of smartphone-based system in combination with nanostructured micro-device for virus detection (i) general view of microfluidic device (ii) Detailed view and process of assay in the system for sandwich virus detection (iii) Structural view and assembly of the optical system. (iv) A general view of the smartphone imaging system design for virus detection (Xia et al, 2019)

FIGURE 6.5 Smartphone-based devices for virus detection. Reproduced from (Samacoits et al., 2021; Xia et al., 2019) with their permission.

It is observed that high sensitivity and specificity can be achieved using the smartphone-based devices for virus detection which tends to be very useful during a viral outbreak. Certainly, such technologies discussed will become more efficient, useful, and accurate with the rapid development of smartphone-based devices and also helpful in the centralized monitoring and treatment of diseases. In conclusion, SIDs have been proved more powerful, hereby showing its application affordable in the field of virus detection, diagnosis, and testing. Their contribution has significantly increase the efficiency and speed of disease detection, diagnosis process with high sensitivity. The widely used application of smartphone devices for detection of virus shows its possibility to be used in remote and resource-less location during pandemic such as COVID-19. The drawback for such technologies is specificity of disease detection, and therefore, a lot of testing and validation process of such devices/technologies are still essentially required before they are openly available to be used by the masses.

6.9 SMARTPHONE-BASED IMAGING SYSTEM FOR FOOD TECHNOLOGY

One of the basic essential requirements of every human being is food and to maintain the quality of food products and prevent the people from any kind of health hazard or sickness, various rules and regulations are enforced by the government. The food technical experts perform the monitoring of contaminants and composition in a food chain by taking the samples from the subject and then analyzing it in food control-based laboratories. However, this approach is costly, non-affordable, and usually time-consuming process. As the growing development of smartphone-based technology to detect bacteria and viruses pathogens, they have also shown capabilities to be used for various detection and analytical applications in quality monitoring of food-based technologies (Coskun et al., 2013; Rateni et al., 2017). Food contamination is widely seen major serious issue to the human kind even for animals also and its ignorance may lead to serious illness and causality. The contamination of milk food is often done with hormones that the people generally give to the animals in order to increase their milk output. Thereby, this kind of issue creates challenges in humans especially in group of children (Ludwig et al., 2012). An effective, affordable, and low-cost portable methodology to screen out at primary stage recombinant bovine somatotropin (rbST)-based contaminants was developed by Ludwig et al. (2012) in milk food in order to detect such hormones rapidly which uses the microsphere-based flow cytometric immunoassay (FCIA) integrated with a smartphone-based platform. In this system, for fluorescence imaging, 3D-printed attachment cell phone module comprised of 12 LEDs each of configuration of (λ = 380 nm); for dark-field imaging, two white LEDs are attached; and to block the scattered excitation light on an optical filter is attached. Though such device was the first device which has combination of both dark-field and fluorescence imaging technology, thereby this kind of device became a new field of imaging especially in food technology. A comparison was made in between this developed assay with a laboratory-based FCIA method and 95% of the samples were predicted correctly using this method. Based on this result, it can be concluded that the accuracy of this model was appreciably close to laboratory-based experimental results, finally sufficient enough for pre-screening process showing the effectiveness and portability of the device (Ludwig et al., 2014). These devices are helpful in supply for everyday use and make effort in bridging the gap between what are the items prepared at laboratories and what are the items used for everyday purposes. Besides use of hormones in food items, some researchers reported that in order to protect the livestock products from diseases and bacterial infections, farmers usually use antibiotics in large amount. The amount of antibiotics used by them is more than prescribed and allowed limit and traces are found in excess amount in various animal products. It has been observed that this factor becomes one of the reasons for the development of rapid antibiotic resistance in most of the human population (Landers et al., 2012). Therefore, a need arises for the rapid detection of these antibiotics to protect the people from diseases and infections.

The omnipresence of smartphones devices equipped with variety of sophisticated sensors, high processing capability, universal portability, all-time network connectivity with reasonable cost and a suitable interface for visible results makes them an auspicious automated tool for non-invasive, low cost, lightweight, and portable quality assessment of food and its product. Additionally, the recent advancements in the field of IoT technology, machine and deep learning algorithms and cloud computing technology have provided an opportunity for making advanced, more powerful and accurate wide-spread, reasonable, and ecological food analytical methods that could be more useful for the process of food production and distribution with better accuracy. A review presented by Kalinowska et al. (2021) mainly focused on the application of smartphone-based methods in the quality assessment and monitoring of food and its products, particularly in such applications in which they are used to detect or analyze the food contaminants, either on their own or in combination with more advanced recent used analytical procedures. In Figure 7.5(a), depicts a view of farm-to-fork use of smartphone-based tools for quality assessment of food and its products. Figure 7.5(b) shows the procedure for measuring and analyzing allergens in food samples with the help of combined smartphone attachment and colourimetric assays. The part-(1) shows the selection of allergen of interest in the given application, (2) shows grounding food sample into a pot, (3) shows the transfer of approx. 5 g of the ground sample to a vessel, (4) shows the powering and mixing the sample with water at 60°C temperature and with extraction solvent,

(5) shows the addition of three drops of the sample solution to the first tube, (6) shows addition of three drops of the control solution to the second tube acting as reference. In part-(7), an observation is taken in which during a 10 min incubation period, both the test and the control tubes are sequentially washed with a conjugate, substrate, and a stop solution, and in (8, 9), the measurement of absorbance of both solutions is taken using a committed smartphone attachment. In part-(10), the qualitative- and quantitative-based test results are shown using smartphone device (Kalinowska et al., 2021).

The authors in (Rateni et al., 2017) have done various studies on the recent advancements and developments in the field of smartphone-based tools for food diagnostic technologies, mainly enhancing smartphone sensing capabilities by highlighting on their custom modules. They have also extended their discussion on the analysis to the food scanning devices that are progressively populating the new technology such as Internet of Things (IoT)-based market, establishing how this recent technology is indeed promising, as the research outcomes are quickly exploited on new start-up industries. Figure 7.5(c) (Coskun et al., 2013) shows a platform for personalized food allergen testing, termed iTube, running on a smartphone-based device and it is able to automatically analyze the colorimetric assays which is performed in test tubes dedicated to sensitive and specific detection of allergens present in food samples. Its part-(i) depicts a view of iTube platform, combining colorimetric assays and a smartphone-based digital reader. The part-(ii) shows the conjunction of the optomechanical attachment with smartphone which is installed on its back side with the dimensions: ~22 mm × 67 mm × 75 mm. Part-(iii) shows the detailed diagram of the same iTube platform with description of each parts (Coskun et al., 2013). Figure 7.5(d) shows a variety of commercial smartphone-based products for diagnosis and analysis of food and its products (Rateni et al., 2017).

A digital image colorimeter was proposed by Masawat et al. (2015). In this work, they have detected analyte of interest, tetracycline in order to determine antibiotic residue in the milk. The ColorConc application enabled with iPhone camera was used to capture the image of the sample solution through a drill hole present inside black-painted box in which the solution of interest was kept inside. The amount of tetracycline detected using this device was in the range of 0.5–10 $\mu g\ mL^{-1}$ having limit of quantification of 1.5 $\mu g\ mL^{-1}$ with large sensitivity and rapidity.

Another smartphone-based biosensing model was developed by (Dou et al., 2016) for the detection of clenbuterol (CLB). CLB is a steroid-type drug, generally used for veterinary purposes and, in some countries, used for the treatment of asthma also. If human takes this drug, various symptoms such as chest pain, dizziness, and increased heart rate are experienced. In this work, different method was proposed in comparison to existing methods as detection process was carried out using immunoreaction. The detection process of the substance was carried out from a layer of immunoglobulin. It was kept inside modified multi-walled carbon nanotubes which comprised a conjunction of screen-printed carbon electrode (SPCE) and a layer of immunoglobulin. This proposed model was capable of detecting CLB in the range from 0.3 unit to 100 ng mL^{-1}. One of the leading causes of food poisoning is contamination of food with bacteria and it may lead very often severe symptoms such as diarrhea and vomiting. The medium of reaching the food contamination to the population is generally through the food vendors and restaurants. Therefore, it becomes necessary to check the cause of it such that the presence of pathogens in food. Most of the detection methods developed so far to detect pathogens in food generally involve first their culturing and then perform various standardized tests for their detection consumes a lot of time. In recent research, smartphone-based devices have shown capability to detect various contaminations in the food. A smartphone-based spectroscopic method was proposed by Liang et al. (2014) to detect microbial-based contamination in beef samples. This process is based on Mie scattering, in which they irradiated the surface of the beef sample with 880-nm near-infrared LED and computed the scatter signal intensities at different angle inclinations (15°, 30°, 40°, and 60°). They quantified the *E. coli* concentrations successfully in the range 101–108 CFU/mL. In this experiment, it is not able to distinguish the similar bacterial species because of non-usage of antibodies (Liang et al. 2014). Another smartphone-based technology was developed by Bueno et al. (2015) in which the presence of foodborne pathogens can be detected in meat sample by observing the presence of three different profiled amine contaminations (isobutyl amine, triethylamine, and isopentylamine). They immobilized the cellulose membrane with five different varieties of Ph-indicators and exposed all of them to each of the amines in order to generate color profiles. They captured the images by using smartphone and quantified using two different methods such as principal component analysis (PCA)-based dimensional reduction and hierarchical cluster analysis (HCA). In this method, the amines were quantified up to 1 ppm which in turn indicates the ability to provide faster detection of pathogens in the food. While it may be the case that certain number of people may not receive any harm due to these pathogens, still it is necessary to detection these pathogens as they can prove it to be harmful for others.

Overall, the role and importance of SIDs cannot be ignored and importantly they can be recognized as a potential tool especially in the field of food technologies which can deal with the severe complications may lead to life-threatening. They are also capable to provide the solution as an efficient, faster monitoring, and extensive measuring tool in order to produce portable as well as cost-effective models.

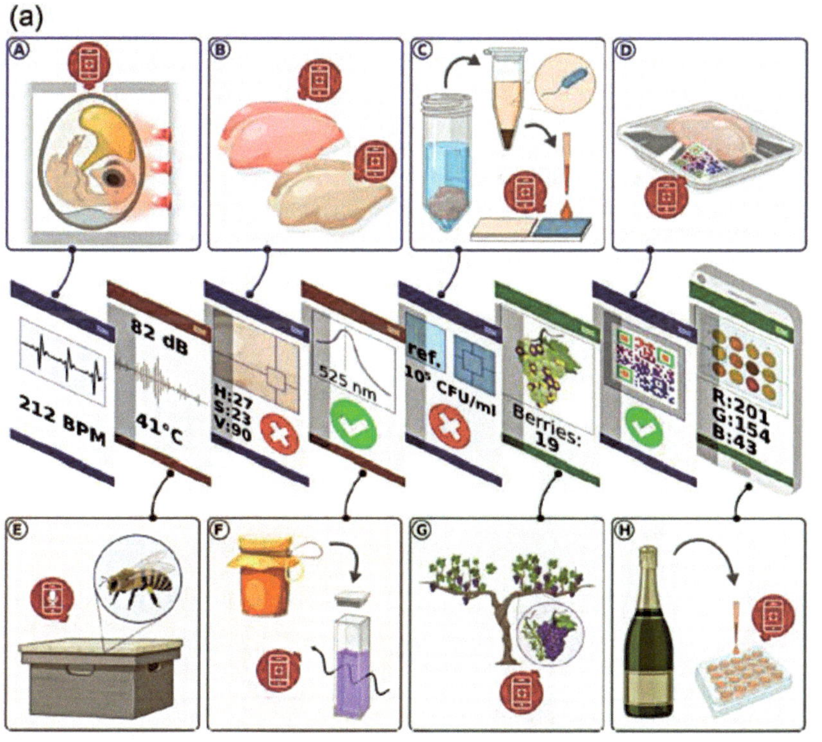

(a) Farm-to-fork use of smartphone-based quality assessment tools for food and its products. Reproduced from (Kalinowska et al., 2021) with their permission.

(Figure 6.6 *Continued...*)

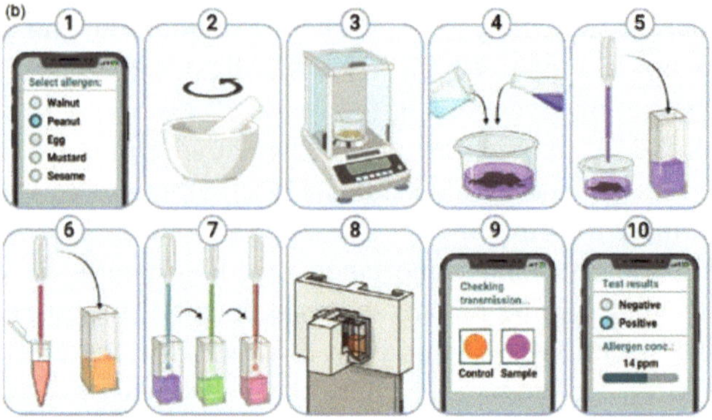

(b) Shows the procedure for measuring and analysing allergens in food samples with the help of combined smartphone attachment and colourimetric assays. The part- (1) shows the selection of allergen of interest in the given application; (2) shows grounding food sample into a pot. (3) shows the transfer of approx. 5 g of the ground sample to a vessel, (4) shows the powering and mixing the sample with water at 60^0 C temperature and with extraction solvent, (5) shows the addition of 3 drops of the sample solution to the first tube, (6) shows addition of 3 drops of the control solution to the second tube acting as reference. In part (7) an observation are taken in which during a 10 min incubation period, both the test and the control tubes are sequentially washed with a conjugate, substrate, and a stop solution, in (8, 9) the measurement of absorbance of both solutions is taken using a committed smartphone attachment. In part-(10) the qualitative and quantitative based test results are shown using smartphone device. Reproduced from (Kalinowska et al., 2021) with their permission.

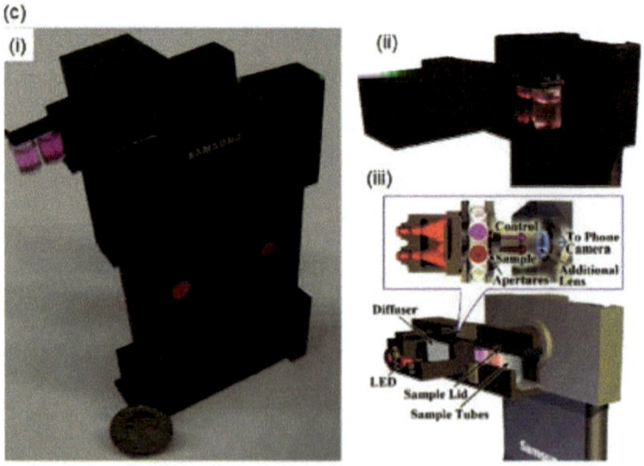

(c) Shows a platform for personalized food allergen testing, termed iTube, running on a smartphone based device and it is able to automatically analyze the colorimetric assays which is performed in test tubes dedicated to sensitive and specific detection of allergens present in food samples. Its part-(i) depicts a view of iTube platform,

(Figure 6.6 *Continued...*)

combining colorimetric assays and a smartphone as a digital reader. The part-(ii) shows the conjunction of the opto-mechanical attachment with smartphone which is installed on its back side with the dimensions: ~ 22 mm × 67 mm × 75 mm. Part-(iii) shows the detailed diagram of the same iTube platform with description of each parts. Reproduced from (Coskun et al., 2013) with their permission.

(d)

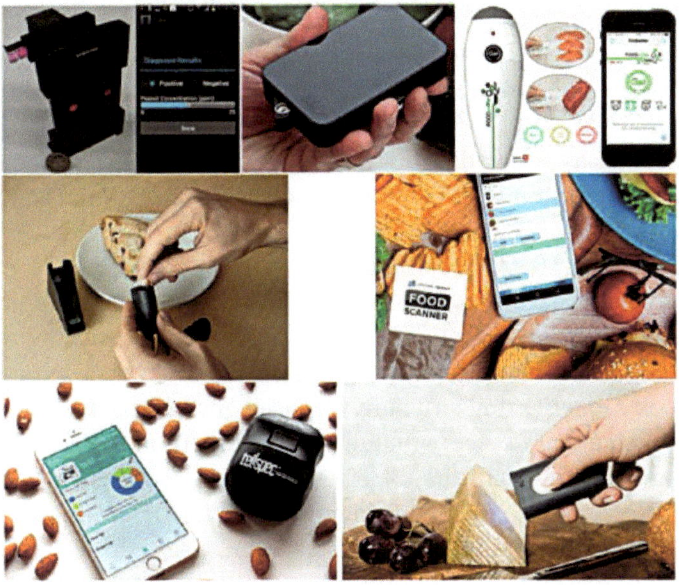

(d) shows a variety of commercial smartphone based products for diagnosis and analysis of food and its products. Reproduced from (Rateni et al, 2017) with their permission.

FIGURE 6.6 Smartphone-based devices for the detection of food contaminations

6.10 INCORPORATING DEEP LEARNING WITH SMARTPHONE-BASED IMAGING DEVICES FOR BIOMEDICAL APPLICATIONS

For the analysis of biological samples, traditionally optical microscopic imaging-based techniques are widely used in the field of bio-optics and biomedical applications. Although this technology is widely used as a standard tool, yet it comprises some limitations like high instrumentation cost, lack of portability, need of expert analyst to analyze the biological samples and their maintenance. On the other side, an alternative solution to overcome these limitations, a smartphone-based imaging technology has become an emerging filed. However, smartphone-based optical imaging system has major drawback of poor image resolution. An efficient image processing method such as deep learning (DL) can resolve this issue (Rivenson et al., 2018) in which multiple layers of neural networks are used for the data abstraction. These techniques require minimum human intervention and provide accurate outputs by automatically exploring the patterns from the data/image. Therefore, in recent research conjunction of smartphone-based microscope systems and deep learning techniques are successfully applied in variety of domains such as from cancer to environmental research (Bornhorst et al., 2019). Convolutional neural network (CNN) algorithm is widely used among various deep learning algorithms as a potential tool in order to improve the image resolution result in detection with better accuracy. An experimental setup was developed in the study done by Rivenson et al. (2018) which consisted of a Nokia Lumia 1020 in combination with CMOS image sensor. This system is also comprised of additional five plastic lenses for visibility along with in-build six lenses composed with smartphone's rear camera as shown in Figure 7.7. In this system, to illuminate the biological sample, a 12 RGB color-based LED ring structure was used and an attachment of 3D-printed optomechanical device with adjustment based on XYZ stage for a given biological sample. In the experiment, the convolutional layer present in the CNN model extracted inherent characteristics of input RGB image for further processing and the linear unit was rectified as an activation function for better result. Initially, multiple network models with the same layered architecture were created for training the model using blood smear, lung tissue, and Papanicolaou samples. Images obtained from a smartphone-based microscope and ×20 resolution images obtained from Olympus IX83 microscope are compared during the training phase and then computation of cost function is performed in each of the iterations which in turn used to modify the network parameters for better learning using a backpropagation algorithm. Further, now analysis of different pathological samples can be done blindly using this network. Additionally, color distortions can also be corrected by using deep learning techniques caused by incoherent light sources used for image acquisition (Rivenson et al. 2018). In similar research, a DL-based CNN model was also developed to identify the sickle cells (to identify disease) from the peripheral blood smear. This model was used to enhance the quality of smartphone images and thereafter, the sickle cells were segmented out from the same model. This model has produced overall accuracy of 98% and, therefore, it has become a potential tool in medical for screening the disease in resource-less areas around the world (de Haan et al., 2020).

Cancer is a kind of severing disease which may lead to death; hence it requires a potential diagnostic tool for early diagnosis. The assessment of cancer can be done using smartphone-based microscopy method in conjunction with DL-based technique for enhancement and classification of sample image. In this direction, smartphone-based microscope was developed by some of the researchers embedded with the android application in order to detect oral cancer in resource-limited remote areas. In this system, a LG android smartphone was used along with an intraoral and it comprises cavity imaging facility. This device is used to perform both bright-field and auto-fluorescence imaging, in which oral cancer is detected at early using auto-fluorescence imaging method by imaging the biomolecules present in it. Further, the oral cancer images are uploaded to cloud servers for automatic process using Wi-Fi to automate the whole process and later pre-trained CNN are used to classify these images and remote specialist diagnose the disease using these outcomes. This system has facility to download the summary report which consists of data uploaded from a smartphone technology. CNN-based diagnostic result and diagnosis report from a specialist. This report can be viewed and downloaded at any time or instant from the online cloud server. They obtained sensitivity and specificity for the proposed model as 0.9259 and 0.8667, respectively, in the case of remote specialists, whereas using DL-based CNN model, they obtained 0.8500 and 0.8875, respectively, (Uthoff et al., 2018). Additionally, a system was developed by Asensio-Cuesta et al. (2019) in which they developed human dynamic reporting service (HDRS)-based application to measure the quality of life of cancer patients, in which the data retrieved from mobile phone sensors of the patients are used to monitor their activities. Furthermore, a CNN model DFU-QNET was developed by Alzubaidi et al. (2019) used for grading the severity of foot ulcers especially in diabetic patients into two different classes such as normal and abnormal. In this work, several other DL-based pertrained networks are also considered in smartphone-based imaging system and trained with different transfer learning methods and their comparative study have been done with the novel models for performance analysis. Additionally, the automatic deep learning-based detection method was used along with smartphone-based imaging techniques to detect drug abuse.

Therefore, a deep learning imaging employed with smartphone-based imaging system has become a powerful tool for detection and analysis in biomedical and mHealth applications. They are very cost-effective, portable, and easy to use technique which may have variety of critical applications to solve many diagnostic problems in the coming days. The smartphone-based imaging produces very promising results when employed with DL-based image processing techniques for detection and analysis, particularly in resource-less remote settings and also during medical emergencies. Furthermore, these smartphone-based microscopes becomes an essential tool when the desired medical assistance and experts are not easily available, can be used to pre-screen and analyze the disease conditions within limited time, hence reducing causality.

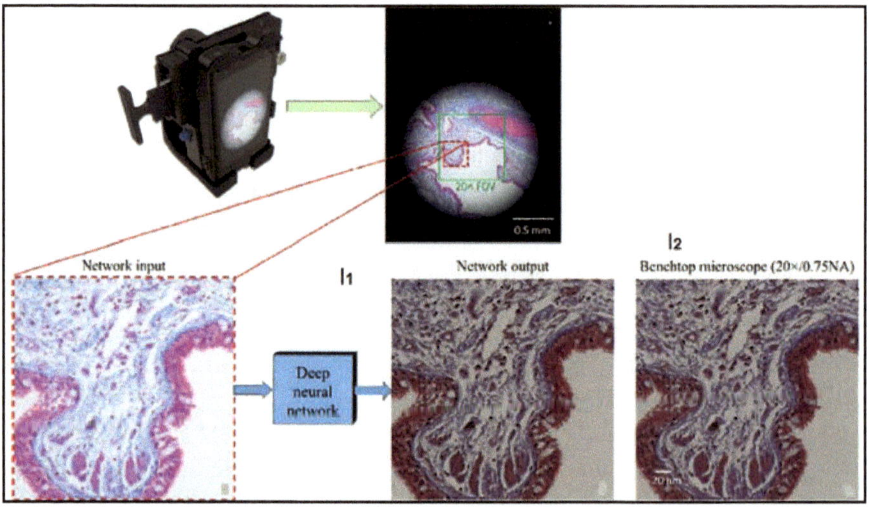

FIGURE 6.7 A view of smartphone-based microscopic imaging system in conjunction with deep leaning based CNN. The output images marked by I1 and I2 shows different images obtained by deep learnin based enhancement technique and benchtop microscopic method respectively. Reproduced from Rivenson et al., (2018) with permission from American Chemical Society (copyright 2018)

6.11 CONCLUSION

Smartphone-based imaging devices (SIDs) have become powerful analytical tools for variety of biomedical and mHealth research applications. A continuous development has been observed under SIDs in combination of different types of technologies such as microscopic and spectroscopic techniques to gain faster acknowledgment in variety of settings in the market. Smartphone-based camera is used as a detection system by most of the biomedical devices which provides better facility to the user to measure variety of metrics such as for colorimetric, fluorescence, luminescence, absorbance, and reflectance-measurements. SIDs have shown interest for advanced research specially in the fields of material science, virology, cell biology, and other related fields to explore, uncover, and discover the unknown information. From the detection and analysis of various disease-causing pathogens to medical science, food technology, and education sector, these devices have shown numerous possibilities for other uses. The ability of smartphones to measure physical quantity has been increased today by embedding new sensor technology and applications with them than it was a decade before. Further, with the availability of several wired and wireless connection technology, provide the facility to the SIDs to record data or information automatically on cloud servers or in turn it can be shared in secure platforms to the experts for prediction analysis. The evergreen features of SIDs such as portability, simplicity, low-cost, and availability of user-friendly smartphone-based applications make them an attractive and useful alternative solution in a variety of fields with possible prospects being incredible. These provide the opportunity of being automated and their advantage is that analysis is much faster and even they can be used without any expert person.

From this chapter, it can be visualized that the SIDs have established to be highly sensitive and rapid policy in biomedical and mHealth applications. The great potential of SIDs in coordination with standard optical microscopy-based techniques, have been observed for hemato-histological-based inspection or detection of bacteria pathogens in samples with high sensitivity and accuracy. To overcome the problem of low accuracy and high complex settings of traditional methods for detection of bacterial pathogens, researchers have integrated SIDs with standard technologies such as fluorescence, LAMP, and autofluorescence technology to detect and quantify the present bacterial load in the biological samples in real-time providing a faster diagnosis and prognosis. These devices integrated with efficient assays have also shown strength to improve the sensitivity of detection of virus and food contaminant as well as reduced detection time. In various research literatures, the smartphone devices have been demonstrated its use for the detection of fruit ripening, detection of content of galactose, and peanut traces present in food items. With the advent of new technologies and their ability to miniaturize complexity of traditional devices such as lenses and lasers, SIDs have emerged as portable, easy to use devices and they can be used as a POC device for variety of biomedical and mHealth applications. Integration of various analytical methods like Raman or Fourier transform-based infrared spectroscopy with smartphone devices will have great applications in human's daily life for visual detection and analysis of bacteria pathogens or contaminants in the samples of food and water to detection of presence of harmful and hazardous chemicals. Amalgamation of standard technology such as optical coherence-based tomography or endoscopy along with smartphone devices have provide an opportunity for faster caring through diagnosis and prognosis using tele-laboratory-based medical services even in small medical clinics. The brightness of the smartphone display is regulated based on the surrounding visibility by using the ambient light sensor which in turn basically a photodiode. In order to detect contaminants in water or liquid food items and monitoring various colorimetric based assays, these devices can be used as a spectrometric-based detection system similar to the standard laboratory-based systems. Further, considering the ability of microfluidic devices to carry out different biochemical assays-based experimentation in POC setting, their amalgamation with SIDs has shown their power for bringing detection and diagnosis process to house settings and resource-less areas. Advent of deep learning-based image processing methods has given the opportunity to implement automated system with SIDs to make the process of detection more accurate and read-outs can be obtained with more efficient and rapid way.

On the other hand, SIDs can be helpful for applications of educational purposes as medium of teaching and learning in remote schools or to carry out analysis based on assays which in turn may eliminate the need of expensive instruments. As rapid increase and easy availability of smartphone connectivity and their increasing use as remote teaching and learning tool, online practical experiments can be performed by using them from their homes which can be monitored by the teachers remotely in critical times of pandemic such as COVID-19. The ability to perform detection of disease, bacteria pathogens, health monitoring, and diagnostics using variety of biological samples with same performance and minimal processing, decides the future scope of SIDs-based analytical and bioanalytical devices. Additionally, it also brings daily health monitoring of general people in their own hands. Using these devices, monitoring of health can be performed regularly which can help in saving a lot of lives from adversaries which often may be caused due to non-symptomatic in nature or delayed onset. Furthermore, they can also be used to detect any food contaminants sitting at restaurants or can help in determining the various contaminations in the food which in turn may help to reduce the problem of allergies. Using such sensitive bioanalytical capabilities of SIDs, on-the-spot tracking of different contamination can be achieved by integrating their GPS data with biosensing data, in which the spread of bacteria pathogens can be measured in the sample. Other application areas such as geology or entomology can also use SIDs, which may help them by providing portable microscopic imaging devices to carry out research in faster way with minimal processing.

Researchers have observed an exponential growth in the development of smartphone-based imaging technologies for the past few decades. Since smartphones have become an essential tool in everyday life, their hardware and processing capability has improved a lot since past decade of 1990s. Now a day, smartphones are easily available with much lesser price and high capability and their display screen and cameras are improving fast year by year in terms of quality, visibility, and sensor sensitivity. They can be easily carried out any remote places in the world due to their characteristics like compactness and easy handling. Further, the capacity of SIDs will be increased with the help of these features. With the advent of modern sensor technology like LIDAR or infrared (IR), it can be integrated with smartphones which might find other possible applications in variety of biomedical fields in future. The only shortcoming of these SIDs is the limited display and sensitivity of in-built smartphone camera in comparison to that of standard CCD or PMT technology. Furthermore, advanced scientific cameras embedded with optical microscopes have comparatively larger sensor size, which in turn receive more light to provide a capability of capturing of sample images better and their background noise is sufficiently reduced; on the other hand, the camera sensors of smartphone devices are small in size due to limited space available in the device and hence suffers from limited resolution, low light intensity, or limited color balance. Additionally, in this system, once the image is captured by smartphone, the built-in image processing is applied on it; as a result, the basic inherent characteristics of the image get changed which in turn causes variation in image properties and hence may increase the risk of disease misdiagnosis. Therefore, a recent deep learning-based technology provides opportunity to be integrated with SIDs which can be trained using images obtained from scientific cameras which in turn can help to acquire similar kind of images using the smartphone. Henceforth, the complete process of image acquisition and analysis becomes much faster and easier for diagnosis with the help of such devices.

Although, such smartphone-based devices embeding with new technologies appear to be more compatible to the traditional devices, yet their real time use in people's everyday life in biomedical and mHealth applications is still uncertain. Moreover, in every year, various research literatures and patents proposing various new technologies integrated with smartphone devices, but very less interest is shown by those researchers in converting their actual research into real-time products. Additionally, a concern is that the power of such devices has been over estimated by the researchers and they do not contribute substantial diagnostic or scientific value. However, if these technologies are successfully integrated with existing smartphones, they promise to transform our lives. Therefore, their performance as POC-based devices can be determined by critically evaluating their analytical performance in resource-less remote settings.

KEYWORDS

- **computer-aided diagnosis**
- **point of care diagnosis**
- **smartphone-based imaging devices**
- **smartphone-based retinal imaging system**

REFERENCES

Ahn, S.; Kang, J.; Kim, P.; Lee, G.; Jeong, E.; Jung, W.; Park, M.; Song, T. K. Smartphone-based Portable Ultrasound Imaging System: Prototype Implementation and Evaluation. In *2015 IEEE International Ultrasonics Symposium (IUS)*, Taipei, Taiwan, 2015, pp 1–4.

Aiello, L. P.; Beck, R. W.; Bressler, N. M.; Browning, D. J.; Chalam, K. V.; Davis, M.; Ferris, F. L. 3rd; Glassman, A. R.; Maturi, R. K.; Stockdale, C. R.; Topping, T. M.

Rationale for the Diabetic Retinopathy Clinical Research Network Treatment Protocol for Center-Involved Diabetic Macular Edema. *Ophthalmology* **2011,** *118* (12), e5–e14.

Alzubaidi, L.; Fadhel, M. A.; Oleiwi, S. R.; Al-Shamma, O.; Zhang, J. DFU_QUTNet: Diabetic Foot Ulcer Classification Using Novel Deep Convolutional Neural Network. *Multimed. Tools Appl.* **2019,** *27,* 1–23.

Asensio-Cuesta, S.; Sánchez-García, Á.; Conejero, J. A.; Saez, C.; Rivero-Rodriguez, A.; García-Gómez J. M. Smartphone Sensors for Monitoring Cancer-Related Quality of Life: App Design, EORTC QLQ-C30 Mapping and Feasibility Study in Healthy Subjects. *Int. J. Environ. Res. Public Health* **2019,** *16* (3), 461.

Ashrafuzzaman, M.; Huq M. M.; Chakraborty, C.; Khan M. R. M.; Tabassum, T.; Hasan, R. Heart Attack Detection Using Smart Phone. *Int. J. Technol. Enhance Emerg. Eng. Res.* **2013,** *1* (3), 2347–4289.

Banerjee, R.; Ghose, A.; Choudhury, A. D.; Sinha, A.; Pal, A. In *Noise Cleaning and Gaussian Modeling of Smart Phone Photoplethysmogram to Improve Blood Pressure Estimation,* 2015 IEEE International Conference on Acoustics, Speech and Signal Processing (ICASSP). Piscataway: IEEE, 2015; pp 967–971.

Barnes, L.; Heithoff, D. M.; Mahan, S. P.; Fox, G. N.; Zambrano, A.; Choe, J.; et al. Smartphone-based Pathogen Diagnosis in Urinary Sepsis Patients. *EBioMedicine* **2018,** *36,* 73–82.

Boehme, C. C.; Nabeta, P.; Hillemann, D.; Nicol, M. P.; Shenai, S.; Krapp, F.; et al. Rapid Molecular Detection of Tuberculosis and Rifampin Resistance. *N. Engl. J. Med.* **2010,** *363* (11), 1005–1015.

Bornhorst, J.; Nustede, E. J.; Fudickar, S. Mass Surveillance of C. Elegans-Smartphone-based DIY Microscope and Machinelearning-based Approach for Worm Detection. *Sensors* **2019,** *19* (6):1468.

Bowler, P. G.; Duerden, B. I.; Armstrong, D. G. Wound Microbiology and Associated Approaches to Wound Management. *Clin. Microbiol. Rev.* **2001,** *14* (2), 244–269.

Bueno, L.; Meloni, G. N.; Reddy, S. M.; Paixao, T. R. L. C. Use of Plasticbased Analytical Device, Smartphone and Chemometric Tools to Discriminate Amines. *RSC Adv.* **2015,** *5* (26), 20148–20154.

Cardiovascular Diseases. https://www.who.int/health-topics/cardiovasculardiseases/ (accessed July 11, 2021).

Carusi, C.; Bernardi, C. An Easy, Efficient, and Safe Method for Intraoperative Digital Photography by Smartphone. *Aesthet. Surg. J.* **2016,** *36* (9), 284–286.

Cesaretti, M.; Poté, N.; Dondero, F.; Cauchy, F.; Schneck, A. S.; Soubrane, O.; et al. Testing Feasibility of an Accuratemicroscopic Assessment of Macrovesicular Steatosis in Liver Allograft Biopsies by Smartphone Add-On Lenses. *Microsc. Res. Tech.* **2018,** *81* (1), 58–63.

Chang, J.; Arbeláez, P.; Switz, N.; Reber, C.; Tapley, A.; Davis, J. L.; et al. Automated Tuberculosis Diagnosis Using Fluorescence Images from a Mobile Microscope. *Med. Image. Comput. Comput. Assist. Interv.* **2012,** *15* (Pt 3), 345–352.

Coskun, A. F.; Wong, J.; Khodadadi, D.; Nagi, R.; Tey, A.; Ozcan, A. A Personalized Food Allergen Testing Platform on a Cellphone. *Lab. Chip.* **2013,** *13,* 636–640.

D'Ambrosio, M. V.; Bakalar, M.; Bennuru, S.; Reber, C.; Skandarajah, A.; Nilsson, L.; et al. Point-of-Care Quantification of Blood-Borne Filarial Parasites with a Mobile Phone Microscope. *Sci. Transl. Med.* **2015,** *7* (286), 286re4.

de Haan, K.; Koydemir, H. C.; Rivenson, Y.; Tseng, D.; Van Dyne, E.; Bakic, L.; et al. Automated Screening of Sickle Cells Using a Smartphone-based Microscope and Deep Learning. *NPJ Digit. Med.* **2020,** *3* (1), 1–9.

Dou, Y.; Jiang, Z.; Deng, W.; Su, J.; Chen, S.; Song, H.; et al. Portable Detection of Clenbuterol Using a Smartphone-based Electrochemical Biosensor with Electric Field-Driven Acceleration. *J. Electroanal. Chem.* **2016,** *781,* 339–344.

English, E.; Hung, A.; Kesten, E.; Latulipe, D.; Jin, Z. In *EyePhone: A Mobile EOG-based Human-Computer Interface for Assistive Healthcar*, 6th International IEEE/EMBS Conference on Neural Engineering (NER) 2013, San Diego, CA, 2013; pp 105–108.

Ganguli, A.; Ornob, A.; Yu, H.; Damhorst, G. L.; Chen, W.; Sun, F.; et al. Handsfree Smartphone-based Diagnostics for Simultaneous Detection of Zika, Chikungunya, and Dengue at Point-of-Care. *Biomed. Microdevices* **2017,** *19* (4):73.

Gaurav, A.; Maheedhar, M.; Tiwari, V. N.; Narayanan, R. In *Cuff-Less Ppg Based Continuous Blood Pressure Monitoring—A Smartphone Based Approach*, 2016 38th Annual International Conference of the IEEE Engineering in Medicine and Biology Society (EMBC). Piscataway: IEEE, 2016; pp 607–610.

Gurcan, M. N.; Boucheron, L. E.; Can, A.; Madabhushi, A.; Rajpoot, N. M.; Yener, B. Histopathological Image Analysis: A Review. *IEEE Rev. Biomed. Eng.* **2009,** *2,* 147–171.

Hameed, S.; Xie, L.; Ying, Y. Conventional and Emerging Detection Techniques for Pathogenic Bacteria in Food Science: A Review. *Trends Food Sci. Technol.* **2018,** *81,* 61–73.

Hartnett, M. E.; Key, I. J.; Loyacano, N. M.; Horswell, R. L.; DeSalvo, K. B. Perceived Barriers to Diabetic Eye Care: Qualitative Study of Patients and Physicians. *Arch. Ophthalmol.* **2005,** *123* (3), 387–391.

Hernández-Neuta, I.; Neumann, F.; Brightmeyer, J.; Ba Tis, T.; Madaboosi, N.; Wei, Q.; et al. Smartphone-based Clinical Diagnostics: Towards Democratization of Evidence-Based Health Care. *J. Intern. Med.* **2019,** *285* (1), 19–39.

Herrick, J.; Bensimon, A. Imaging of Single DNA Molecule: Applications to High-Resolution Genomic Studies. *Chromosom Res.* 1999, 7(6), 409–423. https://doi.org/10.1023/a:1009276210892.

Kalinowska, K.; Wojnowski, W.; Tobiszewski. M. Smartphones as Tools for Equitable Food Quality Assessment. *Trends Food Sci. Technol.* **2021,** *111* (2021), 271–279.

Karakaya, M.; Hacisoftaoglu, R. E. Comparison of Smartphone-based Retinal Imaging Systems for Diabetic Retinopathy Detection Using Deep Learning. *BMC Bioinform.* **2020,** *21* (Suppl 4):259.

Kim, G.; Yoon, C.; Kye, S.-B.; Lee, Y.; Kang, J.; Yoo, Y.; Song, T. K. A Single FPGA-based Portable Ultrasound Imaging System for Point of-Care Application. *IEEE Trans. Ultrason. Ferroelectr. Freq. Control* **2012,** *59* (7), 1386–1394.

Krishna, K. D.; Akkala, V.; Bharath, R.; Rajalakshmi, P.; Mohammed, A. M. In *FPGA based Preliminary CAD for Kidney on IoT Enabled Portable Ultrasound Imaging System*, 2014 IEEE 16th International Conference on e-Health Networking, Applications and Services (Healthcom), Natal, 2014; pp 257–261.

Laksanasopin, T.; Guo, T. W.; Nayak, S.; Sridhara, A. A.; Xie, S.; Olowookere, O. O.; et al. A Smartphone Dongle for Diagnosis of Infectious Diseases at the Point of Care. *Sci. Transl. Med.* **2015,** *7* (273), 273re1.

Lamonaca, F.; Barbe, K.; Kurylyak, Y.; Grimaldi, D.; Van Moer, W.; Furfaro, A.; Spagnuolo, V. In *Application of the Artificial Neural Network for Blood Pressure Evaluation with Smartphones*, 2013 IEEE 7th International Conference on Intelligent Data Acquisition and Advanced Computing Systems (IDAACS), vol. 1. Piscataway: IEEE, 2013; pp 408–412.

Landers, T. F.; Cohen, B.; Wittum, T. E.; Larson, E. L. A Review of Antibiotic Use in Food Animals: Perspective, Policy, and Potential. *Public Health Rep.* **2012,** *127* (1), 4–22.

Li, L.; Liu, Z.; Zhang, H.; Yue, W.; Li, C. W.; Yi, C. A Point-of-Need Enzyme Linked Aptamer Assay for Mycobacterium Tuberculosis Detection using a Smartphone. *Sens. Actuators B Chem.* **2018,** *254,* 337–346.

Liang, P.-S.; Park, T. S.; Yoon, J.-Y. Rapid and Reagent Less Detection of Microbial Contamination Within Meat Utilizing a Smartphone-based Biosensor. *Sci. Rep.* **2014,** *4*, 5953.

Lingen, M. W.; Kalmar, J. R.; Karrison, T.; Speight, P. M. Critical Evaluation of Diagnostic Aids for the Detection of Oral Cancer. *Oral Oncol.* **2008,** *44* (1), 10–22.

Ludwig, S. K. J.; Smits, N. G. E.; van der Veer, G.; Bremer, M. G. E. G.; Nielen, M. W. F. Multiple Protein Biomarker Assessment for Recombinant Bovine Somatotropin (rbST) Abuse in Cattle. *PLoS One.* **2012,** *7* (12), e52917.

Ludwig, S. K. J.; Zhu, H.; Phillips, S.; Shiledar, A.; Feng, S.; Tseng, D.; et al. Cellphone-based Detection Platform for rbST Biomarker Analysis in Milk Extracts using a Microsphere Fluorescence Immunoassay. *Anal. Bioanal. Chem.* **2014,** *406,* 6857–6866.

Masawat, P.; Harfield, A.; Namwong, A. An iPhone-based Digital Image Colorimeter for Detecting Tetracycline in Milk. *Food Chem.* **2015,** *184,* 23–29.

McCracken, K. E.; Yoon, J. Y. Recent Approaches for Optical Smartphone Sensing in Resource-Limited Settings: A Brief Review. *Anal. Meth.* **2016,** *8* (36), 6591–6601.

Muehldorfer, S. M.; Stolte, M.; Martus, P.; Hahn, E. G.; Ell, C. Diagnostic Accuracy of Forceps Biopsy Versus Polypectomy for Gastric Polyps: A Prospective Multicentre Study. *Gut* **2002,** *509* (4), 465–470.

Müller, V.; Sousa, J. M.; Koydemir, H. C.; Veli, M.; Tseng, D.; Cerqueira, L.; et al. Identification of Pathogenic Bacteria in Complex Samples Using a Smartphone based Fluorescence Microscope. *RSC Adv.* **2018,** *8* (64), 36493–36502.

National Kidney Foundation [online]. https://www.kidney.org/news/newsroom/factsheets/FastFacts

Ojha, A.; Banik, S.; Melanthota, S. K.; Mazumder, M. Light Emitting Diode (LED) based Fluorescence Microscopy for Tuberculosis Detection: A Review. *Lasers Med. Sci.* **2020,** *35* (6), 1431–1437.

Olthoff, K. M.; Kulik, L.; Samstein, B.; Kaminski, M.; Abecassis, M.; Emond, J.; et al. Validation of a Current Definition of Early Allograft Dysfunction in Liver Transplant Recipients and Analysis of Risk Factors. *Liver Transpl.* **2010,** *16* (8), 943–949.

Ozcan, A. Mobile Phones Democratize and Cultivate Next-Generation Imaging, Diagnostics and Measurement Tools. *Lab. Chip.* **2014,** *14* (17), 3187–3194.

Panagariya, A. The Challenges and Innovative Solutions to Rural Health Dilemma. *Ann. Neurosci.* **2014,** *21* (4), 125–127.

Peruski, A. H.; Peruski, L. F. Immunological Methods for Detection and Identification of Infectious Disease and Biological Warfare Agents. *Clin. Diagn. Lab. Immunol.* **2003,** *10*(4), 506–513.

Priye, A.; Bird, S. W.; Light, Y. K.; Ball, C. S.; Negrete, O. A.; Meagher, R. J. A Smartphone-based Diagnostic Platform for Rapid Detection of Zika, Chikungunya, and Dengue Viruses. *Sci. Rep.* **2017,** *7,* 44778.

Quero, J. M.; Tarrida, C. L.; Santana, J. J.; Ermolov, V.; Jantunen, I.; Laine, H.; Eichholz, J.; et al. In *Health Care Applications Based on Mobile Phone Centric Smart Sensor Network*, 2007 29th Annual International Conference of the IEEE Engineering in Medicine and Biology Society, Lyon, 2007; pp 6298–6301.

Raja, K. B., Madheswaran, M.; Thyagarajah, K. A Hybrid Fuzzy-Neural System for Computer-Aided Diagnosis of Ultrasound Kidney Images Using Prominent Features. *J. Med. Syst.* **2008,** *32* (1), 65–83.

Rateni, G.; Dario, P.; Cavallo, F. Smartphone-Based Food Diagnostic Technologies: A Review, *Sensors* **2017,** *17,* 1453.

Rivenson, Y.; Ceylan K. H.; Wang, H.; Wei, Z.; Ren, Z.; Günaydın, H.; et al. Deep Learning Enhanced Mobile-Phone Microscopy. *ACS Photon.* **2018,** *5* (6), 2354–2364.

Rodrigues, D. F. M.; Horta, E. T. ; Silva, B. M. C.; Guedes, F. D. M. ; Rodrigues, J. J. P. C. In *A Mobile Healthcare Solution for Ambient Assisted Living Environments,* IEEE 16th International Conference on e-Health Networking, Applications and Services (Healthcom), 2014, Natal, 2014; pp 170–175.

Roy, M.; Jin, G.; Seo, D.; Nam, M.-H.; Seo, S. A Simple and Low-Cost Device Performing Blood Cell Counting based on Lens-Free Shadow Imaging Technique. *Sensors Actuators* **2014,** *201,* 321–328.

Rubin, R.; Strayer, D. S.; Rubin, E. *Rubin's Pathology: Clinicopathologic Foundations of Medicine*. Lippincott Williams & Wilkins: Baltimore, 2018.

Samacoits, A.; Nimsamer, P.; Mayuramart, O.; Chantaravisoot, N.; et al. Machine Learning-Driven and Smartphone-Based Fluorescence Detection for CRISPR Diagnostic of SARS-CoV-2, *ACS Omega* **2021,** *6,* 2727–2733.

Scully, C. G.; Lee, J.; Meyer, J.; Gorbach, A. M.; Granquist-Fraser, D.; Mendelson, Y.; Chon, K. H. Physiological Parameter Monitoring from Optical Recordings with a Mobile Phone. *IEEE Trans. Biomed. Eng.* **2011,** *59* (2), 303–306.

Shabaan, M.; Arshid, K.; Yaqub, M.; Jinchao, F.; Zia, M. S.; Bojja, G. R., Iftikhar, M.; Ghani, U.; Ambati, L. S.; Munir, R. Survey: Smartphone-based Assessment of Cardiovascular Diseases Using ECG and PPG Analysis. *BMC Med. Inform. Decis. Mak.* **2020,** *20,* 177.

Shors, T. *Understanding Viruses*, 3rd ed.; Jones and Bartlett Publishers: Burlington, 2017.

Shukla, S.; Hong, S.-Y.; Chung, S. H.; Kim, M. Rapid Detection Strategies for the Global Threat of Zika Virus: Current State, New Hypotheses and Limitations. *Front Microbiol.* **2016,** *7,* 1685.

Skandarajah, A.; Sunny, S. P.; Gurpur, P.; Reber, C. D.; D'Ambrosio, M. V.; Raghavan, N.; et al. Mobile Microscopy as a Screening Tool for Oral Cancer in India: A Pilot Study. *PLoS One.* **2017,** *12* (11), e0188440.

Thekkek, N.; Richards-Kortum, R. Optical Imaging for Cervical Cancer Detection: Solutions for a Continuing Global Problem. *Nat. Rev. Cancer* **2008,** *8,* 725–731.

Thevenot, J.; L'opez, M. B.; Hadid, A. A Survey on Computer Vision for Assistive Medical Diagnosis from Faces. *IEEE J. Biomed. Health Inform.* **2017,** *22* (5), 1497–1511.

Tian, B.; Qiu, Z.; Ma, J.; De la Torre, T. Z. G.; Johansson, C.; Svedlindh, P.; et al. Attomolar Zika Virus Oligonucleotide Detection based on Loop-Mediated Isothermal Amplification and AC Susceptometry. *Biosens. Bioelectron.* **2016,** *86,* 420–425.

Uthoff, R. D.; Song, B.; Sunny, S.; Patrick, S.; Suresh, A.; Kolur, T.; et al. Point-of-Care, Smartphone-based, Dual-Modality, Dual-View, Oral Cancer Screening Device with Neural Network Classification for Low-Resource Communities. *PLoSOne* **2018,** *13* (12), e0207493.

Vaidya, A. S.; Srinivas, M. B.; Himabindu, P.; Jumaxanova, D. In *A Smart Phone/Tablet based Mobile Health Care System for Developing Countries*, 2013 35th Annual International Conference of the IEEE Engineering in Medicine and Biology Society (EMBC), Osaka, 2013; pp 4642–4645.

Vaish, P.; Bharath, R.; Rajalakshmi, P.; Desai, U. B. In *Smartphone based Automatic Abnormality Detection of Kidney in Ultrasound Images*, 2016 IEEE 18th International Conference on e-Health Networking, Applications and Services (Healthcom), 14–16 Sept. 2016. DOI: 10.1109/Healthcom36776.2016

Vashist, S. K.; Luppa, P. B.; Yeo, L. Y.; Ozcan, A.; Luong, J. H. Emerging Technologies for Next Generation Point-of-Care Testing. *Trends Biotechnol.* **2015,** *33* (11), 692–705.

Wei, Q.; Qi, H.; Luo, W.; Tseng, D.; Ki, S. J.; Wan, Z.; et al. Fluorescent Imaging of Single Nanoparticles and Viruses on a Smart Phone. *ACS Nano.* **2013,** *7* (10), 9147–9155.

Witte, R.; Andriasyan, V.; Georgi, F.; Yakimovich, A.; Greber, U. F. Concepts in Light Microscopy of Viruses. *Viruses* **2018,** *10* (4), 1– 31.

Wu, Y. C.; Kulbatski, I.; Medeiros, P. J.; Maeda, A.; Bu, J.; Xu, L.; et al. Autofluorescence Imaging Device for Real-Time Detection and Tracking of Pathogenic Bacteria in a Mouse Skin Wound Model: Preclinical Feasibility Studies. *J. Biomed. Opt.* **2014,** *19* (8), 085002.

Xia, Y.; Chen, Y.; Tang, Y.; Cheng, G.; Yu, X.; Hongzhang, H.; Cao, G.; Lu, H.; Liu, Z.; Zheng, S.-Y. Smartphone-Based Point-of-Care Microfluidic Platform Fabricated with a ZnO Nanorod Template for Colorimetric Virus Detection, *ACS Sens.* **2019,** *4* (12), 3298–3307.

Yang, K.; Peretz-Soroka, H.; Liu, Y.; Lin, F. Novel Developments in Mobile Sensing based on the Integration of Microfluidic Devices and Smartphones. *Lab. Chip.* **2016,** *16* (6), 943–958.

Yeo, S. J.; Choi, K.; Cuc, B. T.; Hong, N. N.; Bao, D. T.; Ngoc, N. M. Smartphone-based Fluorescent Diagnostic System for Highly Pathogenic H5N1 Viruses. *Theranostics* **2016,** *6* (2), 231–242.

Zhang, K.; Song, L.; Lu, D. In *Design of Remote ECG Monitoring System based on Gprs*, Proceedings of 2011 International Conference on Computer Science and Network Technology, vol. 1. Piscataway: IEEE, 2011; pp 319–22.

Zhu, H.; Mavandadi, S.; Coskun, A. F.; Yaglidere, O.; Ozcan, A. Optofluidic Fluorescent Imaging Cytometry on a Cell Phone. *Anal. Chem.* **2011,** *83* (17), 6641–6647.

Zhu, H.; Sencan, I.; Wong, J.; Dimitrov, S.; Tseng, D.; Nagashima, K.; et al. Cost-Effective and Rapid Blood Analysis on a Cell-Phone. *Lab. Chip.* **2013,** *13* (7), 1282–1288.

Zimic, Z.; Coronel, J.; Gilman, R. H.; Luna, C. G.; Curioso, W. H.; Moore, D. A. Can the Power of Mobile Phones be Used to Improve Tuberculosis Diagnosis in Developing Countries? *Trans. R Soc. Trop. Med. Hyg.* **2009,** *103* (6), 638–640.

CHAPTER 7

Real-Time Health Monitoring Using IoT Sensors

R. K. JARIAL[1], ADARSH DUBEY[2], and ABHINAV DUBEY[3]

[1]*NIT Hamirpur, Himachal Pradesh, India*

[2]*NIT Hamirpur, Himachal Pradesh, India*

[3]*V.B.S.P.U. Jaunpur, Uttar Pradesh, India*

ABSTRACT

Smart healthcare systems are playing a vital role in the medical sector in a big way. The Internet of Things (IoT) is the most powerful technology in the development of ultramodern healthcare systems. IoT in healthcare plays a key role in the real-time health monitoring of patients and facilitates the doctors and hospitals to encompass ultramodern technological tools for evaluating the health condition of their patients through accessing online as well as remote service-providing networks equipped with advanced biomedical instrumentation and sensors.

Smart healthcare monitoring systems with emerging technologies are becoming major concerns of almost every developing nation in the present international arena. With the help of IoT tools and related information technology (IT) interventions in biomedical technology, the exact data required for treatment, and convenient interaction between doctors and patients can be successfully achieved. IoT provides an excellent interactive platform to inconsistent patients for consulting doctors and getting effective responses according to the associated medical care treatment governing issues. In recent years, immense growth potential has been observed wherein

Advanced Research in Electronic Devices for Biomedical and mHealth.
Rajesh K. Kesharwani, Upendra Kumar, Raj K. Keservani (Eds)

advanced application on remote patient monitoring using IoT sensors has proved to be quite convincing and reliable methodology. IoT allows medical devices to collect beneficial data and transfer it to doctors on a real-time mode basis. Almost all modern hospitals, medical care centers, medical research organizations, and laboratories are nowadays trying to adopt these smart IoT technologies for a preferable outcome to circumvent several hurdles that have been standing in this thematic era till the last decade. This chapter describes exhaustive details of several key technical aspects that strive for the purpose of value addition to existing knowledge of all those readers who are interested in specializing in this upcoming field of IoT. Apart from that, several technological breakthroughs, obstructions, and difficulties encountered by applying IoT in health monitoring have also been presented for the benefit of medical practitioners. Another major center of attention that has been taken up in this chapter is its coverage on overview of various IoT medical gadgets that are already in use for certain key areas of health monitoring technologies that if once integrated with IoT systems can open up new application areas for consolidating IoT for not only smart health monitoring systems meant for the comfort of patients located in the remotest part of the world but also they can serve future generations in an ultramodern safer way in quickest possible time.

7.1 INTRODUCTION

Over the past few years, the healthcare industries and manufacturers of medicare instrumentation systems are becoming more and more technologically advanced. Some of these have shown empirically as well as quantitatively more societal sensitive outlooks towards complex health monitoring parameters through careful and comfortable implantation of technologically available modern tools and systems. Try to recall an era in the Indian Context almost 50 years back, when those available healthcare systems were not much advanced. Those healthcare monitoring systems were more time consuming and somewhat more inconvenient for those patients as well. Even, these tools were not enough in numbers to fulfill adequate emergency requirements during a pandemic or similar emergent situations. Therefore, in the modern COVID-19 era, smart care systems equipped with modern infrastructure are the need of the hour to accomplish the demand for a satisfactorily efficient healthcare system in modern times with foolproof inbuilt medicare infrastructure having two- to three-tier level of contingent preparedness (Mukhtar et al., 2021).

Smart medical systems can be created with the judicious application of the Internet of things (IoT), machine learning tools, and artificial intelligence in traditional healthcare systems. IoT plays a crucial role in the medical sector for the purpose of better treatment facilities. These smart models reduce the pressure on hospitals as well as healthcare service providers (Islam et al., 2015). It also reduces the cost of the treatment to provide a better quality of supervision. With the aid of a smart healthcare monitoring system, patients can get fast responses from medical officers/doctors on the medical test reports, and instant expert advice on future medical treatment protocols and hence can get relatively quicker medical healing process at their homes as well as after being hospitalized in modern IoT enabled hospitals (Prithi et al., 2021).

As IoT is an interconnected system having computing devices, apps, sensors, and proper network connectivity for collection and faster transfer of data through these entities, it helps in recording data (patients' physical information) with the help of a variety of sources, such as sensors, mobile phone, email, software, etc.), and transferring them to the healthcare provider through Cloud/Server/Internet Protocol (IP). IoT is becoming a major supportive tool to comply with global communications with the help of innovative protocols and algorithms (Nguyen et al., 2017). The distinctive feature of IoT in smart healthcare modules is to persistently monitor patients by inspecting numerous parameters and conclude good results from the gathered data and constant monitoring. IoT also helps in sharing data and information with specialist doctors, concerned family members, and relatives (Cui et al., 2021). The major application of IoT is in the smart agriculture sector, automobiles, smart homes, smart healthcare, industries, smart parking facilities, etc.

In the context of healthcare applications, wearable sensors or embedded sensors are currently being used to collect physiological data such as temperature, blood pressure (BP), oxygen saturation (SpO_2) level, electrocardiograph (ECG), electroencephalograph (EEG), etc. from the patients' body (Islam et al., 2020). In recent times, the technology that strengthens these attributes is already present, but it is not accessible and affordable by most of the people in developing countries such as India. So, to provide these facilities to each and every citizen of country, Ministry of Health and Family Welfare, Government of India (GOI) is rightly promoting e-health or digital-healthcare ecosystem in the country (Tripathi et al., 2021). The role of government in promoting a smart healthcare system is to make aware that every citizen benefit from these schemes and health systems.

According to the report published in 2013 by Gartner, asserts that over 30 million devices are going to be connected through IoT and it will add up to $2 trillion in global economic values scale in 2020 (Boonsong et al., 2021). Another survey by Allied Market Research Forecast affirms that the IoT healthcare market will extend up to $136.8 billion by 2020 around the globe. According to the e-health market report, it has been prognosticated to expand a compound annual growth rate (CAGR) of 16.5% from 2020 to 2030. This extension is due to swift advancement in the adoption of real-time smart health monitoring systems and an increase in the need for continuous communication in healthcare. Over the past few decades, the growth of IoT-connected devices has increased continuously and it can be predicted that it will continue to increase in the future. Thus, it can be said that IoT plays an important role in the design and development of smart healthcare systems to provide faster healthcare, and better prospects for patient health as well as healthcare professionals not only in India but also at the global level.

7.2 POSITIVE AND NEGATIVE ASPECTS OF IOT

7.2.1 POSITIVE ASPECTS

There are a lot of benefits of IoT in real life. A few of them are listed below:

i. *Easily Approachable*: In the present scenario, essential information from real-time can be accessed very easily; the location of an individual is not a major concern in obtaining information, but the only thing on which it depends are smart devices and network connectivity. For example, to retrieve any useful information we have developed a habit of the natural tendency to either explore it on the internet browser, or we just try to take the help of voice-enabled artificial intelligence or if we need to get an idea about the route for any location, we search it on google map instead of asking an individual.

ii. *Saves time*: As time saving is the key factor for an individual, with the help of the IoT platform an effort made by humans to do any task becomes more efficient and productive, which results in a reduction of time. For example, the Geyser and Toaster will automatically be turned on at the same time when you switch off an alarm in morning.

iii. *Reduces human endeavor*: IoT-connected devices execute a large number of tasks to such an extent that human effort is greatly minimized. This happens as the IoT-connected devices have better communication and interaction with each other.

iv. *Data Monitoring*: It is considered as one of the most important benefits of IoT in real life. With the aid of data monitoring software, beneficial data can be observed and calculated to ensure the quality that fits the occasion. So, by continuously monitoring these data emergency action can be taken on time. For example, indication of low ink in printers, to get information about the quality of air in our homes, smart security systems, SPO_2 level, glucose level in our body, etc.

v. *Saves money by efficient resource utilization*: IoT helps to save money by proper utilization of available resources in our day-to-day lives. For example, by using smart devices like smart lights, smart fans, smart security cameras, smart air conditioning, etc. One can minimize expenditure of money as they are easily accessible and can be controlled by the internet through some programing so they can automatically turn off when not in use.

vi. *Improves quality of life*: Smart IoT technology has changed our living standards as it provides better comfort, high-class facilities, and superior management of resources in our day-to-day life. Thus, it makes our life easier and enhances our comfort level in our way of living.

7.2.2 NEGATIVE ASPECTS

There is significant set of challenges irrespective of its benefits. A few of its challenges are mentioned below.

i. *Insecurity on privacy*:
It is so challenging to store data safely that is reflected by these IoT devices; the issue of cyber security is also a prime concern. Such important aspects should be secured from physical damage

as well as cyberattacks because of their utilization in delicate sections such as medicine and finance. IoT system furnishes essential personal data on various internet platforms, even without the active involvement of the user. Hence, it is necessary to evolve much-advanced security system to prevent the stealing of any important research-related data and misuse of personal data in hands of willful hackers.

ii. *Technical complications:* It looks like IoT devices are executing effortless actions for monitoring data but in actual scenarios, extremely complex technology is being used while developing these IOT devices. During the transferring of data from one system to another, there is a high chance of inaccuracy, and cannot be easily fixed unless one may get it authenticated from reliable experts/sources/consultants and hence it may cause negative outcomes.

iii. *Power dependency and internet connectivity*: At the present time, most of the IoT devices are totally dependent on power and network connectivity to work accurately. Therefore, slight fluctuation in the performance of either of these systems may directly affect the functioning of these devices and this may indirectly result in an error.

iv. *Time consuming and expensive to execute*: These smart systems are expensive as they require extraordinary programing, continuous monitoring, security updates, etc. so for successful implementation and execution of these tasks, there is a need for a skilled team. On the contrary, these systems are time consuming as it depends on internet connectivity.

7.3 APPLICATIONS OF IOT IN REAL LIFE

7.3.1 HOME AUTOMATION

It is also known as smart home or smart house. It uses home automation systems to connect home appliances to an internet to control home appliances such as lighting, and climate entertainment systems and covers home security (access to alarm systems). There are several smart devices that exist in the market now and can be easily installed by the owners themselves for security system and appliances control. Amazon Echo and Google Assistant are such examples of that. Home automation has a high potential for communicating information between family members or friends for our own security leads to energy conservation and good surrounding environmental impact in the future and gives owners a better perspective of their home energy conservation potential after entire end uses.

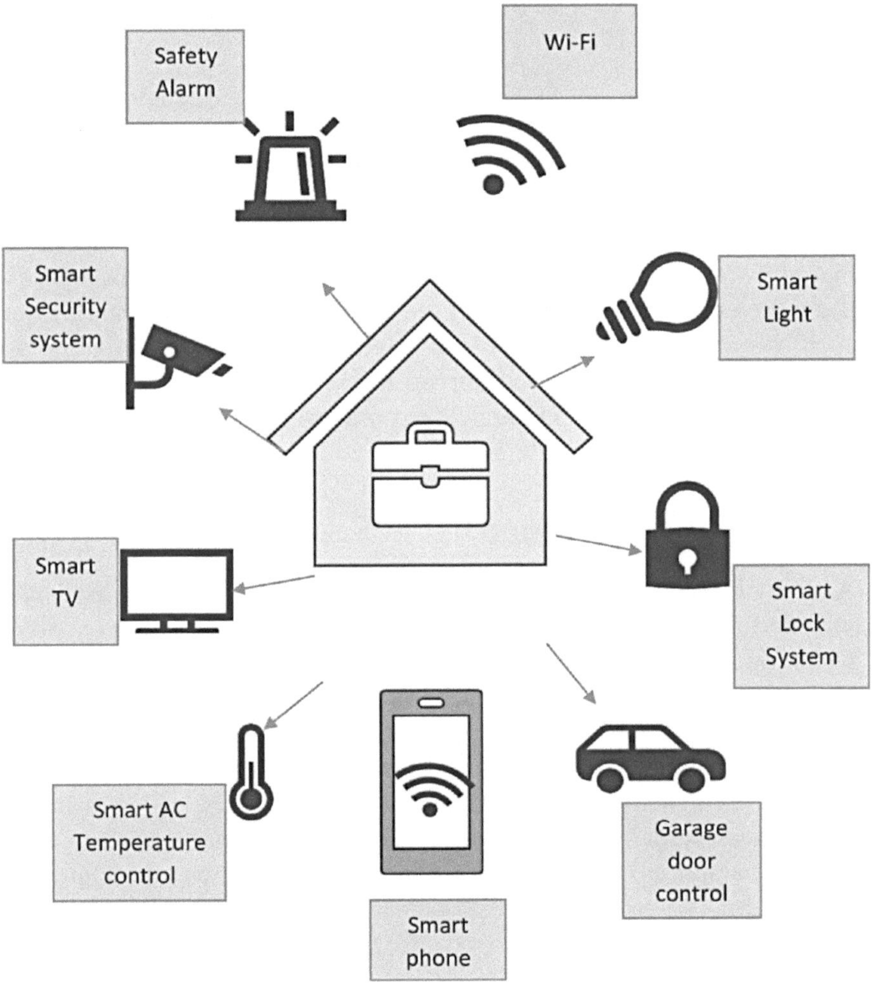

FIGURE 7.1 Structure of smart home.

7.3.2 *SMART HEALTHCARE SYSTEM*

Smart healthcare system can be defined as a medical system that allows medical treatment receivers and healthcare providers to communicate with each other on a common platform and can exchange beneficial information from any location in the globe in real-time with the help of sensors and communication networks. This smart technology helps the physician to analyze patient's data accurately and provide inexpensive and authentic treatment in the smallest possible time span to the great advantage of the patient.

7.3.3 IOT IN AGRICULTURE SECTOR

IoT in the agriculture sector results in smart farming that permits farmers to minimize waste and intensify prolificacy. By using IoT technology farmers can monitor various agriculture parameters such as temperature, humidity, moisture in the soil, climate conditions, state of crops, etc., and these data can be monitored with the aid of several monitoring devices such as agriculture drone, artificial intelligence, sensors, actuators, and network connectivity. It also apprises the required number of pesticides and fertilizers to be used in the field to obtain superior outcomes (Pradhan et al., 2021).

7.3.4 IOT IN SMART CITIES

A smart city is an urban area in which different smart devices are associated with an IoT network to collect and analyze information efficiently, which results in enhanced performance, reduction in cost, optimized resource utilization, etc. These smart technologies, data analyzing tools, and collected data help in achieving energy-efficient and environment-friendly infrastructure and also provide top-quality of government services and improve the living standard of its citizens. A city can be called as smarter if it possesses qualities such as smart governance, smart economy, smart mobility, smart environment, smart living, and smart people (Nguyen et al., 2017).

7.3.5 WEARABLE DEVICES INSTALLED WITH SENSORS AND SOFTWARE

Wearable devices are smart devices that are associated with sensors, microcontrollers, and wireless communication networks. These smart devices are mounted on the consumer's body, clothes, and some other consumer electronic devices (Wan et al.2018). The sensors associated with this smart technology are used to monitor body temperature, heart rate, calorie burn, BP, physical strain, release of certain biochemicals, humidity, SPO_2, motion, etc. Wearable devices perform several tasks such as the following:

i. It collects and monitors information.
ii. Analyze the collected information.
iii. Store information.
vi. Transmit information to the user in real time.

The application of wearable lies in many sectors such as healthcare, agriculture, sports, and navigation systems.

7.3.6 SMART TRAFFIC MONITORING SYSTEM

The majority of today's traffic management systems is not automated and is susceptible to human mistake. This traffic influx is being affected by improper warning system design and the disregard for traffic laws, which is causing overcrowding. Due to overpopulation, growing daily travelers, globalization, and reduced or inadequate highways, traffic monitoring is a major concern in many countries. An automated traffic management system gives you an advantage by ensuring safe public transportation, strong penalties for breaking traffic laws, automated ticketing systems, and innovative traffic-congestion-relieving technologies in major cities around the world. IoT, Artificial Intelligence, computer vision, supervised machine learning, and big data are among the sophisticated tech applications that are delivering real-time answers to traffic management issues. A smart traffic management system includes smart roads, highways, streetlights, enhanced 3D vision cameras, and automated traffic signals.

System objectives for smart traffic management are as follows:

1. Analyze real-time traffic situations to determine which modes of transportation should be prioritized.
2. Ensuring traffic is not congested.
3. Using an automated e-bill payment mechanism to improve traditional ticketing.
4. Speed sensors to alert commuters when they are exceeding the posted speed limit.

5. Install a smart lighting system that saves energy from renewable sources.
6. Ensure that public transportation is safe and reliable.

7.3.7 SMART GRID

The term smart grid refers to a modernized grid that enables a bidirectional flow of electricity, that is, energy can flow either from grid to consumer end or from consumer end to grid. Basically, it is an electrical network that can smartly integrate the performance and behavior of all the consumers that are associated with it.

There are three main layers in each functional domain of an electrical system.

i. Power and energy layer.
ii. Communication and information technology (IT) layer.
iii. Storage layer.

A smart grid has the ability to provide a seamless information interface for the optimum use of electricity to save energy as well as money. It also helps with the selection of the proper time for purchasing electricity. The smart grid offers an opportunity to supply the grid by generating our own electricity either by using Renewable or by distributed generations to save money and conserve energy.

7.3.8 IOT IN INDUSTRIAL AUTOMATION

In automation firms, the IoT has proven to be a major game changer. Companies that use IoT solutions in their industrial automation can gain new benefits. The IoT aids in the development of new technologies that help in solving problems, improving operations and boosting productivity. IoT is defined as the linking of only known electronic things over the internet's data pipeline such as IP, web services, and cloud computing. The IoT has a significant impact on industrial automation, allowing us to use tablets, laptops, smart phones, realistic systems, and cloud data storage, among other things. Engineers and technology suppliers can substantially speed up the creation and delivery of IoT applications by using industrial IoT development kits, which provide a full, high-quality design environment for them. Any development can be swiftly transformed into a production-ready unit with the help of these kits (Dwivedi et al., 2021). The fundamental goal of using the IoT in industrial automation is to be able to replace humans in potentially hazardous working environments and tasks. As of now, the applications have proven to be effective, and the outcomes are optimistic. With the inclusion of IoT for industrial automation, an industrial revolution appears to be on the verge (Darwish et al.,2017).

7.3.9 IOT IN DISASTER MANAGEMENT

IoT devices have the potential to change reactionary disaster management strategies into a forecasting preparedness approach. Sensors, robotics, and autonomous vehicles are examples of IoT technologies that can facilitate improved preparedness and response to natural disasters such as earthquakes, lightning, flash floods, and forest arson or similar disasters. It can also assist in mitigating man-made tragedies such as reactor explosions in power plants or places of stocking weaponry during peace times or similar locations. For predictive analysis, artificial intelligence, and data analytics can be used. These technologies aid in the more accurate prediction of disaster types, severity, and timing of occurrence. As a result, authorities and rescuers/disaster mitigation party will be better equipped to take appropriate action. Forecasting can considerably reduce the losses in terms of both money and saving precious human life.

7.4 STRUCTURE OF HEALTHCARE IOT (HIOT)

The architecture of IoT in medical systems is the combination of numerous technologies such as wireless communication, sensors, data processing, and cloud computing. It can be effectuated by the incorporation of these advanced technologies (Catarinucci et al.,2015). The basic structure of IoT in the healthcare system is furnished in five blocks as follows:

1. Sensor/data collection block.
2. Data transmitting block (via network).
3. Data execution block.
4. Data storing block.
5. Data extracting and learning block.

7.4.1 SENSOR BLOCK

To record the patient's information such as body temperature, pulse rate, BP, ECG, EEG, oxygen saturation (SPO_2) level, the glucose level in the blood, electromyography (EMG), etc. sensors or wearable devices such as motion detection sensor, pressure sensor, temperature sensor, chest strap sensor, smart soles, smart clothing, smart watch, wireless fetal monitoring etc. are used. This is the first layer/block of the structure of IoT in the healthcare system and it acquires components such as ITs, labeling tools [barcode and radio frequency identification (RFID) technology], sensing devices, and gateway devices. The main function of this layer is to sense the patient's physiological parameters to provide better preventive care (Nikolaiev and Timoshenko, 2015).

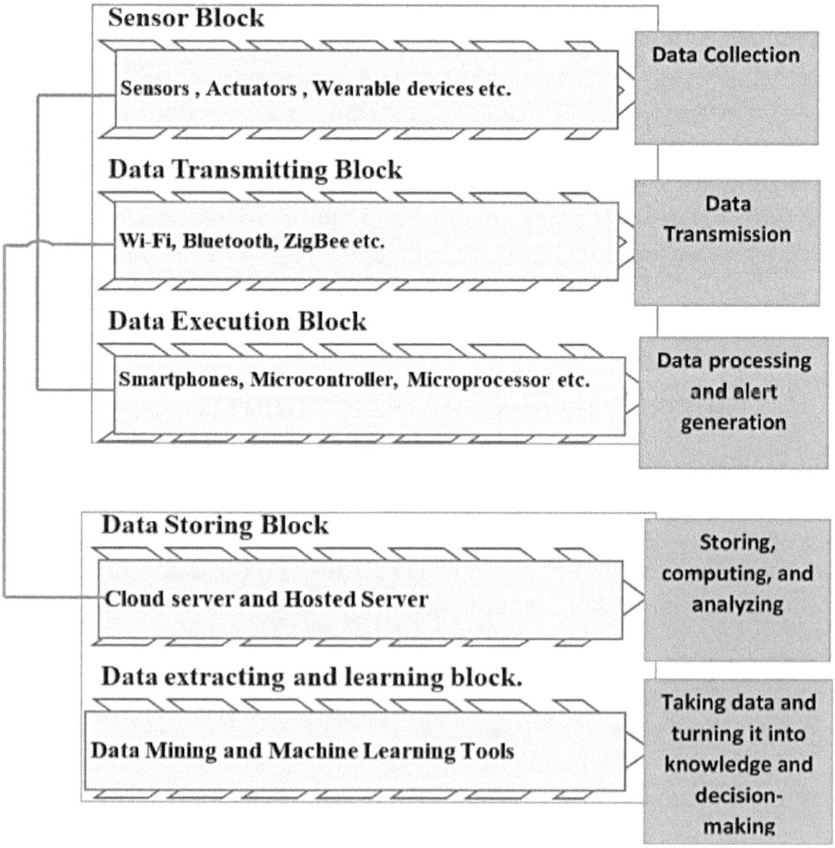

FIGURE 7.2 Structure of HIoT.

7.4.2 DATA TRANSMITTING BLOCK

Data transmission block helps to send patient's beneficial information to executing and storage block with the help of local or global data communication networks such as Bluetooth, Wi–Fi, cellular network, local area network (LAN), wide area network (WAN), etc. to process and store the patient's information in the cloud. Basically, it is the communication between the transmitting layer and the executing layer.

7.4.3 DATA EXECUTING BLOCK

Data executing block is the cerebrum of an IoT system. It involves three main functions as follows:

a. It fetches the patient's data from the transmitting block.
b. Process the fetched data.
c. Transmit it to the storing layer.

In this, the patient's collected information is processed to possess more profound analysis such as making decisions, getting warnings, notifications, etc.

This block consists of the following three main units:

i. Processing unit (smartphones, tablet, microcontroller, microprocessor, etc.)
ii. Hardware platforms (Raspberry Pi, Arduino, etc.)
iii. Operating system or programable unit (Contiki, TinyOS, LiteOS, Android, iOS, etc.)

7.4.4 DATA STORING BLOCK

The large amount of information generated by an IoT system needs sufficient and well-organized storage platform for future analysis. Thus, beneficial data that are transmitted from sensing blocks are stored either in a physical server or in a cloud server.

It performs three main functions as follows:

a) Store information.
b) Access information.

c) Interpret information.

There are many cloud platforms available for storing patient information such as Google Cloud, open IoT, GenI, ThingWorx, etc., and their functions are based on cloud computing technologies. This technology plays an immense role in organizing and conservation of enormous data by shifting it to the cloud. Hence the quality of health data storage systems and their management is being enhanced.

7.4.5 DATA EXTRACTING AND LEARNING BLOCK

This block comprises two tools, that is, data mining and machine learning tools. Data mining tool helps in extracting specific data from a large dataset and discover new trends and potentially useful pattern to predict effective results and decision making. Data mining in healthcare has a significant role as it can help the comprehensive medical insurance company to detect fraud and abuse to provide better healthcare treatment and affordable medical services to patients, customer relationship management, etc. It provides an approach and mechanism to convert large amounts of information which is generated during healthcare transactions into beneficial information, whereas machine learning is a methodology that generates sophisticated algorithms for executing large datasets and providing understandable information to its users. It is the most common subfunction of artificial intelligence.

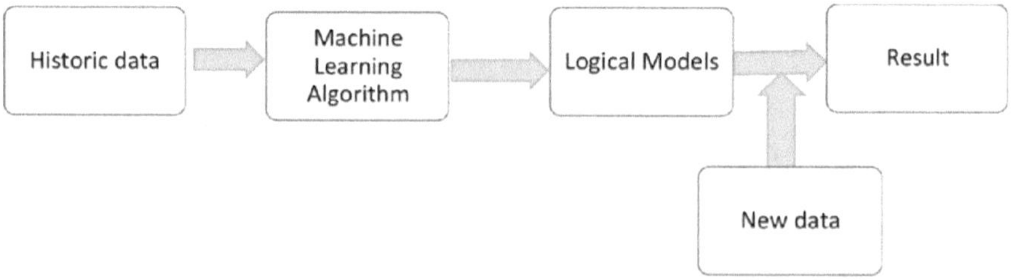

FIGURE 7.3a Functional Block Diagram of machine learning.

It enables computers to automatically learn data and enhance performance from past stored information. Basically, a machine learning tool takes historical data as input and creates the prediction model with the help of a machine learning algorithm, when the system receives new information, estimates new results.

Machine learning has the following three types:

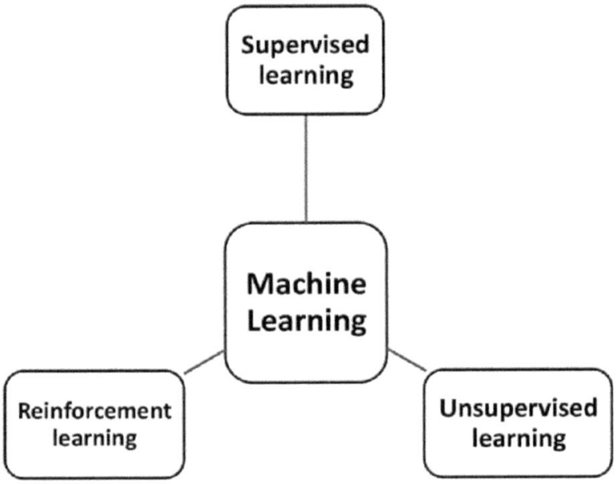

FIGURE 7.3b Types of machine learning.

Supervised learning:

Supervised learning is a sort of machine learning in which machines are taught to predict outcomes using well-labeled training data. The term "labeled data" refers to data that has already been tagged with the appropriate output. The practice of giving input data as well as proper output data to a machine learning model is known as supervised learning.

Unsupervised learning:

The process of teaching a machine to behave on data that has not been defined or labeled is known as unsupervised learning. The machine's goal is to categorize unsorted data based on similarities, patterns, and differences without any prior data training.

Reinforcement learning:

The field of reinforcement learning is included in machine learning. It is all about taking the appropriate procedures to maximize your reward in a given situation. It is used by a variety of software and computers to determine the best feasible action or path in each situation. The solution key is included in the training data in supervised learning, so the model is trained with the correct answer, however in reinforcement learning, there is no answer, and the reinforcement agent selects how to finish the task. In the absence of a training dataset, it will learn from its mistakes.

7.5 IOT TECHNOLOGIES ASSOCIATED WITH HEALTHCARE

The technologies that are adopted to form health IoT systems are very significant, since the utilization of these technologies can amplify the potential of IoT system (Jara et al., 2013). Therefore, to incorporate various medical applications with an IoT system, numerous technologies have been adopted and these can be classified into three broader groups.

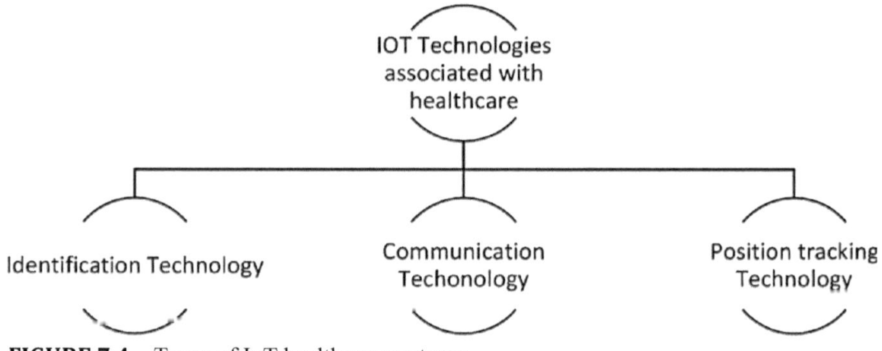

FIGURE 7.4 Types of IoT healthcare systems.

7.5.1 IDENTIFICATION TECHNOLOGY

To access the information of patients at remote locations with the help of sensors-based HIoT system, radio frequency identification (RFID) technology or barcodes are used. The RFID technology is more advanced and better alternative to bar code.

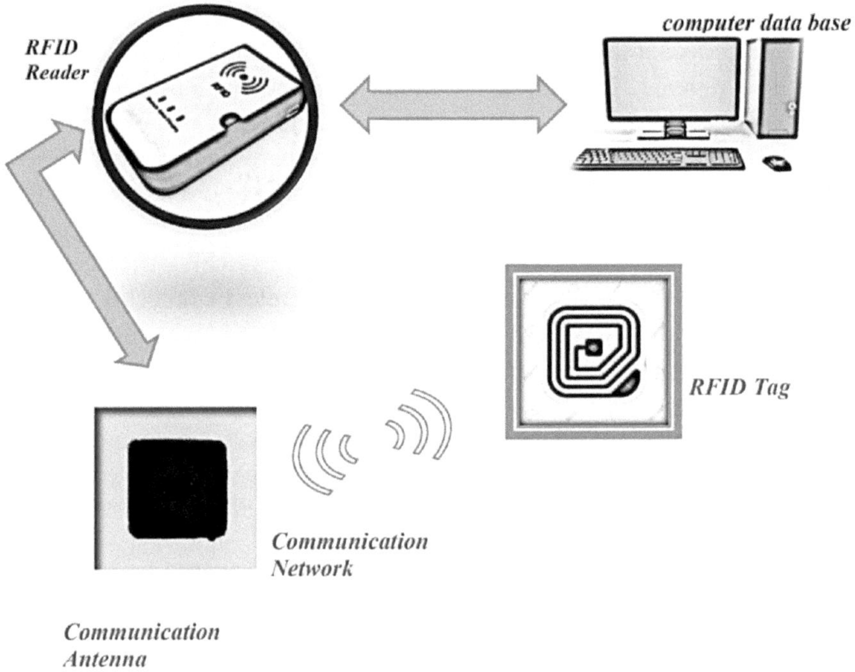

FIGURE 7.5 Working diagram of RFID technology.

RFID reader fetches the information from the RFID tag with the help of a communication network and antenna. It transmits it to a computer database to confirm and permit to access the unique identity of information. Identification leads to the formation of unique identifiers (UIDs) in respect of authorized entities which helps in easily identifying data and apparent exchange of information. A digital UID is generated for every resource associated with the medical system such as hospitals, physicians, caretakers, nurses, medical devices, etc., which helps in the identification of several resources and the relationship between them.

In a practical scenario, a universally unique identifier (UUID) and a globally developed unique identifier (GUID) are developed as two different types of identifiers. These are basically 128-bit numbers that recognize unique information.

7.5.2 COMMUNICATION TECHNOLOGY

This type of technology helps in developing connections between different health IoT systems. Short-range communication and medium-range communication are the classifications of such technology. Short-range communication technology is used to develop connections between objects of limited range such as 10 cm–200 m. whereas medium-range communication technology is used to develop connections between large distant objects. In most of HIoTs, short-range technologies are adopted such as RFID, Bluetooth, Wi–Fi, ZigBee, etc. These technologies provide a wireless connection between two or more medical devices. Bluetooth and ZigBee have the same range of frequency spectrum (2.4 GHz). Bluetooth employs ultrahigh frequency radio waves to communicate. It has a communication range of up to 100 m. The low cost and energy efficiency of Bluetooth are its key advantages. During data transfer, it also assures less interference between connected devices. When it comes to long-range communication in healthcare, this technology falls short. However, ZigBee has a higher communication range compared to Bluetooth. Low power consumption, a rapid transmission rate, and a large network capacity are all advantages of Zigbee (Tao et al.,2018).

Short-range communication (10 cm–200 m) is accomplished via RFID. A tag and a reader make up this system. A microchip and an antenna were used to make the tag. In IoT, it is used to uniquely identify an object or healthcare equipment and by connecting with a tag utilizing radio waves, the reader broadcasts or receives information from the object. Healthcare practitioners can use RFID to rapidly discover and track medical equipment. RFID's key advantage is that it does not require any external power.

A wireless local area network (WLAN) that adheres to the IEEE 802.11 standard is known as wireless fidelity (Wi–Fi). When compared to Bluetooth, it has a wider available bandwidth (around 70 feet). Wi–Fi allows you to set up a network fast and effortlessly. As a result, it is primarily employed in hospitals.

In remote and widely separated geographical places such as rural areas, mountains, peaks, oceans, and so on, satellite communication has proven to be more successful and advantageous than traditional types of communication. The satellite picks up signals from the ground, amplifies them, and then transmits them back to Earth. Around the Earth, there are more than 2000 satellites in orbit to reinforce the process of reliable data transfer for various applications.

7.5.3 POSITION TRACKING TECHNOLOGY

The real-time location system (RTLS) or position tracking technologies are used to monitor and locate an object's position inside a medical organization. It also keeps track of the therapy process by looking at how available resources are distributed. The Global Positioning System—more often known as GPS—is one of the most widely utilized technologies. Satellites are used to track the location of the device. A clean visual range between the object and four separate satellites is required for GPS to recognize an entity, which can be used in healthcare IoT to track the location of an ambulance, a medical professional, caretakers, and patients, and plenty of other things (Lee and Chung, 2009).

The use of GPS is, however, restricted to exterior applications due to the potential for nearby infrastructure to impede communications. A local positioning system (LPS) networking can be useful in these situations. LPS can trace an entity by detecting the radio signal sent by the moving object and sending it to a network of pre-positioned receivers. LPS can also be utilized with a variety of short-range communication technologies such as RFID, Wi–Fi, Zigbee, and so on. Ultrawideband (UWB) radio, on the contrary, is favored because of its superior magnification. This allows the recipient to calculate the time of arrival with precision. GPS, as well as several other high-bandwidth communication technologies, could be used to construct smart health monitoring systems in the future.

7.6 SMART HEALTHCARE MONITORING DEVICES AND THEIR APPLICATIONS

IoT devices open an era of new possibilities for healthcare providers to keep track of their patients, as well as for sufferers to keep track of themselves. As a result, the various wearable IoT devices offer a variety of benefits and challenges for both healthcare practitioners and patients. Wearable sensors, portable gadgets, and medical equipment have become more inexpensive and user-friendly as IoT technology has progressed (Yama et al., 2007). These systems can be used to gather patient data, treat illness, track patients' condition, and send out notifications in the event of a medical emergency. Several HIoTs-based applications are discussed in this section.

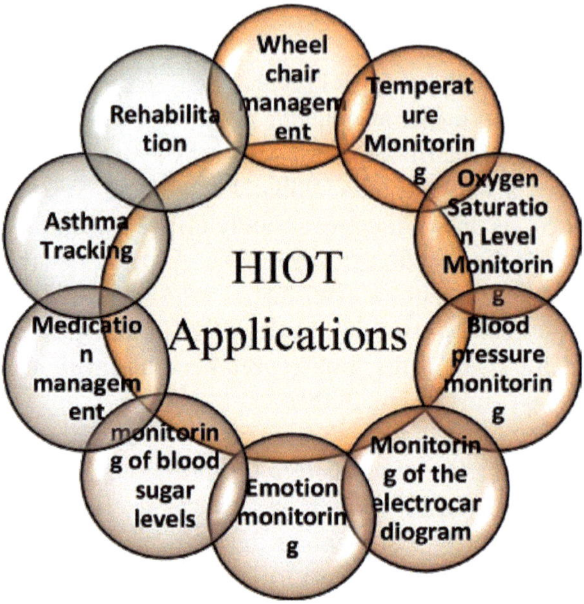

FIGURE 7.6 HIoT-based applications.

7.6.1 HUMAN BODY TEMPERATURE MONITORING

The maintenance of homeostasis is indicated by human body temperature, which is used in various treatment protocols. Under certain conditions, such as trauma, sepsis, and several others, a shift in body temperature can also be a warning indicator. When the body recognizes a bacterial illness, it involuntarily raises its temperature and boosts blood flow to speed up the body's defense actions to fight the infection. To combat an infection, the body can elevate its temperature by 3–5°F, and we don't want to let persistent high temperatures go untreated because they can be harmful to the body. In many disorders, monitoring temperature variations over time aids physicians in making conclusions about the patient's health condition (Banka et al., 2018).

A temperature thermometer affixed to the mouth, ear, armpit, or rectum is the traditional method of measuring temperature. These treatments, however, are constantly hampered by the patient's lack of comfort and the significant risk of infection. However, with the recent advancement of IoT-based technology, numerous solutions to this problem have been presented. An infrared sensor was used to track the core body temperature from the eardrum in a 3D-printed wearable device that could be placed mostly on the ear. A wireless sensing element and a data acquisition unit were installed into the device. The temperature reading is unaffected by the environment or other physical activity in this experiment. Nowadays, using Arduino and Raspberry Pi, a sensor-based temperature monitoring system is created. The temperature data was saved in a database and displayed on a web page that could be accessed from a computer or a mobile phone (Mansor et al., 2013).

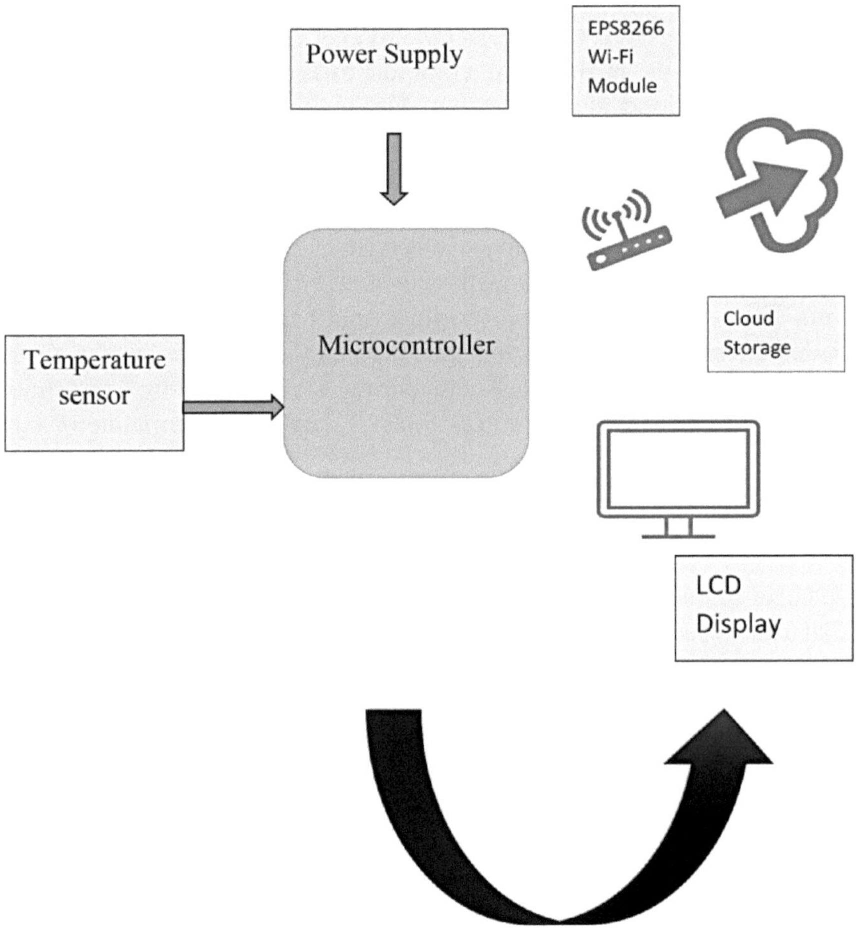

FIGURE 7.7 Block diagram of IoT-based temperature monitoring.

7.6.2 MONITORING OF BLOOD SUGAR LEVELS

Diabetes is a metabolic disorder in which the body's natural blood sugar levels remain elevated for an extended length of time. It is one of humanity's most common illnesses. In the case of diabetes, the function of the pancreas is disturbed, and the B-cell of islet of Langerhans's does not secrete the proper amount of insulin. Mellitus diabetes, insipidus diabetes, and gestational diabetes are the three major kinds of diabetes that are widely observed. Three types of tests can be used to diagnose diabetes: a random plasma glucose test, a fasting plasma glucose test, and an oral glucose tolerance test (Scrugli et al., 2019).

Fingerpicking is the most common method for detecting diabetes, followed by blood glucose testing. Various wearable gadgets for blood glucose monitoring that are painless, pleasant, fast, and ethical have been designed using current advancements in IoT technologies. A noninvasive glucometer based on the IoT has been designed for real-time monitoring of blood glucose levels. A noninvasive persistent glucose monitoring operates by placing a small sensor beneath your skin, typically on your abdomen or arm. The sensor detects glucose in the fluid between your cells, which is called interstitial glucose. Every few moments, the sensor checks glucose levels, and the data is wirelessly transmitted to a display by a transmitter. Some blood sugar level monitors transfer data to a smartphone or tablet directly (Satija et al., 2015).

7.6.3 OXYGEN SATURATION LEVEL MONITORING

A pulse oximeter is a noninvasive method for determining SPO_2 level that can be employed as an important attribute in healthcare analysis. The noninvasive technology avoids the drawbacks of traditional methods and allows for real-time monitoring. Pulse oximetry technology has been enhanced because of the integration of IoT-based technology, and this has demonstrated potential in the healthcare industry. The incorporation of IoT-based technologies has improved pulse oximetry, which has shown significant potential throughout the healthcare sector. Further research led to the development of a noninvasive tissue oximeter that could monitor blood SpO_2 levels, as well as heart rate and pulse parameters, and communicate this data to a server through Bluetooth, Zigbee, or Wi–Fi and based on the fact collected immediate treatment action has been taken (Muthu and Anand, 2020).

7.6.4 ELECTROCARDIOGRAM (ECG) MONITORING

The electrical activity of the heart is represented by an ECG, which depicts the depolarization and repolarization of the atria and ventricles. An ECG is a type of ECG that shows the basic patterns of the heart muscles and can be used to detect various cardiac problems. The traditional monitoring system in clinical practice is the Holter-based ECG monitoring. A Holter monitor is a 12-lead medical gadget that records heart rhythms continuously for 24 or 48 h after being linked to the patient's body through electrodes. Holter is kept in a pocket or a bag around the patient's neck or waist and when the information is successfully recorded the monitor is handed to the physician for proper analysis of recorded information (Serhani et al., 2020).

ECG monitoring has found great potential in the use of IoT technology in the early diagnosis of heart disease. This technology has several different types of equipment for ECG monitoring systems such as mobile devices, wearable devices, and sensor devices, with the smartphone being the most important. Many studies have been proposed on IoT-based ECG monitoring systems that aim to focus on how IoT devices can capture ECG signals and communicate them to a physician in real time through the Internet. In some studies, a wireless data collecting system and receiving processor has been proposed for IoT-based ECG monitoring system that uses real-time search automation method to detect heart abnormalities (Satija et al., 2015. A compact, low-power ECG monitoring system that may be worn on a T-shirt was proposed in another study which collects high-quality ECG data using a biopotential chip and the recorded information was then sent to the end users on a cloud server through Bluetooth or Wi–Fi. A smartphone app is being used to analyze these captured ECG data and can be operated with 5.2 mW of power.

7.6.5 BLOOD PRESSURE MONITORING

The monitoring of BP is one of the most important stages in any medical treatment process. The traditional (sphygmomanometer) method of measuring BP needs at least one skilled person to record the correct BP data. However, the continuous enhancement of IoT and other sensing technologies in healthcare has changed the traditional way of measurement of BP. In some studies, a wearable cuffless device that can detect both systolic and diastolic pressure and save data on a cloud platform has been proposed and its performance was tested on 60 persons to confirm its accuracy. Cloud computing and fog computing have been integrated into an IoT-based BP measurement system for long-term real-time monitoring and storage for future reference (Yang, 2018).

Regular BP checks may be done anywhere, at any time, thanks to the integration of digital BP measurement devices with the IoT. Of course, the results of BP measurements can be directly analyzed by a doctor via a platform such as a web application or a mobile application. BP measuring device with IoT includes cuffs and pumps, sensors and microcontrollers, a network interface, a digital display, and a firebase.

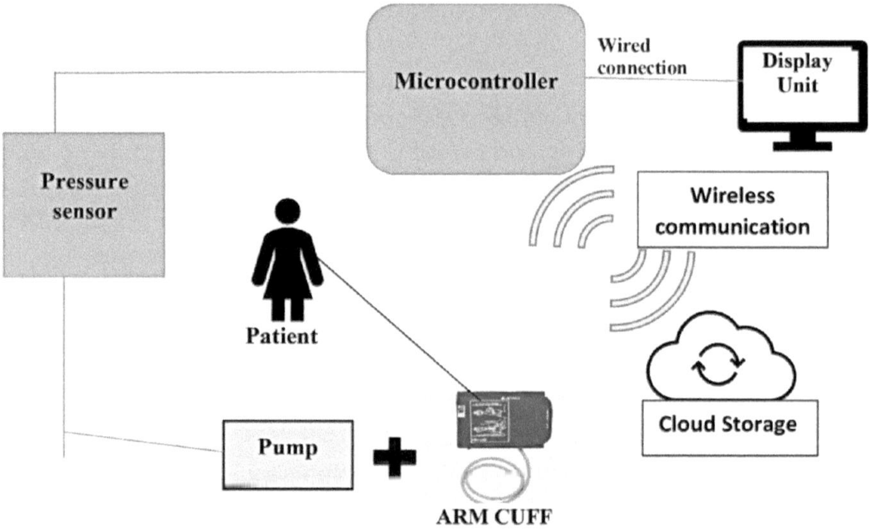

FIGURE 7.8 Block diagram representation of IoT-based BP monitoring system.

After reading the first and last beats, the sensor will calculate the BP. The outcomes of the process will be displayed on the light-emitting diode (LED) display and subsequently communicated to the firebase, where they will be seen in the web application.

7.6.6 ASTHMA TRACKING

Asthma is a long-term disorder that affects the airways and can make breathing difficult. Asthma causes the airways to constrict due to the enlargement of airways. Wheezing, coughing, chest pain, and shortness of breath are all symptoms of this condition. An asthma attack can strike at any time, and at that point, an inhaler or nebulizer is the only thing that can rescue you. Therefore, real-time monitoring of this condition may be required. In recent years, a slew of IoT-based asthma monitoring systems has been presented such as the use of a smart sensor to record respiratory rate was proposed as part of a smart healthcare IoT solution for asthma patients, and such health information was saved on a cloud server that physicians may access for the purpose diagnosis and treatment. In some studies, a researcher presented a respiratory monitoring and warning system that records breathing rates using an LM35 temperature sensor (Gusev et al., 2017).

This can be accomplished by measuring the temperature of air being inhaled and exhaled and the recorded data on breathing was sent to the health center and displayed on the web server. This scheme also generates an alarm and at the same instant warning message is delivered automatically to the patients when a threshold value is achieved. In another study, a proposed system not only monitors and informs patients about their asthma symptoms, but it also advises them on the proper dosage of medicine to take.

7.6.7 EMOTION MONITORING

Emotion tracking is used to ensure a healthy mental state by providing crucial information about a person's emotional condition. It also aids healthcare practitioners in the treatment of mental illnesses such as depression, anxiety, and bipolar disorder. The ability to self-monitor one's emotional state improves one's comprehension of their psychological condition (Migliorini et al.,2015). In some studies, the CNN network is used to assess and categorize a person's mood into six categories.

a. Happy
b. Excited
c. Calm
d. Distressed
e. Angry
f. Sad

Nowadays, IoT integrates cutting-edge technologies into applications and gadgets to measure and display users' everyday mental states and, as a result, influence their behavior patterns. IoT technology allows data on heart rate, BP, and temperature to be collected to determine an individual's emotional state. These emotion-based sensors have a wide range of applications and are quite inexpensive to employ (Prkachin, 2009). Emotions can be sensed remotely using a gadget that generates wireless signals to assist in the measurement of heartbeat and breathing. Without on-body sensors or facial recognition software, the new device, called "EQ-Radio," can tell whether a person is excited, pleased, furious, or depressed with an accuracy of 87%.

7.6.8 MEDICATION MANAGEMENT

In the healthcare industry, medical adherence is a prevalent problem. Patients' bad health problems may be exacerbated if they do not take their medications on time. Therefore, a technique known as brown bag is used for medication management. It is the way to engage with patient's and healthcare professionals to generate accurate and full medication list. These techniques will assist in identifying patient behaviors that may put them at risk for an adverse drug event, such as overdose, underdosing, or missing pills, as well as other crucial contextual elements that may be impeding adherence. In the past, a lot of research has emphasized using IoT to track a patient's prescription compliance (Fei et al., 2017). A smart medical box has been created that can remind patients when it's time to take their medications. The box has three trays, each of which contains medicine for three distinct occasions (morning, afternoon, and evening). Some critical health metrics are also measured by this technology such as blood glucose levels, SpO_2 level, ECG, etc., and the recorded information subsequently transferred to the cloud server to build communication between two end users through a smartphone application.

7.6.9 WHEELCHAIR MANAGEMENT

For people with limited mobility, a wheelchair is an unavoidable aspect of their daily lives. It gives them with both physical and psychological assistance. As a result, new research is concentrating on how to integrate the navigation and tracking system with these wheelchairs. IoT-based technologies are increasingly demonstrating the ability to help in achieving this goal. A potential IoT-based steering system has been developed, which is integrated with a real-time obstacle avoidance system. Using image processing techniques on real-time videos, the steering system can detect obstructions. Wheelchair management has become more engaging and convenient for patients, thanks to the usage of mobile computers. The combination of numerous sensors, mobile technology, and cloud computing resulted in the development of a smart wheelchair. A smartphone app is included in the system to assist patients in interacting with wheelchair and care providers. This also helps care providers to keep an eye on wheelchair from any location (Pham et al., 2018).

7.6.10 REHABILITATION SYSTEM

Physical treatment, in combination with rehabilitation, is beneficial in recovering a patient's functional abilities. The process of rehabilitation entails recognizing the problem and assisting patients in resuming their normal lives. The IoT has a wide range of applications in rehabilitation, including cancer treatment, sports-related injuries treatment, stroke treatment, and other physical disabilities. The use of a multimodal sensor to monitor the patient's walking pattern and evaluate movement parameters has been proposed for a smart walker rehabilitation system. The smart walker used by patients, records several action parameters such as orientation angle, elevation, force, and so on. Doctors have adequately accessed these data and generated diagnostic reports using a smartphone app. Furthermore, by combining a smart wearable wristband, a robotic hand, and a machine learning algorithm, a stroke recovery system was constructed (Chamadiya et al.,2013).

7.7 LIMITATION AND FUTURE CHALLENGES OF IOT IN HEALTH MONITORING

- The primary challenges that require extra consideration when implementing wearables as a separate unit of healthcare are privacy and security. These difficulties can be mitigated to some extent by continuously tracking the activity of wearable devices.

- Information storage can be easily stolen or hacked because of its size and capability.
- In wearable IoT devices, personal calibration is also a prevalent technological difficulty.
- Big data's job is to provide a powerful footprint for storing vast amounts of data, however, outliers can occasionally lead to disastrous consequences for a single user.
- In IoT-based systems, interoperability is a major challenge that requires attention to provide viable solutions.
- Sensor devices that are small and inexpensive are required to collect data in the healthcare platform.
- Sensor devices need small antennas to prevent interference, save energy, and improve transmission dependability.
- In the healthcare industry, low-cost sensor devices with no side effects are essential.

7.8 CONCLUSIONS

In the current chapter, a brief description of the proliferation aspects of the IoT healthcare system has been examined, including a detailed examination of the structure of the HIoT system, its components, and the interaction between these components. This chapter includes details on the current scenario of healthcare services that have investigated IoT-based technologies. The IoT has provided researchers with an almost limitless number of predictions about how the healthcare industry will change due to better use of medical devices, better quality of care, and lower medical costs. IoT-enabled devices are expected to grow in popularity, according to a healthcare market forecast. Sensors were not brought in to replace medical doctors rather, they were brought in to help them do their jobs more efficiently. Energy efficient robust and cost-effective IoT-enabled gadgets and sensors are being designed and developed nowadays by leading global medicare companies to provide a preventive and proactive health monitoring system, rather than a reactive treatment in which the patient is diagnosed only when they are sick. Despite the fact that in recent times this industry has experienced a higher boom, it needs to be investigated carefully to overcome current limitations and challenges of the modern era to transform traditional health monitoring systems into more fruitful effective IoT-based healthcare systems for human endeavor.

KEYWORDS

- **Internet of Things (IoT)**
- **Electrocardiograph (ECG)**
- **Electroencephalograph (EEG)**
- **Artificial Intelligence**
- **Computer Vision**
- **Supervised Machine Learning**
- **Healthcare Internet of Things**
- **Radio Frequency Identification (RFID)**
- **Universally Unique Identifier (UUID)**
- **Real-time Location System (RTLS)**

REFERENCES

Banka et al. Smart Healthcare Monitoring using IoT. (2018).

Boonsong et al. Contactless Body Temperature Monitoring of in-Patient Department (IPD) Using 2.4 GHz Microwave Frequency via the Internet of Things (IoT) Network. *Wireless Pers Commun.* **2021**.

Catarinucci, L. An IoT-Aware Architecture for Smart Healthcare Systems. *IEEE Internet Things J* **2015,** *2* (6), 515–526,

Chamadiya, B.; Mankodiya, K.; Wagner, M.; Hofmann, U. G. Textile-Based, Contactless ECG Monitoring for Non-ICU Clinical Settings. *J. Ambient Intell. Humaniz. Comput.* **2013.**

Cui, M.; Baek, M.; Soo, S.; Crespo.; González, R.; Premalatha, R. Internet of Things-Based Cloud Computing Platform for Analyzing the Physical Health Condition. **2021,** 1233–1247.

Darwish, A.; Hassanien, A. E.; Elhoseny, M.; Sangaiah, A.; Muhammad K. The Impact of the Hybrid Platform of Internet of Things and Cloud Computing on Healthcare Systems: Opportunities, Challenges, and Open Problems. *J. Ambient Intell. Human. Comput.* **2017,** *10* (10), 4151–4166.

Dwivedi, R.; Mehrotra, D.; Chandra, S. Potential of Internet of Medical Things (IoMT) Applications in Building a Smart Healthcare System: A Systematic Review., *J. Oral Biol. Craniofacial Res.* **2021**.

Fei; Jiang, Y.; Zhi, H.; Dong, Y.; Li, H.; Ma, S.; Wang, Y.; Dong, Q.; Shen, H.; Wang, Y. Artificial Intelligence in Healthcare: Past, Present and Future. *Stroke Vasc. Neurol.* **2017,** *2* (4), 230–243.

Gusev, M.; Stojmenski, A.; Guseva, A. ECGalert: A Heart Attack Alerting System. In *Proceedings of the 9th International Conference, Skopje, Macedonia*, 18–23 September 2017.

Impact of Internet of Things on Industrial Automation. https://www.plantautomation-technology.com/articles/impact-of-internet-of-things-on-industrial-automation

Impact of IoT on Industrial Automation. https://www.hiotron.com/iot-and-industrial-automation/(**2013**)

IoT-Based Smart Tracking of Body Temperature for Healthcare, MosChip. https://moschip.com/blog/iot/IoT-based-smart-tracking-of-body-temperature (accessed 23 Jan 2018).

Islam, M.; Rahaman, A.; Islam, R. Development of Smart Healthcare Monitoring System in IoT Environment. *SN Comput. Sci.* **2020,** *1* (185), 1–11.

Islam, S. M. R.; Kwak, D.; Kabir, M. H.; Hossain, M.; Kwak K. The Internet of Things for Health Care: A Comprehensive Survey**.** *IEEE Access* **2015,** *3*, 678–708.

Jara, A. J.; Zamora-Izquierdo, M. A.; Skarmeta, A. F. Interconnection Framework for mHealth and Remote Monitoring Based on the Internet of Things. *IEEE J. Sel. Areas Commun.* **2013,** *31*, 47–65.

Lee, Y. D.; Chung, W. Y. Wireless Sensor Network Based Wearable Smart Shirt for Ubiquitous Health and Activity Monitoring. *Sens. Actuators B Chem.* **2009,** *140*, 390–395.

Mansor, H.; Shulkor, A.; Meskam, S.; Rusli, M.; et al. Body Temperature Measurement for Remote Health Monitoring System. In *The IEEE International Conference on Smart Instrumentation, Measurement, and Applications*, 26–27 Nov 2013, Kuala Lumpur, Malaysia, 2013; pp 1–5.

Migliorini, M.; Mariani, S.; Bertschy, G.; Kosel, M.; Bianchi, A. M. Can Home-Monitoring of Sleep Predict Depressive Episodes in Bipolar Patients? In *Proceedings of the 2015 37th Annual International Conference of the IEEE Engineering in Medicine and Biology Society (EMBS), Milano, Italy*, 25–29 August 2015; pp 2215–2218.

Mood-Detecting Sensor Could Help Machines Respond to Emotions. IEEE spectrum. https://spectrum.ieee.org/mooddetecting-sensor-could-help-machines-respond-to-emotions (accessed 20 Sept 2016).

Mukhtar; Hamid; Rubaiee, S.; Krichen, M.; Alroobaea, R. An IoT Framework for Screening of COVID-19 Using Real-Time Data from Wearable Sensors. *Int. J. Environ. Res. Public Health* **2021,** *18* (8), 4022.

Muthu; Anand, B. IoT Based Wearable Sensor for Diseases Prediction and Symptom Analysis in Healthcare Sector. *Peer-to-Peer Networking and Applications* **2020,** *13* (6), 2123–2134.

Nguyen, H. H.; Mirza, F.; Naeem.; M. A.; Nguyen, M. A Review on IoT Healthcare Monitoring Applications and a Vision for Transforming Sensor Data into Real-Time Clinical Feedback. In *2017 IEEE 21st International Conference on Computer Supported Cooperative Work in Design (CSCWD)*; IEEE, April 2017; pp 257–262.

Nikolaiev, S.; Timoshenko, Y. Reinvention of the Cardiovascular Diseases Prevention and Prediction Due to Ubiquitous Convergence of Mobile Apps and Machine Learning. In *Proceedings of the 2015 Information Technologies in Innovation Business Conference (ITIB)*, Kharkiv, Ukraine, 7–9 October 2015; pp 23–26.

Pham, M., Mengistu, Y., Do, H.; Sheng, W. Delivering Home Healthcare Through a Cloud-Based Smart Home Environment (CoSHE). *Fut. Gen. Comput. Syst.* **2018,** *81*, 129–140.

Pradhan, B.; Bhattacharyya, S.; Pal K. IoT-Based Applications in Healthcare Devices. *J. Healthcare Eng.* **2021,** *21*, 2040–2309.

Prithi, S.; Poongodi, T.; Sumathi, D.; Suresh, P. Chapter 23—Real-Time Remote Health Monitoring Using IoT Sensors. In *Electronic Devices, Circuits, and Systems for Biomedical Applications*; Academic Press, **2021**; pp 481–501.

Prkachin, K, M. Assessing Pain by Facial Expression: Facial Expression as Nexus. *Pain Res. Manag.* **2009,** *14* (1), 53–58.

Satija, U.; Ramkumar, B.; Manikandan, M. S. A Simple Method for Detection and Classification of ECG Noises for Wearable ECG Monitoring Devices. In *Proceedings of the 2nd International Conference on Signal Processing and Integrated Networks SPIN, Noida, India*, 19–20 Feb 2015.

Scrugli, M. A.; Loi, D.; Raffo, L.; Meloni, P. A Runtime-Adaptive Cognitive IoT Node for Healthcare Monitoring. In *Proceedings of the ACM International Conference on Computing Frontiers* **2019,** CF 2019–Proceedings, Alghero, Italy, 30 April–2 May 2019.

Serhani; Adel, M.; El Kassabi, H. T.; Ismail, H.; Navaz, A. N. ECG Monitoring Systems: Review, Architecture, Processes, and Key Challenges. *Sensors* **2020,** *20* (6), 1796.

Tao, X.; Huang, T.; Shen, C.; Ko, Y.; Jou, G.; Koncar, V. Bluetooth Low Energy-Based Washable Wearable Activity Motion and Electrocardiogram Textronic Monitoring and Communicating System. *Adv. Mater. Technol.* **2018,** *3*, 1700309.

Tinnakornsrisuphap, T.; Billo, R. E. An Interoperable System for Automated Diagnosis of Cardiac Abnormalities from Electrocardiogram Data. *IEEE J. Biomed. Health Inform.* **2014,** *19*, 493–500.

Tripathi, S.; Prakash, K.; Balas, V.; Mohapatra, S.; Nayak, J. *Electronic Devices, Circuits, and Systems for Biomedical Applications*; Academic Press , 2021.

Wan, J.; Al-awlaqi, A. A. H.; Li, M. Wearable IoT Enabled Real-Time Health Monitoring System. *J. Wireless Commun. Netw.* **2018**. https://doi.org/10.1186/s13638-018-1308-x

Wikipedia Contributors. Remote Patient Monitoring. *Wikipedia, The Free Encyclopedia.* https://en.wikipedia.org/w/index.php?title=Remote_patient_monitoring&oldid=1058551441 (accessed 23 Jan 2022).

Wikipedia Contributors. Unsupervised Learning. *Wikipedia, the Free Encyclopedia.* https://en.wikipedia.org/w/index.php?title=Unsupervised_learning&oldid=1065886298 (accessed 23 Jan 2022).

Wikipedia Contributors. Wearable Technology. *Wikipedia, the Free Encyclopedia.* https://en.wikipedia.org/w/index.php?title=Wearable_technology&oldid=1067088614 (accessed 23 Jan 2022).

Yama, Y.; Ueno, A.; Uchikawa, Y. Development of a Wireless Capacitive Sensor for Ambulatory ECG Monitoring Over Clothes. In *Proceedings of the Annual International Conference of the IEEE Engineering in Medicine and Biology, Lyon, France*, 23–26 August 2007; pp 5727–5730.

Yang, G. IoT-Based Remote Pain Monitoring System: From Device to Cloud Platform," *IEEE J. Biomed. Health Inf.* **2018,** *22* (6), 1711–1719. doi: 10.1109/JBHI.2017.2776351

CHAPTER 8

IC Design: An Approach of Study in Bio-Medical and mHealth Care Applications

ROHIT SRIVASTAVA[1], ASHUTOSH SINGH[1], UPENDRA KUMAR[2], DIWAKER YAGYASEN[1], and HIMANSHU KUMAR SHUKLA[1]

[1]*Department of CSE, BBDITM, Lucknow, Uttar Pradesh, India*

[2]*Department of CSE, IET Lucknow, Uttar Pradesh, India*

ABSTRACT

In today's era of mobility and portability, IC's are playing a vital role in the development of modern electronic devices. In this chapter, the author is going to elaborate and trying to describe the designing of ICs in the area of Biomedical and mHealth applications. As it is well known to all of us that a very huge quantity of portable and wireless medical appliances are being consumed in hospitals and health care centers for the diagnosis and treatment of patients. In order to design such appliances, the role of ICs is very important from low energy consumption and cost-effective point of view.

In this modern era of electronics engineering under discipline of biomedical applications, enormous devices are designed which are entrenched inside the human body in order to remove the introduction of medical instruments and apparatus for easy survival and treatment of patient. It is also very helpful in order to reduce the use of high dose drugs which are having high side effects by replacing the orthodox treatment policy with electro-therapeutic process. This mode of treatment is very helpful to maintain future options of treatment along with safety of lives of patients.

Advanced Research in Electronic Devices for Biomedical and mHealth.
Rajesh K. Kesharwani, Upendra Kumar, Raj K. Keservani (Eds)

Since it is very difficult to perform because of low frequency signals of human body are also associated with a lot of noise and attenuation. In such circumstances, there is a huge trade-off between energy and attenuation. There is also a challenging task to make the devices practically portable for practically and easily adaptations.

In this chapter, the author is trying to describe some modern techniques which are adapted in order to design in the area of biomedical and mHealth applications which are currently being used for designing of ICs with low strength, low frequency, and noisy human body signals. This chapter also includes a multiparameter, human body signal monitoring, and processing technique.

8.1 INTRODUCTION

It has been observed that integrated circuits are very important for construction of widely adapted electronics appliances because of their rapid growth in application of biomedicals and mHealth. In the age of 1948, ICs were introduced as a semiconductor device with the integration of limited transistors. But after a decade ahead, the capacity of ICs was increasing with a revolutionary change in integrated circuits by introducing some complementary transistors in order to make it capable for signal processing device. From the age of 1959, the regular improvement and research in the field of modern electronics engineering have opened a new scope of engineering after almost 25 years, known as integrated microsystem (Li et al., 2013).

This phase of research has introduced microelectromechanical system (MEMS) which provided the capability of constructing the devices with very small size, least weight, and low power consumption.

IMC have provided better and effective solutions for the complex problems in the field of biomedical which cannot be solved previously. Currently, the use of CMOS (complementary metal oxide semiconductor) in biomedical and mHealth application is very significant for implantation in the body. These are designed in such a way to provide a satisfactory, reliable, and capability of error checking requirements by associating with lifesaving implantable medical equipment (Chiu et al., 2013).

8.1.1 CLASSIFICATION AND DESIGNING STEPS OF IC

It is well known to all of us that integrated circuits are the instances of digital circuits which works on specific value of voltage and operates on two distinct values zero and one. These values are sometimes considered as true and false as well as high and low. Before the use of digital circuits there was a very vast use of analog circuits which was used in various areas like signal processing as well as in sensor-based devices, etc.

In the case of classification of integrated circuits, it is clear that the ICs are formed with the help of logic gates and their classification can be done on the basis of number of counts of logic gates per chip.

On the basis of capacity of logic gates following types of ICs are designed:

Small-Scale ICs which contains almost minimum of three and maximum up to 30 logic gates and it is generally called as SSI.

The second variant of IC has more capacity and is called as Medium-Scale ICs (MSI) and which contains minimum of 30 and maximum of 300 logic gates per chip.

The third generation of IC is known as Large-Scale ICs (LSI) and it contains which contains minimum of 300 and maximum of 3000 logic gates per chip.

The latest and most popular technology associated with 3000 and more logic gates per chip is called as Very Large-Scale ICs (VLSI), and it is the most adapted technology for complex operations.

8.1.2 STEPS INVOLVED IN DESIGNING OF IC FOR BIO-MEDICAL APPLICATIONS

The most required parameter for designing the ICs for biomedical and mHealth applications are low size, low weight, and long life. Since the use of IC has made the implantation of medical devices very feasible for human bodies. The process of implantation was very typical for the patient aspect because of its heavy size and short battery life. We can easily understand this term by having an example of pacemaker which was used in case of heart failure. The basic drawback of this implantation was limited duration of battery for its working. This was a very tough process because the pacemaker was implanted inside the human body and its battery was associated outside of the body because of its heavy size and weight and short battery life.

But nowadays, it has become very feasible for patients to get implanted because of its small size and better functioning and long life.

With the help of this example it is clear that the use of ICs in Biomedical and mHealth applications have given a new revolution to the medical science for treatment and diagnosis of patients with lots of advantages (Cha et al., 2014).

8.1.2.1 SOME BASIC STEPS FOR DESIGNING OF IC ARE LISTED AS BELOW

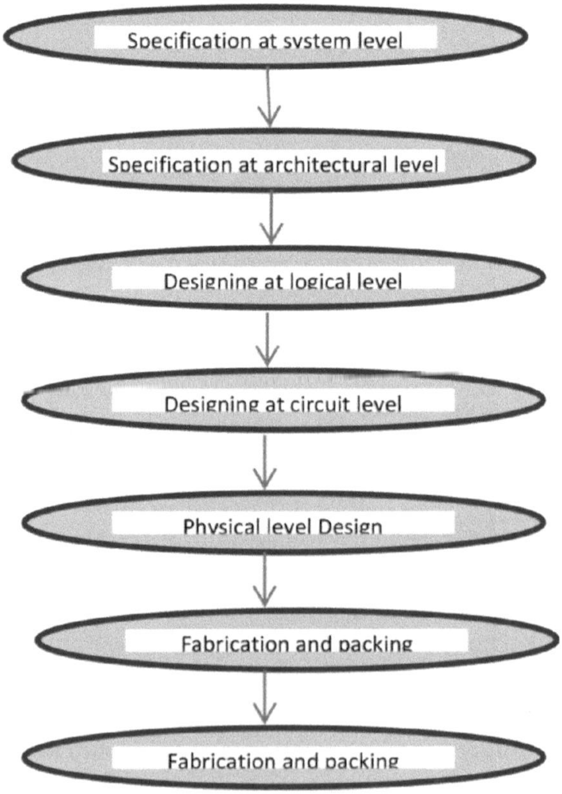

FIGURE 8.1 Steps required for designing of IC.

8.2 PREVIOUS PROGRESS IN DESIGNING OF IC FOR BIO-MEDICAL APPLICATION

8.2.1 *ELECTRONIC FEATURES AND THEIR ASSIMILATION USING SILICON*

In the previous decade, these strategies were applied for the treatment of asymmetrical heart beats, such as bradycardia (heart beat gets very slow) or tachycardia (heart beat gets very fast). Instead, Nowadays, such type of implantable devices be responsible for therapy to treat several diseases. Stirring fresh solicitations in neurological stimulation which is applied for the treatment of sleep apnea, pain managing, Parkinson's disease, epilepsy, bladder controller, gastrointestinal complaints, several autoimmune diseases, and psychological disorders, such as obsessive compulsive disorder (OCD). This system of implantation has provided an exact quantity of dose and interval supply of drugs in order to treat more effectively with patient's conditions along with reducing the side effects.

There are described some common functions of implantable ICs which are supporting biomedical implantation on the basis of some criteria, such as front-end (sensing and simulation), storage element, processing element, intercommunication, and power management.

The sensing and stimulation sections of an implantable IC can be referred to collectively as the analog front-end (AFE).

The output of this implanted device is considered as simulation or delivery of therapy, for example, in multiple cases, the response can be recorded on the base of sensing, such as rate of heart beat and level of sugar in blood and blood pressure.

Storage unit or memory is very important for any implantable device. Memory for the IC may be determined in two basic types; one is volatile and second is nonvolatile. In this regard, few nonvolatile memories are single time or multi-programmable, including flash and EEPROM. Flex Memory technology is also introduced in such type of applications. This can be configured as a high speed write, high-endurance EEPROM or a data or program flash memory.

All the processing and decision-making is done by the CPU or sometimes considered as brain of implantable integrated circuit. It is also referred as a microprocessor which is responsible for the execution of the program memory and maintains the register contents for controlling the AFE.

There is also required communication between implantable device and any external controlling device for initial setting up of the implantable device because of monitoring and controlling purpose.

It is also very important to manage power supply in implantable device and this can be possible by making use of specific battery or use of super capacitor.

8.2.2 DESIGN PARTITIONING AND SILICON TECHNOLOGIES

Since it has been discussed previously that small size and less power consumption are the basic parameters for constructing the implantable devices, in such a scenario, there is required a maximum level of integration on a single small chip.

Partition is a very typical task in ICs, which means that grouping of features or electronic blocks together into a single silicon die or an IC. This process is not only critical for implantable devices but also in every application area of IC Designing.

At last, performance issues and risk analysis is necessary to be done while partitioning a design. Process of integration of a complete system into a single unit (chip) of silicon is considered as integration of sensitive AFE devices and noisy digital circuits on a single silicon chip. This causes noise issues which may lead to degrade the performance of analog unit. Since it is discussed that a complete digital system are elevated for gate concreteness and limited processing steps in order to reduce the cost so in general analog features should not be present in a pure digital-oriented process (Harrison et al., 2003).

Similarly, the process for the implantable IC optimizing analog requisitions does not allow providing the desirable density of gates for integration. This may degrade the performance of an IC which is larger than the required size and so the process of design partitioning of the IC should take into deliberation the availability of silicon technologies.

8.2.3 SIGNAL PROCESSING IN BIO-MEDICAL

This technique was implemented for wireless endoscopy in which image compression was applied with less complexity of lossless image compression approach. In this particular architecture, a Bayer color filter array generally known as CFA was used, and it was implemented to access the raw data from an image-sensing device and to store it inside static RAM after filtering. Further, this stored image was compressed using JPEG-LS compression method. Again, the compressed image was stored in static RAM in order to provide better quality of image communication. The synchronous accessed by CMOS sensor (image) contains both straight and perpendicular output along with pixel clock outcome. This is generally used to obtain the actual position of pixel in the form of row and column number. In accordance with the synchronous signal, a controlling device of JPEG-LS is used to decide that which specific pixel is need to be filtered or not in order to implement lossless image compression (Cheng et al., 2015).

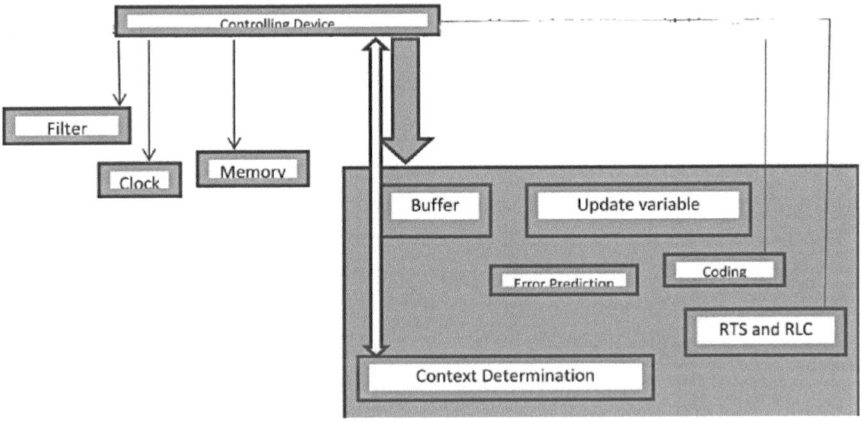

FIGURE 8.2 Image compression encoder architecture for JPEG-LS using VLSI.

Here, architecture of image compression using VLSI was proposed by Prof. Z. H. Wang with his team in 2005.

In Figure 8.3, the architecture proposed a combined signal VLSI CMOS sensor for image compression represented by Figure 8.3 (a). This architecture is basically used to compute a block of matrix and convolution transformation of image of every video frame along with a digital and programmable kernel of size 8 × 8 pixels which is directly associated with focal plane. It uses an algorithm for multiplying analog to digital converter in order to apply spatial calculations, whereas the array of pixel is read out along with quantization in parallel (Akhavian et al., 2009).

In this approach, the kernel coefficient C is multiplied with the signal provided by the pixels having sequence of most significant bit to least significant bit. A multiplexer is used to access the output which is associated with binary weights with a weight decreasing factor of 2 in every repetition of cycle. A circuit implementation was performed for matching the weight of pixels with the corresponding signal.

This is properly defined in the Figure 8.3 (b) which shows a column signal path from the pixel to the accumulator (Li et al., 2013). A multi-sampling of the same pixel containing two frame of memory is allowed. A single amplifier is used to combine the functionality of a pixel followed with a gain stage unit. A programmable bank of capacitor feedback bank is applied to perform accumulation over vertical adjacent pixels. Finally, by programming the gain, the process of matching of output with the size of block matrix is performed (Yayu et al., 2015).

8.2.4 BIOMEDICAL IMPLANTATION FOR SENSING BRAIN SIGNALS

An approach for sensing Brain Signals was proposed by "AlirezaKarimi-Bidhendi" with the help of a front-end constructed with block of BSA. It was capable for sensing and amplifying signal of brain at microvolt level. It was a completely implantable circuit and the front-end for signal gaining with very light watt consumption or microwatt level front-end. This AFE was designed with the help of differential amplifiers, buffers for output and serialize biased in WI region (Zou et al., 2013).

The outcome received from array was multiplexed in time in order to provide a better management for I/O cable by sinking wires count. A non-overlapping clock generator was also introduced along with serializer which produces M-phase clock signals with 1/M cycle of duty (Ong and Cruz, 2012).

After reducing noise and power, decadence provides a strict design trade-off in acquisition front-end regarding implantation system. If it is observed at the device level, it is clear that designing of transistors should be in a manner that it may operate in a region that generates least consumption of power at a given IR Noise enforced by a very low accessible power of ECoG signal. It is also clear that metal oxide semiconductors transistors are in WI region obtains highest gm/IDs ratio, which provides maximum power efficiency in exchange with minimum operation and maximum bandwidth.

8.2.5 ADVANCEMENT IN BIO-MEDICAL IMPLANTATION USING MICRO-ELECTRONICS

In this section, we will have a discussion about advancement in Biomedical implantation with the help of microelectronics. The basic aim is specified here about neural recording and replication circuit which are suitable for the process of construction in latest silicon technologies and biotelemetry techniques for data and energy transfer. Here, multiple techniques and circuit designing strategies are followed for neural memory storage on a chip in order to reduce the bandwidth necessity for wireless transfer link. Another section has discussed the advancement in neural simulation and application of inductive coupling.

It has been discussed previously that frequency and amplitude of neural signals are very low. For instance, the amplitude of ENG in region of 1 μV is limited between 300Hz and 5 kHz. Hence, it must be considered that circuit with amplification of neural signals should associate with low noise working and low consumption of power in order to increase battery life for a long time in the case of biomedical implantation. Another approach for monitoring cardiac parameters like electrical activity is discussed where loop recording method for implantation is applied.

The process of neural signal amplification is done with help of clock-based strategy because the problem of noise is generally controlled by flicker (1/f) in CMOS which is relatively a very high frequency of the ratio of multiple of tens of kilo Hertz (Ward et al., 2013).

8.2.6 USE OF SIGNAL MODULATING TECHNIQUE IN BIO-MEDICAL

There is applied one more technique for the acquisition of brain signals known as chopper techniques which is applied to amplify the weak signals received from brain using signal modulation technique. This strategy provides the capability to design the amplifiers with saturated and high percentage of common mode rejection. In this technique, the input signal of the amplifier is amplified after the modulation of square wave signal of with frequency "f" which is greater than the frequencies of base band. These chopping signals may be represented by Figure 8.4. Furthermore, the highly converted signals are amplified and filtered through band pass (Pabboji et al., 2020).

At the time of sampling phase, the auto zero-technique was observed where the configuration of amplifiers is done as a buffer called unity gain and the sampling of input noise was carried out. The sampled noise was subtracted from the frequency which was higher than 1/f frequency of noise and this selected sample was very much interrelated with the immediate noise and also with the noise of low frequency which is considered to be canceled. An analysis in depth was done of auto zero-technique in which it was observed that a drawback occurs in this technique which shows that the frequency with high amplitude including noise is creased back into baseband where the increment occurs in noise floor. In order to remove this drawback, a neural amplifier with band pass micropower capability was used to implement auto zero-feature along with the capability of variable gaining.

8.2.7 NOISE REDUCTION WITH CONTINUOUS TIME APPROACH

Another technique has been introduced in order to reduce the noise by using a clock circuit. Previously there were associated various problems related to high frequency intrusion and clock feed. Including this, the complication and power feeding of the designed circuit is increased due to use of circuits of high frequency exchange. Another approach of continuous time technique was introduced which was highly deployed in designing neural amplifiers. This circuit design was generally a coupled OTA-based neural amplifier along with capacitive feedback capability. This circuit was designed around a sole phase OTA in CMOS approach. Here, the ratio of capacitors locates a midpoint of band gain of response received from band pass. In this approach, the input is capacitive attached with C1, and because of this any offset of D.C. from the electrode-t, the interface issue was resolved. In such a scenario, C1 must be constructed too small to reduce the attenuation of signal, the subtraction of transistors M_a-M_d should be implemented in metal oxide semiconductor pseudoresisters along with a sufficient high incremental resistance in order to allow the cutoff frequency of highly passing input filters needed to be deployed and the low cutoff frequency should be deployed as multiplication of C2 and metal oxide semiconductor pseudoresister which was implemented by M_a and M_b.

8.2.8 IMPLEMENTATION OF NEURAL STIMULATORS

In this section, we see the use of neural stimulator which is implied to the nerves in order to rise up the working abilities. In such scenario, a minimum of two electrodes are needed to generate the flow of current. The arrangement of electrodes is done in approach monopolar or bipolar configuration. In both the approaches, the acting electrode is physically situated close to the nerve to get stimulation. In the case of monopolar stimulation, the uninterested electrode is kept in distance from the working electrodes. In the case of bi-polar stimulation, the indifferent electrode is kept close to the working electrode.

In case of voltage simulation, the outcome of a stimulator is voltage rather than the current. So the magnitude of the current is provided to the t-issue electrodes which are completely based on inter-electrode impedance. So it considers very typical to limit the certain amount of charge which is applied to the load due to alterations in impedance. In such type of system, the stimulators operate on electrodes with an order of voltage stages by charging the capacitance of metal of electrode. This provides a waveform of voltage which comes near to the waveform at the electrodes in the case of applying pulses of current (Zhang et al., 2011).

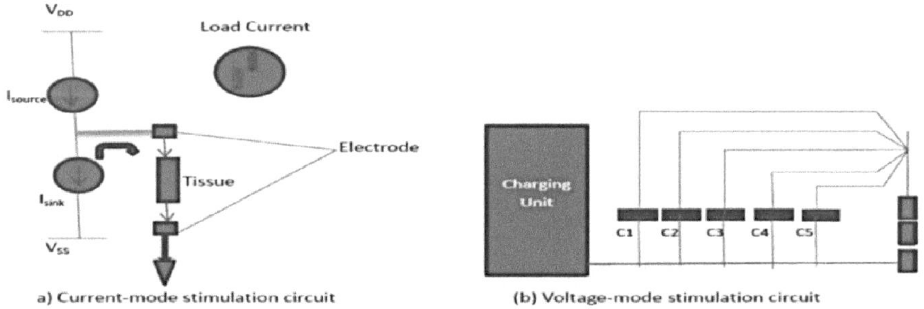

FIGURE 8.3 Design of voltage and current mode simulation circuit.

8.2.9 DESIGNING PROCESS OF IC AS FRONT-END FOR BIOMEDICAL MONITORING

In the case of designing of integrated circuits, it is very important to choose appropriate technology which is needed to be applied. This is very effective for taking decisions in designing throughout the remaining process. In the case of analog designing of analog integrated circuits, the designers regularly attempts to pull down their process regarding decrement in dimension, cost, and performance speed. In the case of designing of biomedical integrated circuits, this is completely opposite to design with the same parameters. This can be explained using following descriptions.

Limitation in carrier frequency is one of the important parameter in which comparing with latest chips being used in communication of high speed data, the breakdown in frequency is generally caused by two factors, the first factor is analyzed by requirements for digital processing due to their very low frequency acquisition in biomedical signal monitoring, and this is why these circuits do not require clocking with speed. The second factor is considered because power refinement is done to the radio frequency carrier, which is also very low. This can be observed that the frequencies with high amplitude are not sufficient efficient for power transfer because of high-energy absorbing capacity of human body's capacity. There is also no requirement for too much fast technology (Cha et al., 2014).

Requirement for high voltage is also very effective in such scenario which may affect the designing process of integrated circuits. It may be described by the inductive link mechanism where L1 shows the primary coil and L2 shows the secondary or implanted coil. There exists a coupling factor which is represented by k where L1<k<L2; and this may be equated by the link equations mentioned as below:

$$V1 = j\omega L_1 I_1 + j\omega k\, (L_1 L_2 I_2)^{1/2} \tag{8.1}$$

$$V2 = j\omega L_2 I_2 + j\omega k\, (L_1 L_2 I_1)^{1/2} \tag{8.2}$$

These equations show the relationship between main and subordinate voltages and current across the coils.

It is considerable that the alteration between coupling factors may enforce another higher voltage V_2, which is basically considered as a violation in degrading the factors of designing the standard integrated circuit mechanisms. The technology which is adapted preferably is a matured process with additional downfalling in voltage. In the case of requirements of high performance ratio for digital and analog integrated circuits, it is still conceivable to make use of two dissimilar schemes where the mature technology is applied in frontend integrated circuits and less matured scheme is applied in designing of analog and digital processing with more operational chips. In such type of cases, both integrated circuits can be loaded to construct a system in package (SIP) and multi-chip module

(MCM) (Nair et al., 2015). In such designing aspects, only the front-end integrated circuits are expanded. A high voltage allowance over 0.35 m process is chosen and the limits of breakdown are expanded to 80 V.

8.2.10 BATTERY-ENABLED IMPLANTATION

In some special case of implantation, application of batteries was exhilarated. For instance, implantation which contains restricted working time period or life and they are extended after reintegration. In such scenario, really, use of battery is very important for increasing the life of implantable biomedical devices for E-health monitoring purpose along with replacement facility of battery (Ko et al., 2012). In some cases of implantation like pacemaker which does not only perform reflexive monitoring but also gives a life protecting pacing activity which needs the application of a regular source of power supply.

In the case of orthopedic implantation system an additional power may be acceptable in order to avoiding the use of battery. The basic and primary coil of the inductive link system is searched out using a type of E-driver because of its greater efficiency (Bu et al., 2009).

In such type of system, the incoming radio frequency waves are firstly refined to a partial stable DC voltage and voltage with temperature independency up to 3.3 V, which is able to provide a minimum of 50 mW of power which is sufficient to power a strain gauge-enabled implantation.

The process of rectifying the RF carrier is refined to achieve a DC voltage and merging the refinement elements on a chip produces a problem of constructing a parasitic diode from substrate toward a node. In reality, the lowest potential on chip is linked with the substrate. The terminal goes down under the ground stage at the time when a half-wave rectifier is situated in between one of the terminal of the basic coil and the voltage controlling device. The only external component called a stabilization capacitor required needed to be placed after the rectifier in order to reduce the asynchronous voltage.

There is also a possibility to contrivance the capacitor on chip density with only 1.5 nF/mm^2 which may not so much efficient in the use of high-cost die area. Such type of stabilization capacitor in the single outer system entity with a minimum of 0402 size SMD capacitor of 100 nF($1 \times 0.5 \times 0.15$ mm).

Another process called rectification has been realized like a cataract of both a pre-regulator and a regulator. The succeeding elements are protected from unknown and higher voltage by introducing a pre-regulator to the remedied signal. Using this approach, the elements that are comparatively much smaller in the die-area with low voltage can be considered to practice for use. One more benefit of using a pre-regulating device is the reality that a partially stable voltage of DC is also obtained whose amplitude is limited within the range of 4–5 V, while the voltage of input coil moves up to more than 10 V because of the effects of loading and alterations in coupling. Hence, the device following the regulator looping is much easier compatibility with DC input. Additionally, the pre-regulator devices provide the substantial increment in PSRR limited up to 36 dB. Where a higher range of Power Supply Rejection Ratio is not considered as basic concern in stimulator-based implantation and it is also important there to apply a continuously monitoring approach where the quality of incoming analog signal is directly related with the noise of supply (Zhang et al., 2011).

Telemetry was also an approach for short time implantation in which low power consumption and transmitters with low bandwidth are constructed and packed with the help of Hysol Epoxy along with silicon used for medical applications. In this scheme, glass capsules and Macorceramic flat boxes were deployed for the purpose of long-term implantation system. Generally, the volume of the device is within the range of 1 $cm^3$and its power consumption level is between milliwatts and microwatts. These are generally deployed for the purpose of monitoring and diagnosis in biomedical applications. These approaches are implemented in psychological research by applying small animal models, biological study system, monitoring systems for patients and reaction and growth of treatment.

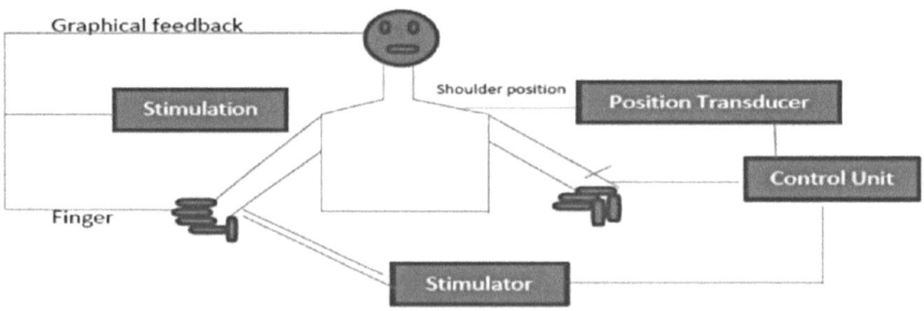

FIGURE 8.4 Design of telemetry based implantation.

8.2.11 CONTROL SYSTEM FOR ELECTRONIC IMPLANTATION SYSTEM

Various implantation system are existing such as pacemaker and electromyography (EMG) for hand prosthesis which involves an additional feedback circuit in order to monitor the exact position of the response of stimulation for adjustment of commanding signal. In the case of EMG system, telemeter controlling system is applied for monitoring the command execution. There are various examples like paralyzed limb controlling approach for lower and upper boundaries, infusion control for drug and many more controlling systems are applied in the field of biomedical implantation system in order to improve the treatment process of patients. Some efforts were also made to deploy some commanding and demonstrative project, but it has taken too much time as many years to get implemented. An example is shown of arm aid system and that was slightly in real implantation. In the same manner, a demonstrating project for limb movement controlled by EMG was introduced. In between telemetry unit called K-6 was implanted inside the Dr. Vodovink's skin and the EMG signals were transmitted from his shoulder's muscle were delivered to a frequency modulator receiving terminal which was nearby the command signal and another same technology was implanted inside the muscles of the dog's rear legs. The signal of Dr. Vodovink was being used for low and high movement of the dog's leg. Just like these experiments, some other similar research were done in order to control the speed of a motor. Such types of projects have shown the existence of a thought-controlled device or also known as brain-oriented controlling system (Andreas et al. 2014).

8.2.12 DESIGNING SCHEMES FOR ELECTRONIC IMPLANTABLE DEVICES

In the case of designing of tiny implantable circuits, some parameters should be taken into consideration like power consumption, low weight, small size, long life time, and many more. Generally, the heavy weighted and large size devices face the problem of long-lasting power supply and also do not get well-suited with human body. These are the highly complex situations which are being faced from initialization till today. Because of the advancement in LSI and MEMS, it became very helpful to achieve this level of implantation. It includes the interface electronics with radio frequency joint may be designed to get small size and low weight. Never the less various schemes were developed in recent periods which may be interesting for today's requirements.

Some examples like modulated RF pulse stage scheme are considered to highly reduce the power consumption by the factor which is slightly different from the duty cycle. Another approach of applying tunnel diode to share the voltage of battery with the transistors where implementation of two channel telemetry circuit has been deployed where 1.35V battery is shared by transistors and tunnel diodes arranged in series.

8.2.13 ISSUES AND CHALLENGES ASSOCIATED WITH BIO-MEDICAL IMPLANTATION

There are some basic issues, and challenges are associated with biomedical implantation is considered as problem of long-lasting power supply where the implantable device contains small battery with minimum internal impedance for rapid charging and temporary current at output. The power supply factor is an organization of battery which includes super capacitor and thin film of lithium. This is very helpful to increase the performance in order to meet out the current requirement of the power storage for long time (Teng et al., 2008).

Another issue which was observed in biomedical implantation is considered as small packaging by using MEMS. The basic functionality of packaging of implantable devices is to keep the human body secured from device being implanted. There are some primary needs and challenges for keeping the implantable body secured which include the issue of using toxic material for implantation, interface-related issue of implantable devices which may harm the surrounding tissues of body, temperature of implantable interface is also a typical parameter which should be normally compatible with human body temperature. Rather than these issues, one more factor is observed as a gravity of implantable device which must be near to its adjacent areas.

8.2.14 WIRELESS IMPLANTATION USING HIGH POWER RECEIVER IC

In previous research approaches, it was observed that somewhere there is a drawback in biomedical implantation just because of failing in receiving high power for implementation of wireless-oriented bio-medical implantation in order to reduce chronic power supply issue. In order to restrict the tempted voltage basically low voltage strategies are deploys limiter devices and regulators with shunt are generally ineffective techniques for power point of view. For restricting the drawback of voltage limitation and for improving the competency of power there is also given an approach to develop such IC which may work as high power receiver on the basis of phase dejected scheme. This scheme may have acquisition of 30 volts and includes a partially alive rectifier, series regulator, and voltage reference generator. A battery management circuitry is also introduced which provides a safe implant chargeable battery on the basis of analog controlling system (Li et al., 2013).

8.3 CONCLUSIONS

In this chapter, the author has given some reviews regarding the importance of integrated circuits in the field of biomedical implantation system. This was observed that biomedical implantation was very useful and provided a revolutionary change in traditional treatment process. Some facts and information were also provided which have enlightened the designing strategy of some implantable devices. In this chapter, the author has also mentioned about the issues and challenges associated with biomedical implantation in terms of long-lasting life, small size, and weight. Rather than these analysis, some future scope of research is also provided in this scenario. As it is well known that as per the current requirements, the use of wireless implantation is more in demand along with wireless charging facility. This is somewhere achieved but not applicable in every area of implantation. Finally, the author wants to conclude with the result that the role of integrated circuits is very important in the field of biomedical and mHealth applications which have provided a security to human bodies to get protected themselves by using harmful drugs in the case of organ failure. Biomedical implantation has provided a revolutionary change in the treatment policy and provided a better approach to save the lives of patients.

KEYWORDS

- **micro electromechanical system (MEMS)**
- **complementary metal oxide semiconductor (CMOS)**
- **obsessive compulsive disorder (OCD)**
- **multi-chip module (MCD)**
- **electromyograph (EMG)**
- **power supply rejection ratio (PSRR)**

REFERENCES

Akhavian, A.; Judy, M.; Sodagar, A.M. Anti-Logarithmic Quantization for Data Reduction in Multi-Channel Intra-Cortical Neural Recording Implants, Accepted for presentation at the IEEE-EMBS International Conference on Biomedical and Health Informatics, 2012.

Andreas, D. Advances in Microelectronics for Implantable Medical Devices. *Hindawi Pub. Corp. Adv. Electron.* **2014,** *2014*, Article ID 981295.

Bu, L. P.; Cong, P.; Kuo, H. I.; Ye, X. S.; Ko, W. H. Micro Package of Short Term Wireless Implantable Microfabricated Systems. In *Proceedings of the IEEE EMBC Annual Conference* 2009; pp 6395–6399.

Cheng, Y.; Li, Y. The Design of Integrated Circuit for Biomedical and mHealth Application. In: *Mobile Health. Springer Series in Bio-/Neuroinformatics*; Adibi, S., Eds., Vol. 5; Springer: Cham. https://doi.org/10.1007/978-3-319-12817-7_23

Chiu, H. W.; Chuang, J. M.; Lu, C. C.; Lin, W. T.; Lin, C. W.; Lin, M. L. In Situ Measurement of Tissue Impedance Using an Inductive Coupling Interface Circuit. *IEEE Trans. Biomed. Circ. Syst.* **2013,** *7*, 225–235.

Harrison, R. R.; Charles, C. A Low-Power Low-Noise CMOS Amplifier for Neural Recording Applications. *IEEE J. Solid-State Circ.* **2003,** *38*, 958–965.

Ko, W. H. Early History and Challenges of Implantable Electronics. *ACM J. Emerg. Technol. Comput. Syst.* **2012,** *8* (2), 9. Article 8.

Li, Y. T.; Peng, C. W.; Chen, L. T.; Lin, W. S.; Chu, C. H.; Chen, J. J. J. Application of Implantable Wireless Biomicrosystem for Monitoring Nerve Impedance of Rat After Sciatic Nerve Injury. *IEEE Trans. Neural Syst. Rehabil. Eng.* **2013,** *1*, 121–128.

Nair, V. V.; Choi, J. R. An Integrated Chip High-Voltage Power Receiver for Wireless Biomedical Implants. *Energies* **2015,** *8*, 5467–5487. https://doi.org/10.3390/en8065467

Ong, J. M.; Cruz, L. da. The Bionic Eye: A Review. *Clin. Exp. Ophthalmol.* **2012,** *40*, 6–17.

Pabboji, A.; PullaRao, B. Integrated Circuit Design for a Biomedical Device. *J. Interdisc. Cycle Res.* **2020,** *XII* (VIII), 978.

Teng, X. F.; Zhang, Y. T.; Poon, C. C.; Bonato, P. Wearable Medical Systems for p- Health. *IEEE Rev. Biomed. Eng.* **2008,** *1*, 62–74.

Ward, C.; Henderson, S.; Metcalfe, N. H. A Short History on Pacemakers. *Int. J. Cardiol.* **2013,** *169* (4), 244–248.
Zou, X. D.; Xu, X. Y.; Yao, L. B.; Lian, Y. A 1-V 450-nW Fully Integrated Programmable Biomedical Sensor Interface Chip. *IEEE J. Solid-State Circ.* **2009,** *44*, 1067–1077.

CHAPTER 9

Experimental Setup and Analysis of Energy Harvesting Systems for Low Power Biomedical Applications: Lab-on-Chip Application of Impedance Micropump and Microfluidic Logic Gate

KAMAL KISHOR UPADHYAY[1], SHUBHAM SHUKLA[2], DEEPIKA AGRAWAL[1], SUDHAKAR PANDEY[1], and NARENDRA KUMAR SHUKLA[3]

[1]*Department of Information Technology, NIT Raipur, Raipur, Chhattisgarh, India*

[2]*Department of ECE, KIET Ghaziabad, Uttar Pradesh, India*

[3]*Department of ECE, University of Allahabad, Prayagraj, Uttar Pradesh, India*

ABSTRACT

One of the biggest challenges in the evolution era of the Internet of Things is power supply. Battery-powered medical equipment is often used to provide low-power electrical power. However, their charging costs are usually high. This chapter proposes energy harvesting from the environment and storing the energy from various sources. This study reviews the various aspects of the development of biomedical implants. It aims to provide a comprehensive view of the various methods and technologies involved in the development of these devices. The chapter describes the

Advanced Research in Electronic Devices for Biomedical and mHealth.
Rajesh K. Kesharwani, Upendra Kumar, Raj K. Keservani (Eds)

experimental and modeling verification of linear models, electromagnetic energy harvesters, that are prompted by a low-frequency random gradual forced movement or an exogenous acceleration. The system is designed to be used in biomedical and wearable electronic devices. The concept of a double-structure harvester is that it maintains a large magnetic flux gradient in each component while reducing the force exerted between the fixed and moving parts. An external acceleration pulse was used to study the effects of this structure on the system's dynamics and electrical power output. The development of biosensors has gained tremendous attention due to their wide use in the field of biomedicine and healthcare. Biosensors are being widely used in the detection of various diseases and their monitoring of human health. In this chapter, we focused on the development of the battery-less system for biomedical applications: (1) micropump and (2) microfluidic Fredkin gate. Both systems are powered by energy harvested from the electromagnetic waves present in the environment.

9.1 INTRODUCTION

Direct energy conversion is used by energy harvesting systems to create electric power from their surroundings as Billinghurst and Starner (1999) suggested in their research. Implantable biomedical devices are now powered by a few cables, which can lead to skin infections, pain, and other problems for patients. Implantable biomedical devices are now powered by batteries that are already in place in the body. Batteries, on the other hand, have a set energy density, a finite lifespan, chemical side effects, and a big physical bulk. Consequently, Beeby and Tudor (2006) discussed about white energy. Pereyma (2007) devised several strategies for generating power for implanted electronic devices. Traditional gadgets are less comfortable and safer than those powered by collected energy because of their shorter lifespan. Khaligh et al. (2010) suggested energy from the surrounding environment is an effective solution to wireless sensor energy concerns. Infrared radiant energy is one of the scavenge-able energies, solarthermal energy, geothermal temperature gradients, and combustion are examples of thermal energy, kinetic energy (KE) (wind waves, gravity, vibration, and body motion), radio frequency (RF) radiation energy and wireless transmission energy (inductive and capacitive coupling). Harvesting energy from human or natural sources has been offered as a feasible alternative. Many scholars (Wise et al., 2004) have uncovered potentially useful solutions and incorporated them in a review paper. Many publications give evaluations on a specific form of categorized capturing KE from physiological motion, vibration, or piezoelectric material for biomedical implanted devices, or wireless energy harvesting transmission (Torres and Rincón, 2010) using thermal (Wojciech, 2010) and solar energy from environmental sources as described in Schmidt and Scott (2011). Researchers (Paulo and Gaspar, 2010) and Jaeseok et al. (2011) investigated the use of biomedical sensor nodes that are powered by human-body movements. This survey of the literature on biomedical implantable energy harvesting is comprehensive. Biomedical implanted devices and wireless telemetry devices are used to examine and categorize all kinds of energy harvesting to provide a thorough understanding of the challenges and problems encountered, and suitable solutions are devised.

This chapter consists of three major parts: one is the introduction, general methods of energy harvesting and a related literature survey. The second part focuses on the development of such kind of circuitry which generates usable power from the electromagnetic (EM) and RF waves presented over there in the environment. The last section of this chapter reflects the application part of the harvested energy. Here in this chapter, we have taken two examples which are manufactured by us and driven by harvested energy, that is, micropump for perfusion and microfluidic Fredkin logic gate.

9.2 METHODS

There are two types of implantable biomedical devices. An example of a human body-powered gadget is one that is covered in the secondary forest. The second kind is powered by renewable energy and is surrounded by the secondary forest. As shown in Figure 9.1, there are many different types of energy harvesting technologies that may be employed in the applications of biomedical.

9.2.1 HUMAN ENERGY HARVESTING

Kinetic and thermal energy are generated by human actions. The amount of power generated by various body functions varies (Stamer, 2011). About 1630 mW of electricity is generated by sprint walking and motion, whereas sleeping produces 81 mW. Even when the temperature outside changes, the human body preserves its heat. The metabolic processes required for energy generation can continue even when the ambient temperature is quite low because of this characteristic. Because of this, two forms of energy are produced: As a result, kinetic and thermal energy harvesting from human body activities are the focus of this section's research.

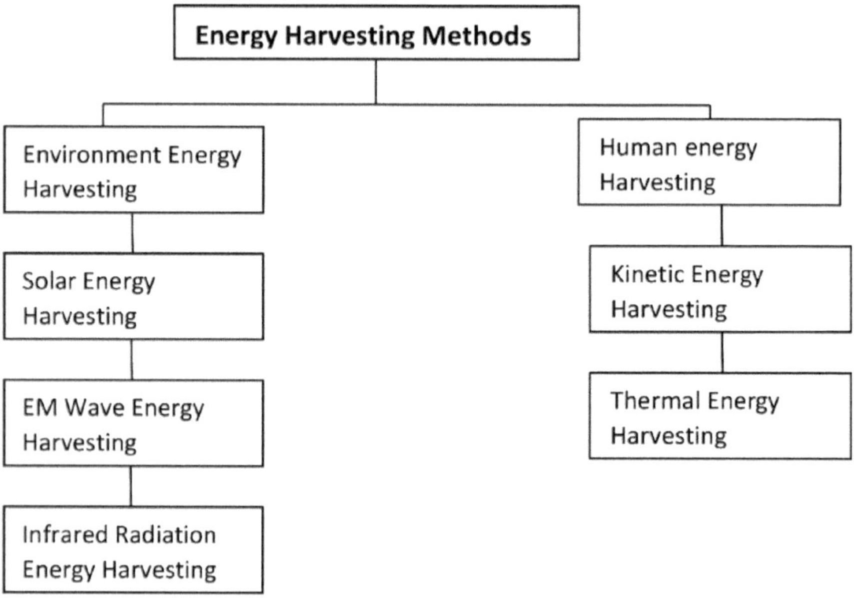

FIGURE 9.1 Different energy harvesting methods.

9.2.2 KINETIC ENERGY

Implantable biomedical devices have a bright future because of the potential energy that comes from human body activities. KE is a wide energy source that is available for energy harvesting devices used by humans and the environment. Mitcheson et al. (2008) discussed about various transducers for converting KE into electrical piezoelectric, magnetic induction generator, and electrostatic transduction processes are all examples of energy.

9.2.3 PIEZOELECTRICITY

The Curie brothers made the initial discovery of the piezoelectric effect in 1880. They discovered that when materials are mechanically stretched, an electrical polarization occurs in direct proportion to the strain exerted. To transform mechanical motion into electrical energy, we employ the piezoelectric effect. Figure 9.2 depicts the conversion flow chart, whereas Figure 9.3 depicts the corresponding plan. MIT's Media Lab built the first human walking-based energy harvesting system in 1990, a wearable electronic applications that convert human motion into energy (Romero et al., 2009). In 1998, a spring magnetic generator in the shoe heel generated roughly 1 W of energy, according to Paradiso et al. (1998). It is only for patients who can walk properly that can utilize this prototype, despite its ability to produce electricity. In 2001, Shenck and Paradiso (2001) added piezoelectric components to the shoes in two places: the heel and the toes. There are 8.35 mW and 1.4 mW outputs from this design prototype, respectively. This prototype on the contrary is limited in terms of power output and only those who are able to walk correctly should utilize it. Kornbluh (2002) compressed piezoelectric components in a boot heel to enhance findings.

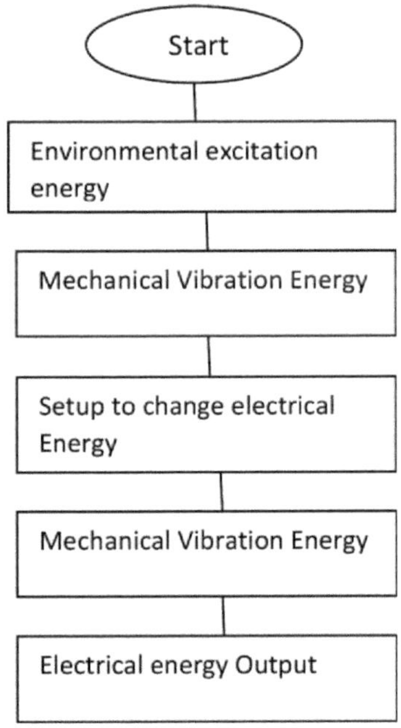

FIGURE 9.2 Stepwise procedure for energy harvesting.

Despite the fact that Ramsay and Clark (2001) deliver additional power, this prototype suffers from the same limitations as those stated in Sohn et al. (2005) and Platt et al. (2005). Electrical energy is created when mechanical pressure is applied to piezoelectric materials. Ramsay and Clark used normal blood pressure changes to power a square PZT-5A up to at max 2.3 W of energy. Hong et al. (2007) investigated blood pressure fluctuations using circular and square plates made with polyvinylidene fluoride.

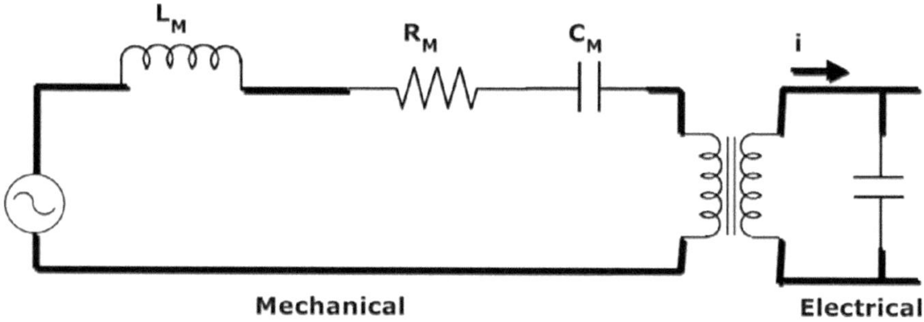

FIGURE 9.3 Piezoelectric conversion.

To create 4.85 mW, Platt et al. (2005) used piezoelectric ceramics with orthopedic implants. To create 1.2 mW, Woodson and Melcher (1968) used knee replacement implants integrated with piezoelectric ceramics. Shaban et al. (2010) created 1.89 mW generated by ceramic piezoelectric plates in implants for the knees.

9.2.4 *ELECTROSTATIC ENERGY*

Electrostatic generators convert mechanical vibrations into electrical energy. They can generate electricity with a fixed charge or a steady voltage. An electrostatic generator can be built with a variable micro-machined capacitor. This system can produce 8 W of power and is capable of controlling an external charge. Electrostatic transducers that use variable capacitors can generate current through the force exerted by an external force. They can also operate under a fixed charge or a dynamic potential.

9.2.5 MAGNETIC INDUCTION GENERATOR

Mechanical generators are divided into two types: relative motion and rigid body motion. The former uses relative motion (Meninger et al., 2001), while the latter uses the force of the weight on the generator. Although both types can generate EM energy, they can also be vulnerable to vibration. Human walking is used to demonstrate employed EM VDRG constructed to create 410 μW of electricity (Amirtharajah et al., 1998). A novel VDRG was created using EM MEMS technology to produce 10.2 μW of power at 2.1 V DC utilizing the input frequency of 64 Hz (Li et al., 2001). Tashiro et al. (2000) utilized the same prototype as in to generate 0.3 W of power using a 4-MHz excitation input. Ashiro et al. (2002) built an axial flux generator to generate energy using EM signals on a planar coil. A gear-shaped planar coil with a ring-attached eccentric weight makes up this generator (Miao et al., 2006).

9.2.6 ENVIRONMENTAL ENERGY HARVESTING

The first wireless power transmission definition system depicts a device that releases electrical energy from one place and collects it at another location in the atmosphere of the Earth without the usage of cables or another medium of support. In the late 1950s, a microwave-powered helicopter system pioneered RF power scavenging in outer space. Later, power harvesting or energy scavenging was defined as a strategy for collecting energy from the external environment by employing various mechanisms such as thermoelectric conversion, vibrational stimulation, solar energy conversion, and pressure gradients.

Environmental bio-energy harvesting (EEH) is a technology for powering biomedical equipment that captures infrared and other low-grade ambient energy sources: sunshine and transmission of energy across the air and converts it into useable electrical energy for implanted devices (Renaud et al., 2008). As a result, EEH devices have the potential to be battery replacements that have been inserted. They may also be used to power a variety of implanted and wearable medical equipment in the future.

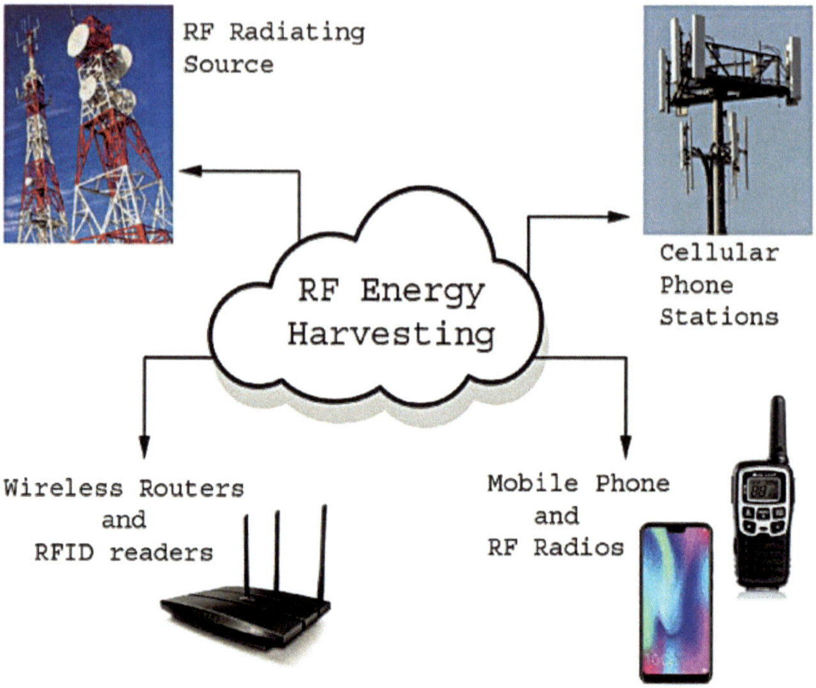

FIGURE 9.4 General diagram of energy radiation sources.

9.2.7 ELECTROMAGNETIC WAVE ENERGY HARVESTING

To offer low-power electronics for a variety of applications, such as wireless monitoring devices and sensors, electromagnetic energy harvesters (EMEHs), it may mechanically act to create electrical power, are intensively investigated since a few decades. Biomedical applications, such as powering different wearable gadgets with human-motion EH (Miao et al., 2006) or bio-implantable systems (Renaud et al., 2008) that collect the human heart's and diaphragm's power (Elfrink et al., 2009), are also being studied actively. To monitor physiological indicators and send data wirelessly at a modest rate, a power of about 500 W is necessary. Hosaka (2003) suggested energy-harvesting EMEHs may be found in several locations throughout the body. The forced displacement and perceived acceleration might be unpredictable and irregular for every harvester. To meet this power goal while also minimizing the harvester's overall volume, to optimize each component of the harvester, a simulation canvas should be constructed, allowing a fair comparison of alternative harvester shapes, and eventually validating the complete system in its real-world setting. EMEHs are typically preferred to rival technologies like piezoelectric and electrostatic when the available space is confined and bigger than a few cm^3 because of their better yield and the already existing production technique and equipment. EMEHs have the advantage of being conceptually simple because of their strong connections to commonly utilized methods for EM conversion, when similar devices are used for energy harvesting purposes methods for EM conversion. Additionally, the efficiency of EM EHs with slow forced movement excitation is poor, and the collected energy is no longer a viable option with alternative technologies like electrostatic energy harvesters that do not rely on rapid and erratic motions. Natural accelerations that subject energy harvesters to broad excitation frequencies might be another factor in their design. In EM EHs, there are two major approaches to deal with these issues. The first is to utilize head-to-head permanent magnets to increase the magnetic field's gradient and reduce the step. The alternative is to employ a trigger location that is multistable, a rapid movement when the forced displacement is significant enough.

When these two approaches are used together, it is possible to cause by adding an external slow movement to the system as mentioned in Equation (9.1), a fast oscillating movement via a quickly changing magnetic field (for EHs that rely on the use of force directly) or by applying an increase in the system's speed from outside sources (for inertial EHs). Because of this, the induced electromotive force is proportional to the position-time (velocity) fluctuation and the position-dependent variation in magnetic flux density.

$$\mathrm{EMF} = -N_{\mathrm{coil}} \frac{\mathrm{d}\varphi_{\mathrm{core}}}{\mathrm{d}y} \frac{\mathrm{d}y}{\mathrm{d}t} \tag{9.1}$$

The number of turns in the winding is denoted by N_{coil} and φ_{core} which represent the average magnetic flux in the coil's center section.

Furthermore, harvesters are most commonly employed in limited regions where the EH's size is a restriction. Scaling a generator's size by a factor S results in EM energy collected scaling by a factor of S^3 and S^4 (Rinderknecht et al., 2005). Permanent magnets used in EM generators degrade drastically when downsized (Dongeum et al., 2011) and the number of turns on magnetic coils must be decreased to meet the restricted amount of available space. As a result, precise numerical models that can accurately predict the energy generation and efficiency of the impedance micropump and microfluidic logic gate in a Lab on Chip application are essential. The system's behavior is critical for achieving optimal performance step. In year 2014, C. Luni et al. studies on EM harvesters concentrate on finding out more about the magnetic flux collected by the coils is optimized (Luni et al., 2014). This chapter emphasizes the need of doing further research adjusting the magnetic force generated by the core's shape. It is necessary to alter and adjust the system's dynamics as a result of its power efficiency in relation to its surroundings.

9.3 DESIGN AND GEOMETRY OF THE EM WAVE ENERGY HARVESTER RECEIVER BOARD

We know from Ampere's law that the magnetic field created by a collection of densely wrapped wires is dependent on the net current flowing through them. As long as the live and neutral wires are close enough, the magnetic fields they create should cancel each other out and keep the circuit safe. However, it is worth noting that EM energy can be found in ordinary living and working environments owing to the distance between live and neutral wires or to ground loop imbalances. According to previous research, the ambient magnetic field in houses varies between 0.01 and 10 G near appliances and usually reaches 100 G in enterprises using large electrical gear. Our studies showed that the cancellation of magnetic fields is practically nonexistent when the wires are separated by more than a few inches. The magnetic field may be used as an electrical energy source if the sensor equipment is strategically placed and designed well. Some of the cables in a typical office building carry currents of 5–10 A (Khot et al., 2020), which is common for office buildings. The design process begins with the first step process is to figure out if the harvesting system will be employed in a near-field or a far-field application. Near-far field and near-infinite field boundaries are defined in a variety of ways and use the tiny antennas definition (the diameter $d \ll$ wavelength). Figure 9.5 depicts a simplified field region plot and computation, with R2 representing the estimated far/near field border. Due to the harvesting system's 7-cm target distance, frequencies exceeding 1-GHz are used in the far-field zone. For this reason, the Friis equation (9.2) is used to estimate the receiving power when free space propagation is assumed.

$$P_{RX} = P_s G_s G_r \left(\frac{\lambda_{air}}{4\pi r} \right)^2 \tag{9.2}$$

where P_s represents source power, G_s represents the gain of source antenna, G_r is the gain for the receive antenna, λ shows the transmission wavelength, and the distance between the transmit and receiving antennas is represented by r. Because the source and receive antennas are both directional, they must be aligned for the best transmission power. Because of biological tissue's limited form factor, rectifier efficiency, and transmission frequency, the antenna is set to function at 4 GHz. Antenna and inductor design are combined in the on-chip antenna. A high-frequency structure simulator (HFSS) was used to simulate the loop antenna to maximize gain and the necessary inductance to resonate with the capacitance of the rectifier. The antenna was made out of top copper metal (Lachaux et al., 2021) that was 2 m thick (M8). Due to the antenna being placed on the chip's edge, proximity meta-HFSS simulation includes antenna measurement effects and bond pads. As a result, the radiation pattern is skewed (less omnidirectional) and the resonance frequency is somewhat shifted. This can be described as follows: the additional substrate coupling capacitance and the random floating metal that alters the direction of magnetic field lines. To determine the viability of the suggested energy harvesting system, we must first calculate the average power that can be collected from magnetic fields originating from AC power lines, microwave ovens, and TV transmitting towers. We carried out tests under strict supervision to see how much power could be extracted from different configurations of current-carrying conductors and inductors in the magnetic field generated by the conductors.

Removing or extending the life of batteries may be as simple as using RF wireless power harvesting (WPH). The bulk of low-power remote-sensing devices and embedded technologies now use battery power. In reality, batteries have a limited lifespan and must be replaced on a regular basis. Through the use of power harvesting methods, systems and equipment may become self-sufficient in terms of the energy required for operation, resulting in an infinite operational lifespan. As a result, the need for electricity maintenance will be minimal (Zislin and Rosenfeld, 2018).

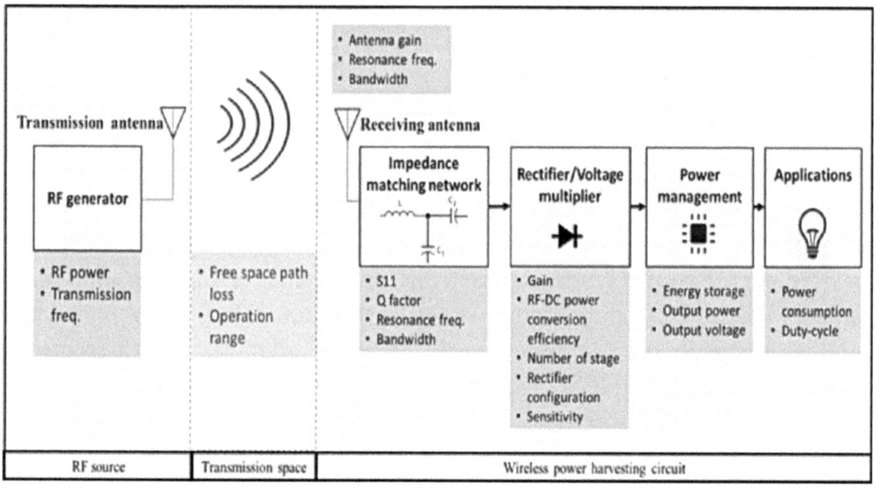

FIGURE 9.5 Block diagram of radio frequency (RF) energy harvesting system.

9.4 EXPERIMENTAL SETUP

Figure 9.6 shows the experimental setup. We utilized two parallel wires on a graded flat board to power ten 100-W light bulbs in series. A current of 8.4 A passes through the conductors when the entire load is applied. For the sake of our research, we looked at a variety of inductors. Table 9.1 displays the inductors' specifications. The chapter's findings are based on experiments with two inductors having inductances of 15 H and 4.50 H, respectively. Separate experiments were carried out on each inductor to avoid magnetic coupling (Ottesen, 2003).

In this chapter, we show you what happened in the following tests:

- Measured the induced voltage on the inductors at various distances from a pair of wires, where the distance between the conductors is quite great (>15 in).
- Induced voltage may be measured by altering the supply load.
- Maintain a spacing of 1 in between the conductors and the inductors and measure the fluctuation of the induced voltage along with the height of the inductors from the plane of the conductors.
- Check the voltage produced on the inductor when a group of wires passes through a metal conduit often seen in structures.

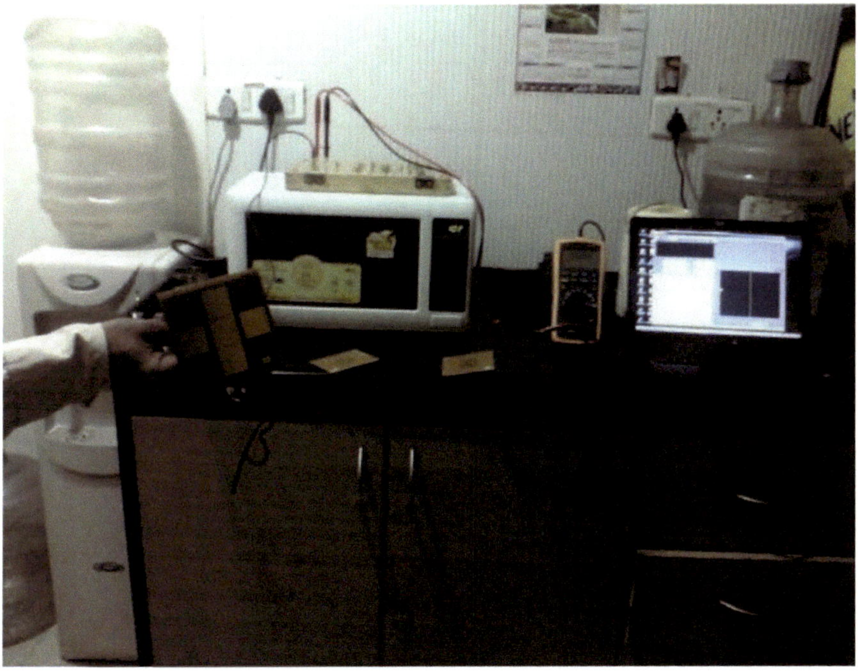

FIGURE 9.6 Experimental setup of energy harvesting system.

Using an inductor in an alternating magnetic field, we can quantify how much power is being taken from it. With a matched impedance load, the power drawn from a source is near to its maximum. The inductor serves as the voltage source in our system and drives a sensor gadget. Figure 9.6 shows an oscilloscope snapshot of voltage between two inductors connected in series between two parallel cables carrying 8.4 A of current in the opposite direction (corresponding to 1000 W load). The inductor's terminal RMS voltage is depicted in the figure's upper right corner.

The configuration is essentially an integrated component comprising a few minor components. The first part of this experiment is to find the proper location for energy harvesting because the intensity of EM waves varies as per the location and place. The first task of this experiment is to find a suitable place where the intensity of EM waves should be maximum. This phenomenon is known as field sensing and mapping. Field mapper (RF meter) is used for the above-said purpose as shown in Figure 9.7.

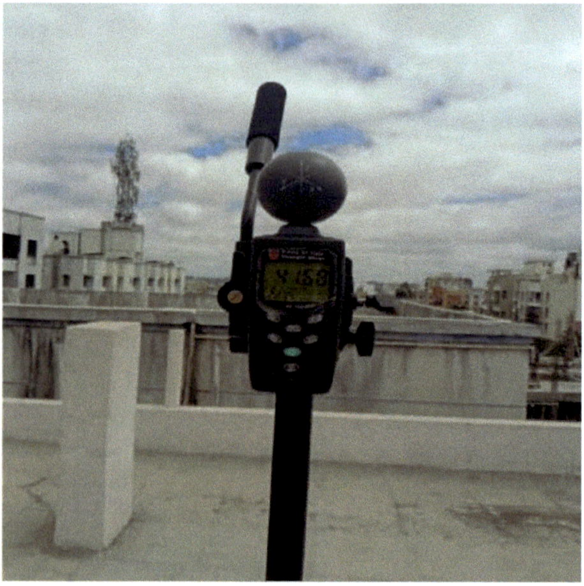

FIGURE 9.7 Field mapping device (RF meter).

The first step is to map the vicinity RF field using hand-held RF meter in both polarization, using MATLAB-based code postprocess the field versus locations like as shown in Figure 9.8.

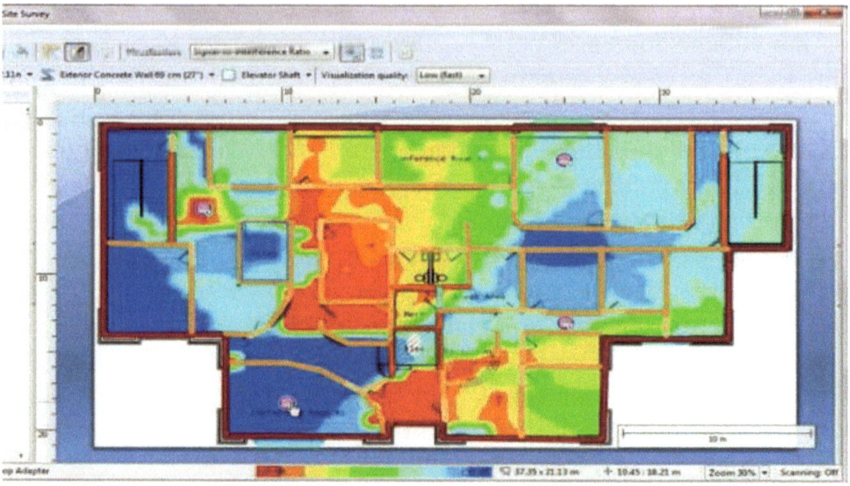

FIGURE 9.8 (a) MATLAB result for EM wave intensity of RF wave detected by RF meter.

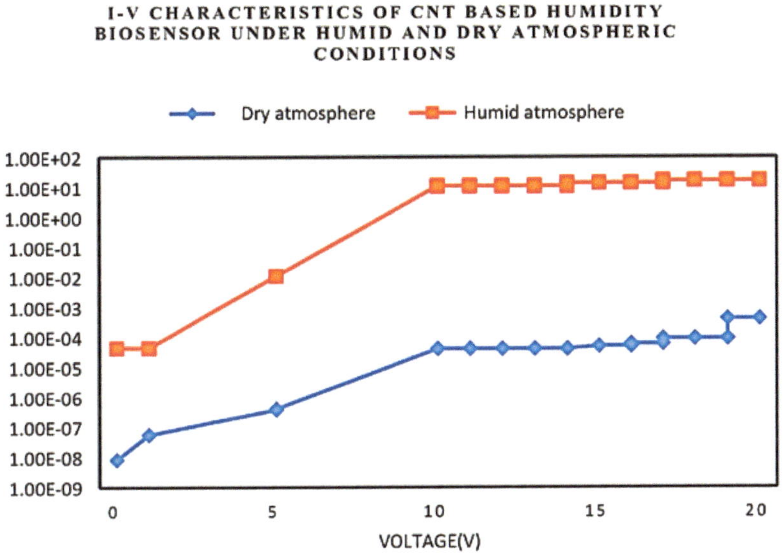

FIGURE 9.8(b) Current and voltage rating in different atmospheres.

9.5 EXPERIMENT OBSERVATIONS

RFWPH system design requires an understanding of EM waves. Depending on the distance, frequency, and conductivity of the surroundings, EM waves behave differently. To get the greatest outcomes, the designer must choose appropriate EM wave parameters based on the application's specifications. Figure 9.9 displays the transmitting and receiving part of the proposed design. When a signal travels through free space, it experiences free-space path loss (FSPL), which is a loss of power. To calculate FSPL, you will need to know things like antenna gain, wave frequency, and transmitter-to-receiver distance.

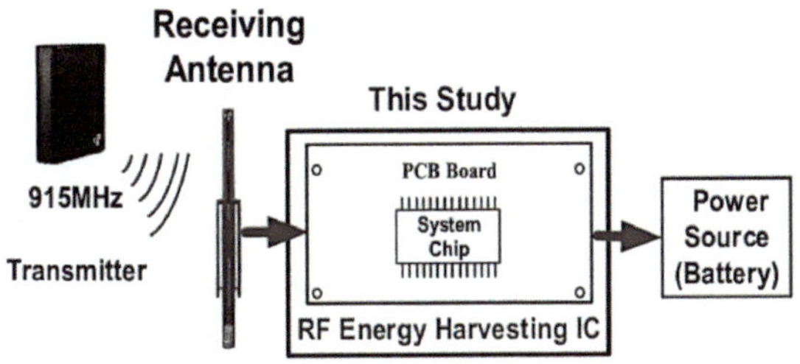

FIGURE 9.9(a) Schematic diagram of energy harvesting.

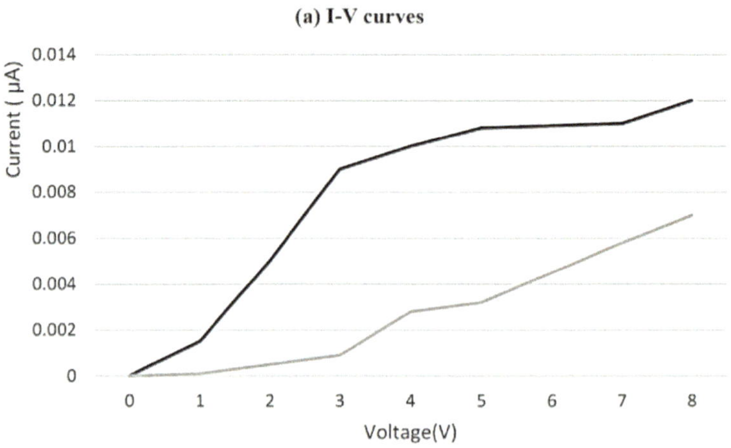

FIGURE 9.9(b) Current and voltage rating extracted from the environment.

Figure 9.10 shows the actual experimental board which are used for energy harvesting; this module has a small antenna part to receive EM waves and many different small modules to process the harvesting energy in usable power. Multiband antenna is used to collect the RF energy. The array of the Schottkey diode converts to DC voltage. DC to DC booster will raise this up to 4.25 V. Supercapacitor and battery used to store and reuse the voltage for WSN.

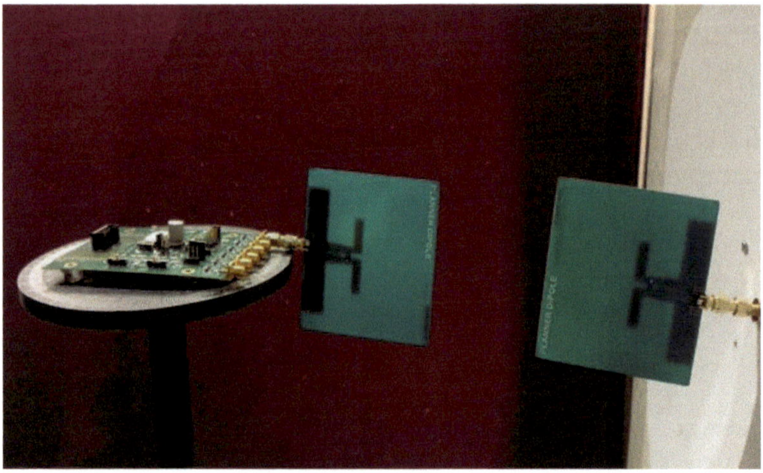

FIGURE 9.10 Energy harvesting board.

The behavior of EM waves changes with the distance between the transmitting antenna and the receiver. Far-field and near-field features are separated into these two categories. While the pattern of EM waves is consistent at a distance, the electric and magnetic components are highly powerful and independent, so one can have an advantage over the other. When speaking about the near-field and far-field regions, the term "Fraunhofer distance" (Eq. 9.3) refers to the space between the two. The Fraunhofer distance is described as follows:

$$d_F = \frac{2D^2}{\lambda} \tag{9.3}$$

where d_F is the Fraunhofer's distance, D is the maximum dimension of the radiator (or diameter of the antenna), and λ is the wavelength of the EM wave. For a WPH design to be effective, a number of parameters must be assessed. The evaluation merits vary based on the application. In spite of this, important variables like efficiency, sensitivity, operating distance, and output power are established as benchmarks so that you may make meaningful comparisons between them. Tradeoffs do occur, however, such as between the distance an operation may be operated before losing overall efficiency. In addition to this benefit, other production auxiliary variables such as a low-cost, fabrication process maturity and availability of manufacturing in quantity are also crucial.

9.6 APPLICATION IN BIOMEDICAL FIELD

9.6.1 APPLICATION 1: IMPEDANCE MICROPUMP

As per the above discussion, we are able to generate power from the environment. Now we are going to design a system that will work by using the power generated by the harvesting system. The next section will describe the 3D-printed micropump. It is a small size of device that will use for the purpose of flow in blocked veins. The controlled pumping of fluids by micropumps is well known in the microfluidics field. These pumps may be utilized both in small and large fluidic systems and are classified as valveless pumps because of their small size. This micropump would be used in cell culture and tissue engineering microfluidic systems to provide nutrients and remove waste (Lachaux et al., 2021). Using injection molding or 3D printing, the impedance pump may be quickly and cheaply produced. It is easy to mass produce because of its straightforward design and absence of intricate parts. Adjustment of basic factors such as the excitation frequency or tapping position may vary the direction of the flow along with giving a very flexible range of flow outputs. Such features make the impedance micropump ideally suited to a number of applications ranging from point-of-care (POC) devices, drug-toxicity testing, organ-on-a chip, and drug administration with finely regulated flow rates. During the last few years, there has been tremendous progress in 3D printing technology making them more dependable and accurate than ever. SLA 3D printers use near UV lasers and photocurable resins to 3D print items and may provide higher resolutions of 30–50 μm in their 3D printed products. SLA 3D printers are readily available. Digital light processing (DLP) 3D printers employ a UV LCD screen to 3D print things. Impedance micropump components created using CAD software and printed with a DLP 3D printer give accurate structural details every time. In recent years, the field of organ-on-a-chip (OOC) microfluidics has gained a lot of attention and is a popular issue for researchers. These OOC microfluidic chips include human cells because they simulate the microenvironment outside the human body, which offers more precise findings than animal models (Cheng and Wu, 2012). For perfusion and circulation of culture medium, this low-cost tiny impedance micropump may be utilized as a little heart linked to a cell-based microfluidic chip. It is possible that peristaltic pumps may be utilized in place of more traditional, larger pumps, as demonstrated in a study by Khot, M. Ibrahim, and colleagues, who built a 3D cell culture platform and used it for drug-toxicity testing and perfusing culture medium using one. They created a microfluidic system for drug toxicity assessment by combining PMMA and polydimethylsiloxane (PDMS), seeded the HT29 cell line, and growing 3D spheroids inside the microfluidic channels (Valveless, 2003). Using their custom-made setup (Lachaux et al. (2019) have demonstrated a novel microfluidic device or oxygenating blood sample using their syringe pump, which proves the crucial role of pumps in the microfluidic domain and the needs to develop low-cost alternatives that consume low power, are small in size, and have low operational costs.

9.6.1.1 MATERIALS AND METHODS

9.6.1.1.1 3D Design and Operation of Impedance Micropump

It is important to keep in mind while developing the impedance micropump that its assembly should be straightforward and easy to handle.

Additionally, the pump base, tapping mechanism, and tubing holder are all modular components of the micropump. Before being included in the micropump design, components such as a miniaturized DC motor and a tapper head are properly sized. The impedance micropump components are designed using Google Sketchup 2020, as shown in Figure 9.11. Once the design is completed, it may be imported in the steriolithography (.stl) format, which is also necessary for 3D printing. The final design after 3D printing resulted in an extremely compact device of (22 mm × 10 mm × 11.7 mm) volume comprising all the electromechanical components except for the microcontroller unit.

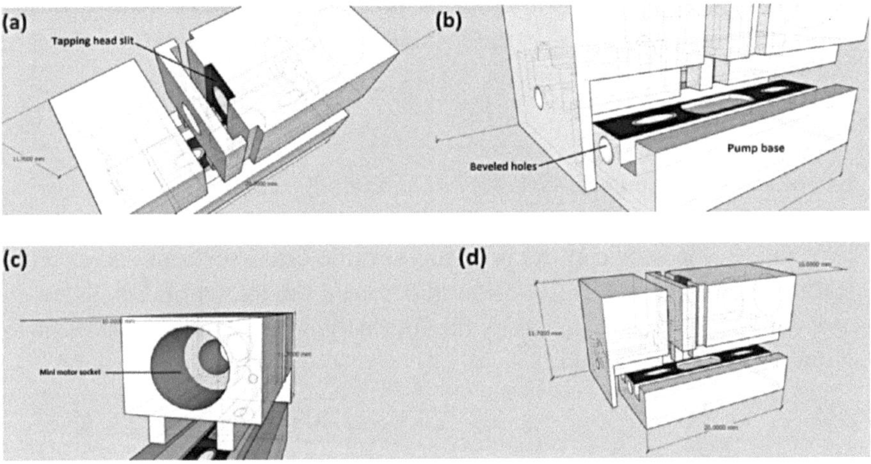

FIGURE 9.11 3D designs made on Google Sketchup 2020: (a) view showing slit where tapper-head moves, (b) where pump and tubings sit and the (c) miniature motor socket. (d) Full design.

Components of the main impedance pump include a compressible unit made of elastic PDMS that is attached end-to-end to comparable PTFE rigid material tubings but is somewhat flexible and sealed using resin-based glue after which can be fitted into the 3D-printed impedance micropump components. Viscosity affects were discussed by Cheng and Wu (2012) in their research while the flow rate within the Impedance micropump has been discussed by Nguyen et al. (2019) as discussed in Equations (9.4) and (9.5). It may be calculated by connecting the elastic boundary shear stress to the mean (axial) flow and utilizing continuity and momentum equations as follows:

$$\frac{\partial A}{\partial t}+\frac{\partial(Au)}{\partial x}=0 \tag{9.4}$$

$$\frac{\partial u}{\partial t}+\frac{\partial}{\partial x}\left(\frac{P}{\rho}+\frac{u^2}{2}\right)=\boldsymbol{F} \tag{9.5}$$

where x is the elastic tube's length, t is the passage of time, A is the elastic tube's cross-sectional area, and u is the cross-sectional mean flow velocity. The transmural pressure is given by P, while the density is given by ρ. Because of friction between the fluid and elastomer tube wall, F is referred to as the quasi-viscous source. It is possible to express a fully formed laminar flow as discussed in the following equation:

$$\boldsymbol{F}=-\frac{8\pi v u}{A} \tag{9.6}$$

where v is the kinematic viscosity (Zhang et al., 2016).

The fluid interaction among flow to the elastic tube wall is determined by a relation in between the pressure and the cross-sectional area, with a state equation, $P = P(A)$. Relation in between the transmural pressure and cross-sectional area as stated by the linear theory of elasticity is discussed in the following equation:

$$P-P_0=\frac{8}{3}E_L\left(1-\sqrt{\frac{A0}{A}}\right)E_L \tag{9.7}$$

9.6.1.2 FABRICATION PROCESS

Before constructing the impedance micropump, all the components were accurately measured with a digital vernier calliper. For the design of the micropump's 3D components, engineers used Google Sketchup 2020, a 3D-designing platform. There are three elements to an impedance micropump. A 3D (.stl) file that has been designed must be exported and sliced using 3D printing G.code slicing software after it has been completed. . The UV photocurable resin was 3D printed with Anycubic Photon Zero. A UV LCD screen on the DLP 3D printer allows it to project a slice of the 3D-designed item, which it then uses to 3D print the required design. Light projections to the z-axis build plate are made possible by using UV photocurable resin poured into a resin vat on the 3D printer's optically transparent base. The UV projection instantaneously cures the projected area on the build plate submerged in the resin vat and rises to the predetermined *z*-axis thickness, resulting in the perfectly produced 3D object. The linear tapping action of the tiny tapper head, which is performed by a reciprocating mechanism or what is also known as the Scotch and Yoke mechanism, drives the designed 3D impedance micropump. The small motor shaft must have some eccentricity to create a miniature reciprocating mechanism with the appropriate linear displacement. A liner displacement of 0.5 mm is required for this impedance micropump, and a little bend in the tiny motor's shaft is used to introduce the shaft and make it eccentric. A 0.5-mm stainless steel sheet is used to make an 8-mm × 3-mm tapper head with a 1-mm × 0.5-mm slot in the middle for inserting the eccentric shaft of the tiny motor to actuate it linearly as illustrated in Figure 9.12.

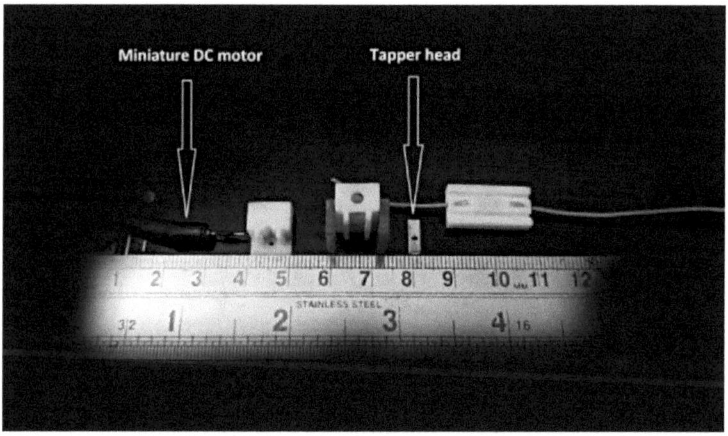

FIGURE 9.12 All 3D printed parts with miniature DC motor metal and tapper head.

Compressible elastic tubings (PDMS) and certain similar stiff tubings make up the bulk of the main impedance pump (PTFE). Compressible PDMS tubing was made in the lab using a stainless steel smooth wire with a cross-sectional diameter of 0.5 mm. PTFE tubing had previously been obtained. To begin minor crosslinking, PDMS is produced in the normal 1:10 ratio and kept at room temperature for at least 1 h. One hour after the stainless steelwire has been soaked, the sections are cut into 5 cm lengths and dipped into the PDMS elastomer. They are then dried for 20 min in a hot-air oven without turning it on to remove the extra elastomer. After 20 min, the oven is preheated to 100° and left for 30 min to fully cross-link the PDMS elastomer. Once the elastomer has been cross-linked, the elastomer covering may be readily removed with sufficient oil lubrication, as illustrated in Figure 9.15a. The next step is to cut PDMS tubings into 1 cm lengths and PTFE tubing into two sections each 10 cm long. The impedance micropump is now complete with the PDMS tubing connected end-to-end to the PTFE tubing using resin-based adhesive.

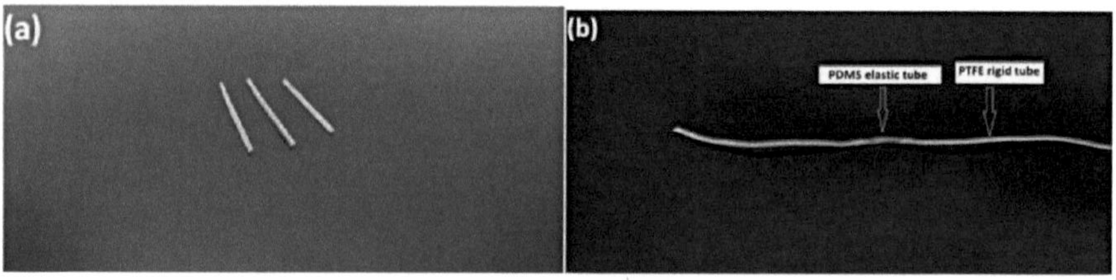

FIGURE 9.13 Fabricated (a) PDMS elastic tubing and (b) impedance micropump tubings.

9.6.2 APPLICATION 2: MICROFLUIDICS LOGIC GATE

Microfluidic technology has evolved substantially in the recent several years, and numerous theoretical research and devices that are based on applications have been developed. It is a field of biology, optics, medicine, and chemistry are only a few examples. Yang et al. (2018) created a microfluidic binary logic device. Microfluidic devices can deal with fluid volumes as tiny as a few hundred nanoliters (Mosadegh et al., 2010). As a result, this is a key component of today's microfluidic devices such as analytical technologies such as POC and lab-on-a-chip. Electrical applications have also inspired microfluidics to integrate numerous fluid handling components, cell separation, biosensors, and manipulation, and medicine administration are just a few examples, in addition to undertaking progressive research to uncover new biological applications (Gong et al., 2016). As examples, microchannels can be employed as pipelines or as active components in valves (Whitesides, 2006), mixers, and pumps (Raghu, 2013). Fluidic transistors (Cheikh and Lakkis, 2016), droplet manipulation, fluid diodes (Zhang et al., 2017), and pneumatic switches have been demonstrated. Electronics may be a viable paradigm for the future creation of functional nanoscale microfluidic devices. Several papers have investigated and analyzed the electric-fluidic analogy. Because their simplified formulations are so close, Poiseuille and Ohm's laws may be compared. To address the energy needs and irreversibility of a standard logic gate, Fredkin and Toffoli (Oh et al., 2012) presented a new form of logic gate named "Fredkin gate" (F-gate). The value of a control signal changes, this gate opens and closes its two output signals (Figure 9.14a). The logical inputs (C, A, B) and outputs (C', A', B') are crucial components in the experimental setup and analysis of energy harvesting systems for low power biomedical applications, specifically in the Lab on Chip application of Impedance micropump and microfluidic logic gate. These inputs and outputs are central to the control and monitoring of the microfluidic logic gate and impedance micropump, which play a pivotal role in regulating fluid flow and logical operations in microfluidic systems. Figure 9.14a depicts the basic Fredkin gate. When the control input signal (C) is engaged, it switches outputs A′ and B′. When C as a control signal is turned off (0: logic low), there are no A′ or B′ output signals (A, B). When

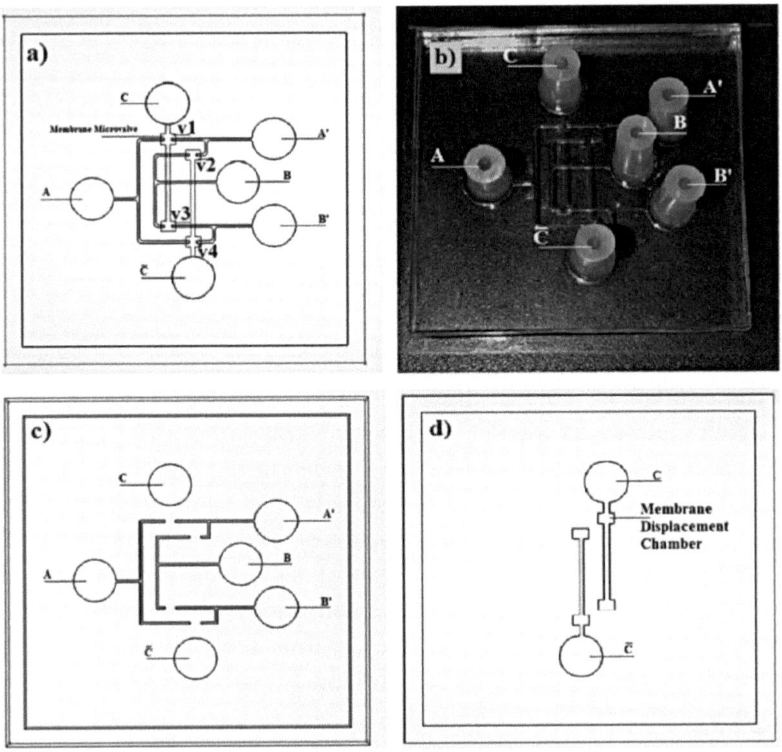

FIGURE 9.14 Design of flexible membrane microvalves for the Fredkin gate in microfluidics (a) assemble design of top and bottom (b) Fredkin gate (c) mold design top (d) bottom layer.

Source: Adapted from Ref. [43]

(1: logic high) is activated, the following happens, signals from the input are crossed across. According to the following Boolean connections, the Fredkin gate's influence on signal C determines signals A and B

TABLE 9.1 Fredkin Gate Truth Table.

Input			Output		
C	**A**	**B**	**C′**	**$A' = A\bar{C} + B\bar{C}$**	**$A' = A\bar{C} + B\bar{C}$**
0	0	0	0	0	0
0	0	1	0	0	1
0	1	0	0	1	0
0	1	1	0	1	1
1	0	0	1	0	0
1	0	1	1	1	0
1	1	0	1	0	1
1	1	1	1	1	1

C is equal to C′. If C is 0, B′ equals B and A′ equals A. If C = 1:B′ = A; A′ = B, then A′ = B.

As a result, the equation for the Fredkin gate may be generalized C is defined as C′s complement (not C).

$$A' = A\bar{C} + BC \tag{9.8}$$

$$B' = AC + B\bar{C} \tag{9.9}$$

The equivalent table of the Fredkin gate may be created by utilizing the gate's outputs as inputs. This demonstrates that the Fredkin gate is unreversible. As a result, unlike logic gates in the classical sense, it can function backward to recover the signals that were originally entered, making it informationally nondissipative. These definitions are based on the inversion of Equations (9.8 and 9.9), which Fredkin and Toffoli provided (Zaidon et al., 2006). These definitions, on the other hand, have been used in other comparable articles, and we feel they are more suited to our research. The Fredkin gate, as previously indicated, is a computationally universal gate. As a result, it is possible to use a Boolean function with only a few Fredkin gates and significantly less hardware complexity (Ajdari, 2004). Flip-flops and other sophisticated functions may be simply shown. The Fredkin gate provides two extra outputs than typical logic gates, which we can utilize or ignore.

9.6.2.1 *MICROFLUIDIC CHIP FABRICATION*

The microfluidic chip is made up of four membrane microvalves as well as control channels that connect the input and exit channels. Three layers were employed to make this device. The outermost layer houses the circular openings that enable access to the channels and the inlet–outlet channels. All channels have a 300-m cross-section, and each path has been meticulously planned to be exactly the same length (26 mm) to keep the hydraulic resistance constant. The next stratum is a 90-m-thick membrane layer. At the bottom are deflection chambers, control channels, and a membrane to cover everything. Each control channel has two-membrane deflection chambers and is 600 mm wide and 500 mm thick (2.1 mm in length, 1.5 mm in width, and 0.5 mm in thickness). The replication molding of two PDMS layers with a control and inlet–outlet microchannel network onto master molds made of 3D-printed plastic resulted in the creation of a microfluidic Fredkin gate. Each layer was 3 mm thick. Molds were created in SolidWorks (D2S, France) and printed on Vero White Plus printing material with a ProJet HD 3000 (3D Systems, USA). The upper master mold layer was coated with peroxide-cured silicone tubes (P#96400-14, Cole-Parmer, Canada), which were used to link the main and control channels' inlets and outputs.

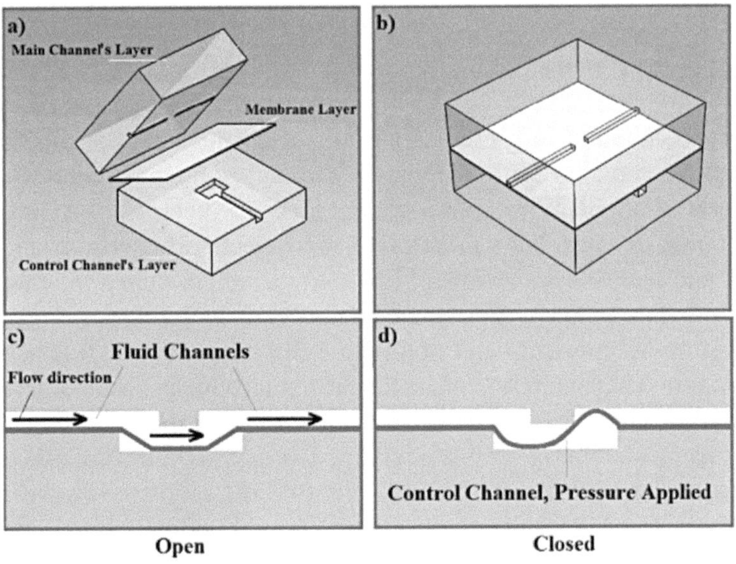

FIGURE 9.15 Schematic diagram of membrane microvalve.

The master molds were poured using PDMS prepolymer and cured at 75°C. The process was repeated for another 2.5 h to guarantee that the silicone tube and solidified PDMS were securely linked. On a silicon wafer, a PDMS membrane layer with a thickness of 90 m was created with the use of a spin coater and the formula used. A needle was used to puncture the bottoms of the tubes in the PDMS layer on top to get access to the channels. To avoid corrosion, surface passivation is essential plasma treatment from activating the solid interconnections that span the main channels (Supplementary Fig. S1). Normally, these components would connect to the bottom layer membrane during the plasma bonding process; however, this is not the case. Oil was used to wet the mesas on the metal's surface during the passivation process. Using oxygen plasma, the membrane layers and the top PDMS layer were bonded together (Harrick Plasma, USA, Plasma Flo PCD-FMS with plasma cleaner PDC-001-HP). For the control tubes of inlets to punch through the membrane and reach the bottom layer, they must first punch through the membrane; we needed them to punch through the membrane. Another punching operation is going on here. After aligning and attaching the PDMS layer at the bottom (the control layer) between the other two layers, a membrane was sandwiched, according to the supplied construction. For stability, the complete device is mounted to a sliding of glass (35 mm × 50 mm, Fisher Scientific, USA).

9.7 CONCLUSION

Battery technology advancements and electronics power requirements are not keeping up with the rising demands of many wireless sensor networking applications. As a result, there has been a lot of interest in developing devices that can extract useful electrical energy from current environmental sources. Ambient EM energy, temperature gradients, vibration, and other kinds of motion are examples of such sources. This chapter shows how to construct and optimize a full experimental test bench and simulation environment, miniaturized micropump, and microfluidic design of Fredkin logic gate. In this work, a simple modular design valveless impedance micropump is developed as an alternative to conventional pumps and micropumps for OOC microfluidic chip-based applications. The experimental results show normal growth of cells inside the OOC microfluidic chip while connected to the impedance micropump and no cellular detachment was observed inside the microfluidic chip while performing perfusion and circulation of culture media. Due to its lightweight and miniature design, it can be easily placed along with the OOC microfluidic chip inside the incubator. Its modular design makes it easy to assemble. At a later stage, it can be fully automated while maintaining its compact size. The micropump design can be further altered to make it so miniature that it could be fabricated on the OOC microfluidic chip itself.

KEYWORDS

- **electromagnetic**
- **electromagnetic energy harvesters**
- **environmental bio-energy harvesting**
- **organ-on-a-chip**
- **microfluidic**
- **radio frequency**
- **energy harvesting**

REFERENCES

Adams, M. L.; Johnston, M. L.; Scherer, A.; Quake, S. R. Polydimethylsiloxane Based Microfluidic Diode. *J. Micromech. Microeng.* **2005,** *15* (8), 1517–1521. DOI: 10.1088/0960-1317/15/8/020.

Ajdari, A. Steady Flows in Networks of Microfluidic Channels: Building on the Analogy with Electrical Circuits. *C. R. Phys.* **2004,** *5* (5), 539–546. DOI: 10.1016/j.crhy.2004.02.012.

Almouahed, S.; Gouriou, M.; Hamitouche, C.; Stindel, E.; Roux, C. Self-Powered Instrumented Knee Implant for Early Detection of Postoperative Complications. In. *Proceeding of the 32nd Annual International Conference of the IEEE (EMBS). Buenos Aires, Argentina*, Buenos Aires, Argentina, 2010; pp 5121–5124. DOI: 10.1109/IEMBS.2010.5626199.

Ashiro, R. N.; Kabei, K.; Katayama, Y.; Ishizuka, F.; Tsuboi, K.; Tsuchiya, B. Development of an Electrostatic Generator That Harnesses the Ventricular Wall Motion. *Int. J. Jpn. Soc. Artif. Organs* **2002,** *5*, 239–245.

Beeby, S. P.; Tudor, M. J. White Energy Harvesting Vibration Sources for Microsystems Applications. *Meas. Sci. Technol.* **2006,** *17*, 175–195.

Billinghurst, M.; Starner, T. Wearable Devices. New Ways to Manage Information. *IEEE J. Mag. (Comput.)* **1999,** *329* (1), 57–64.
Cheikh, M.; Lakkis, I. Microfluidic Transistors for Analog Microflows Amplification and Control. *Microfluids Nanofluids* **2016,** *20* (6), 91. DOI: 10.1007/s10404-016-1754-x.
Cheng, S.; Wu, Z. Microfluidic Electronics. *Lab Chip* **2012,** *12* (16), 2782–2791. DOI: 10.1039/c2lc21176a.
Dongeum, H.; Geraldine, A. H.; Donald, E. I. From Three Dimensional Cell Culture to Organ on Chips. *Trends Cell Biol.* **2011,** *21* (12), 745–754.
Kornbluh, R. Electroelastomers: Applications of Dielectric Elastomer Transducers for Actuation, Generation, and Smart Structures. In *Proceeding of Smart Structures and Materials (SPIE)*, San Diego, 2002; pp 254–270.
Elfrink, R.; Kamel, T. M.; Goedbloed, M.; Matova, S.; Hohlfeld, D.; Andel, V. Y.; Schaijk, V. R. Vibration Energy Harvesting with Aluminum Nitride-Based Piezoelectric Devices. *J. Micromech. Microeng.* **2009,** *19* (9), 094005.
Gong, H.; Woolley, A. T.; Nordin, G. P. High Density 3D Printed Microfluidic Valves, Pumps, and Multiplexers. *Lab Chip* **2016,** *16* (13), 2450–2458. DOI: 10.1039/C6LC00565A.
Hong, C.; Chen, J.; Chun, Z.; Zhihua, W.; Chunsheng, L. Power Harvesting With PZT Ceramics. New Orleans. *The Int. IEEE Symposium on Circuits and Systems (ISCAS)*, 2007; pp 557–560.
Hosaka, H. Personal Electric Power Generation Technology for Portable Information Equipamention. *Micro Mechatron.* **2003,** *47* (3), 38–46.
Jaeseok, Y.; Shwetak, N.; Patel, M.; Reynolds, S.; Gregory, A. D. Design and Performance of an Optimal Inertial Power Harvester for Human-Powered Devices. *IEEE Trans. Mob. Comput.* **2011,** *10* (5), 669–683.
Khaligh, A.; Peng, Z.; Cong, Z. Kinetic Energy Harvesting Using Piezoelectric and Electromagnetic Technologies—State of the Art. *IEEE Trans. Ind. Electron.* **2010,** *57* (3), 850–860. DOI: 10.1109/TIE.2009.2024652.
Khot, M. I.; Levenstein, M. A.; de Boer, G. N.; Armstrong, G.; Maisey, T.; Svavarsdottir, H. S.; Andrew, H.; Perry, S. L.; Kapur, N.; Jayne, D. G. Characterising a PDMS Based 3D Cell Culturing Microfluidic Platform for Screening Chemotherapeutic Drug Cytotoxic Activity. *Sci. Rep.* **2020,** *10* (1), 15915. DOI: 10.1038/s41598-020-72952-1.
Lachaux, J.; Hwang, G.; Arouche, N.; Naserian, S.; Harouri, A.; Lotito, V.; Casari, C.; Lok, T.; Menager, J. B.; Issard, J.; Guihaire, J.; Denis, C. V.; Lenting, P. J.; Barakat, A. I.; Uzan, G.; Mercier, O.; Haghiri-Gosnet, A. M. A Compact Integrated Microfluidic Oxygenator with High Gas Exchange Efficiency and Compatibility for Long-Lasting Endothelialization. *Lab Chip* **2021,** *21* (24), 4791–4804. DOI: 10.1039/d1lc00356a.
Luni, C.; Serena, E.; Elvassore, N. Human-on-Chip for Therapy Development and Fundamental Science. *Curr. Opin. Biotechnol.* **2014,** *25*, 45–50. DOI: 10.1016/j.copbio.2013.08.015.
Meninger, S.; Mur-Miranda, J.; Amirtharajah, R.; Chandrasakan, A. P.; Lang, J. H. Vibration to Electric Energy Conversion. *IEEE Trans. Very Large Scale Integr. Syst.* **2001,** *9* (1), 48–53.
Miao, P.; Mitcheson, P. D.; Holmes, A. S.; Yeatman, E. M.; Green, T. C.; Stark, B. H. MEMS Inertial Power Generators for Biomedical Applications. *Microsyst. Technol.* **2006,** *12* (10–11), 1079–1083. DOI: 10.1007/s00542-006-0152-9.

Mitcheson, P. D.; Yeatman, E. M.; Rao, G. K.; Holmes, A. S.; Green, T. C. Energy Harvesting from Human and Machine Motion for Wireless Electronic Devices. *Proc. IEEE* **2008,** *96* (9), 1457–1486. DOI: 10.1109/JPROC.2008.927494.

Mosadegh, B.; Kuo, C. H.; Tung, Y. C.; Torisawa, Y. S.; Bersano-Begey, T.; Tavana, H.; Takayama, S. Integrated Elastomeric Components for Autonomous Regulation of Sequential and Oscillatory Flow Switching in Microfluidic Devices. *Nat. Phys.* **2010,** *6* (6), 433–437. DOI: 10.1038/nphys1637.

Nguyen, N. T.; Wereley, S. T.; Shaegh, S. A. M. *Fundamentals and Applications of Microfluidics*; Artech House: Norwood, MA, 2019.

Oh, K. W.; Lee, K.; Ahn, B.; Furlani, E. P. Design of Pressure-Driven Microfluidic Networks Using Electric Circuit Analogy. *Lab Chip* **2012,** *12* (3), 515–545. DOI: 10.1039/c2lc20799k.

Ottesen, J. T. Valveless Pumping in a Fluid-Filled Closed Elastic Tube-System: One-Dimensional Theory with Experimental Validation. *J. Math. Biol.* **2003,** *46* (4), 309–332. DOI: 10.1007/s00285-002-0179-1.

Paradiso, J.; Kymissis, J.; Kendall, C.; Gershenfeld, N. *Parasitic Power Harvesting in Shoes. IEEE Int. Sym. Wrbl. Co.* **1998,** *24*, 132–139.

Paulo, J.; Gaspar, P. D. Review and Future Trend of Energy Harvesting Methods for Portable Medical Devices. In *Proceedings of the World Congress on Engineering (WCE)*, London, UK, 2010; pp 1–6.

Pereyma, M. Overview of the Modern State of the Vibration Energy Harvesting Devices. In *Proceeding of the International IEEE Conference on Perspective Technologies and Methods in MEMS Design (MEMSTECH)*, Ukraine Lviv-Polyana, 2007; pp 107–112. DOI: 10.1109/MEMSTECH.2007.4283437.

Platt, S. R.; Farritor, S.; Garvin, K.; Haider, H. The Use of Piezoelectric Ceramics for Electric Power Generation within Orthopedic Implants. *IEEE/ASME Trans. Mechatron.* **2005,** *10* (4), 455–461. DOI: 10.1109/TMECH.2005.852482.

Raghu, S. Fluidic Oscillators for Flow Control. *Exp. Fluids* **2013,** *54* (2), 1455. DOI: 10.1007/s00348-012-1455-5.

Ramsay, M. J.; Clark, W. W. Piezoelectric Energy Harvesting for Bio-MEMS Applications. In *Proceeding of the Smart Structures and Materials (SPIE)*, Newport Beach, CA, 2001; pp 429–438.

Renaud, M.; Karakaya, K.; Sterken, T.; Fiorini, P.; Van Hoof, C. V.; Puers, R. Fabrication, Modelling and Characterization of MEMS Piezoelectric Vibration Harvesters. *Sens. Actuat. A* **2008,** *145–146*, 380–386. DOI: 10.1016/j.sna.2007.11.005.

Rinderknecht, D.; Hickerson, A. I.; Gharib, M. A Valveless Micro-Impedance Pump Driven by Electromagnetic Actuation. *J. Micromech. Microeng.* **2005,** *15* (4), 861–866. DOI: 10.1088/0960-1317/15/4/026.

Romero, E.; Warrington, R. O.; Neuman, M. R. Energy Scavenging Sources for Biomedical Sensors. *Physiol. Meas.* **2009,** *30* (9), R35–R62. DOI: 10.1088/0967-3334/30/9/R01.

Schmidt, C. L.; Scott, E. R. Energy Harvesting and Implantable Medical Devices—First Order Selection Criteria. In *Proceeding of the Int. IEEE Conf. of Electron. Devices Meeting (IEDM),* Washington, US, 2011; pp 1051–1054. DOI: 10.1109/IEDM.2011.6131529.

Shenck, N. S.; Paradiso, J. A. Energy Scavenging with Shoe-Mounted Piezoelectrics. *IEEE Micro* **2001,** *21* (3), 30–42. DOI: 10.1109/40.928763.

Sohn, J. W.; Choi, S. B.; Lee, D. Y. An Investigation on Piezoelectric Energy Harvesting for MEMS Power Sources. *J. Mech. Eng. Sci.* **2005,** *219* (4), 429–436. DOI: 10.1243/095440605X16947.

Stamer, T. Human-Powered Wearable Computing. *IBM Syst. J.* **1996,** *5*, 618–629.

Tashiro, R. N.; Kabei, K.; Katayama, Y.; Ishizuka, F.; Tsuboi, K.; Tsuchiya, B. Development of an Electrostatic Generator That Harnesses the Motion of a Living Body. *Int. J. Jpn. Soc. Mech. Eng.* **2000,** *43*, 916–922.

Torres, E. O.; Rincón, G. A. A 0.7-µm BiCMOS Electrostatic Energy-Harvesting System IC. *IEEE J. Mag.* **2010,** *45* (2), 483–496.

Whitesides, G. M. The Origins and the Future of Microfluidics. *Nature* **2006,** *442* (7101), 368–373. DOI: 10.1038/nature05058.

Wise, K. D.; Anderson, D. J.; Hetke, J. F.; Kipke, D. R.; Najafi, K. Wireless Implantable Microsystems: High-Density Electronic Interfaces to the Nervous System. *Proc. IEEE* **2004,** *92* (1), 76–97. DOI: 10.1109/JPROC.2003.820544.

Wojciech, M. B. Thermal Integration of Combustion-Based Energy Generators by Heat Recirculation. *Rynek Energy* **2010,** *91* (6), 108–115.

Woodson, H. H.; Melcher, J. R. *Electromechanical Dynamics*; Wiley: New York, NY; Vol 1, 1968.

Yang, S. H.; Youn, J. R.; Song, Y. S. A Microfluidic Binary Logic Device Using Inertia-Elastic Particle Focusing. *Curr. Appl. Phys.* **2018,** *18* (9), 975–981. DOI: 10.1016/j.cap.2018.05.012.

Zaidon, N.; Nordin, A. N.; Ismail, A. F. Modelling of Microfluidics Network Using Electric Circuits. In *IEEE Regional Symposium on Micro and Nanoelectronics (RSM)*, 2015; pp 1–4. DOI: 10.1109/RSM.2015.7354954.

Zhang, J.; Yan, S.; Yuan, D.; Alici, G.; Nguyen, N.; Ebrahimi Warkiani, M.; Li, W. Fundamentals and Applications of Inertial Microfluidics: A Review. *Lab Chip* **2016,** *16* (1), 10–34. DOI: 10.1039/C5LC01159K.

Zhang, Q.; Zhang, M.; Djeghlaf, L.; Bataille, J.; Gamby, J.; Haghiri-Gosnet, A. M.; Pallandre, A. Logic Digital Fluidic in Miniaturized Functional Devices: Perspective to the Next Generation of Microfluidic Lab-on-Chips. *Electrophoresis* **2017,** *38* (7), 953–976. DOI: 10.1002/elps.201600429.

Zislin, V.; Rosenfeld, M. Impedance Pumping and Resonance in a Multi-vessel System. *Bioengineering (Basel)* **2018,** *5* (3), 63. DOI: 10.3390/bioengineering5030063..

CHAPTER 10

Analysis and Application of Power Amplifiers in Biomedical Instrumentation

NEEVATIKA VERMA[1], SAURABH KUMAR[2], and NITESH TIWARI[3]

[1]*Department of Electrical Engineering, Delhi Technological University, New Delhi, India*

[2]*Department of Electrical Engineering, Engineering Degree Division, Institute of Engineering and Rural Technology, Prayagraj, India*

[3]*Department of Electrical Engineering, Madan Mohan Malaviya University of Technology Gorakhpur, Uttar Pradesh, India*

ABSTRACT

Bio-amplifiers are crucial to medical implants like hearing aids, pacemakers, and other implantable devices. Thus, signal amplification is a critical component of any biomedical measurement system. Bioelectric measurements are typically low level, ranging from microvolts to millivolts. As a result, amplification is required to improve the measurement's resolution and sensitivity by increasing the input signal's level to satisfy the needs of recording or display systems or to match the range of the analog-to-digital converter. This chapter explains the characteristics of several power amplifiers, such as carrier, chopper, isolation, differential, and instrumentational amplifiers. For biomedical instrumentation, the instrumentational amplifier is the most preferred. These amplifiers are analyzed using various circuit design strategies and production methodologies. Many techniques, including level shifting, cascade, and multistage

Advanced Research in Electronic Devices for Biomedical and mHealth.
Rajesh K. Kesharwani, Upendra Kumar, Raj K. Keservani (Eds)

amplifiers, have been used to reduce power consumption and achieve high-gain and common-mode rejection ratio (CMRR) and are discussed in this chapter. This chapter highlights the advancements in bio-amplifiers in CMRR, voltage gain, noise level, and bandwidth.

10.1 INTRODUCTION

Biomedical instrumentation encompasses developing new devices and procedures that tackle medical and health-associated problems by integrating recent biology, medicine, and engineering advancements. These are done to enhance human health via cross-disciplinary procedures that integrate the design concepts of medicine and biology and engineering principles for healthcare purposes (Bajoria et al., 2011). A biomedical instrumentation system comprises an amplifier, transducer, and associated signal conditioning circuit. Biological/bioelectric signals in humans, such as EEG, ECG, and heartbeat rate, are typically weak signals (a few mV to 100 V) that must be amplified. Although operational amplifiers (Op. Amps) can be utilized, instrumentation amplifiers (I.Amps) are the most common choice for achieving the desired results. CMRR must exceed 90 dB, and voltage gain must exceed 80 dB, according to AAMI. As a result, the I.Amp is frequently employed for signal amplification (Burt and Zhang, 2006). Low dc offset, high CMRR, high gain, and small size are among the characteristics of I.Amp also offer the amplification process with the accuracy and stability it requires. I.Amp must have a high CMRR, low input-referred noise voltage, low dc offset, and low-power consumption. Designing circuits with such low power consumption and little noise has been a complex problem for a long time. CMOS technology is used to make these amplifiers (Chow and Wang, 2007). The IC was fabricated utilizing CMOS techniques such as TSMC, BSIM3V3, and SIMC processes employing 90 nm, 160 nm, 0.35 m, and 0.18 m fabrications, depending on the size and area needed of the device. Thus, the primary goal of various fabrication technologies is to decrease the power consumption, the number of transistors utilized (to minimize chip area), and the thickness of the IC chip to maximize gain without compromising the I.Amp's essential properties. Different strategies for low-power bio-amplifiers are given in this chapter. The following is how the rest of the chapter is structured: the requirement for a biological amplifier is described in Section 10.2, types of amplifiers used in biomedical measurement and their applications are presented in Section 10.3, varied amplifier performance and findings are shown in Sections 10.4–10.6, and the conclusion is offered in Section 10.7.

10.2 BASIC REQUIREMENTS FOR BIOLOGICAL AMPLIFIERS

In general, biological/bioelectric signals have low amplitude and frequency. As a result, biosignal amplifiers are developed to increase the amplitude level. The outputs of these amplifiers are analyzed further and appear as ECG, EMG, or other bioelectric waveforms. These amplifiers are referred to as bio-amplifiers or biomedical amplifiers. The biological amplifier's essential requirements are as follows (Denison et al., 2007):

- The biological amplifier's input impedance should be high. The value range is between 2 MΩ and 10 MΩ, depending on the application. When the impedance is higher, the signal is less distorted.
- The input circuit must be protected when electrodes pick up biopotentials from the human body. Every bio-amplifier should contain isolation and safety circuits to safeguard patients from electrical shocks.
- The amplifier's voltage gain should be more than 100 dB because the output of a bioelectric signal is in the millivolt (mV) or microvolt range (μV).
- A constant gain should be maintained throughout the whole bandwidth range.
- A bio-output amplifier's impedance should be very low.
- Drift and noise should be absent in a decent bio-amplifier.
- The amplifier's CMRR should be more than 80 dB to avoid interference from the common-mode signal.
- For each measurement, the biogain amplifiers should be calibrated.

10.3 TYPES OF AMPLIFIERS AND THEIR APPLICATION IN BIOMEDICAL MEASUREMENT

Any biomedical measurement would be incomplete without signal amplification. Because bioelectric measurements are often low level, that is, microvolt-level (μV) measurements, amplification is requisite to increase the measurement's resolution and sensitivity to satisfy the needs of recording/display systems or to match the range of the analog-to-digital converter. Some of the amplifiers utilized in biomedical measurement applications are discussed.

10.3.1 CARRIER AMPLIFIERS

Transducers that require an external source of excitation are employed with carrier amplifiers. High gain, small drift, extremely low noise, and the possibility to use resistive, inductive, or capacitive transducers are just a few of their characteristics.

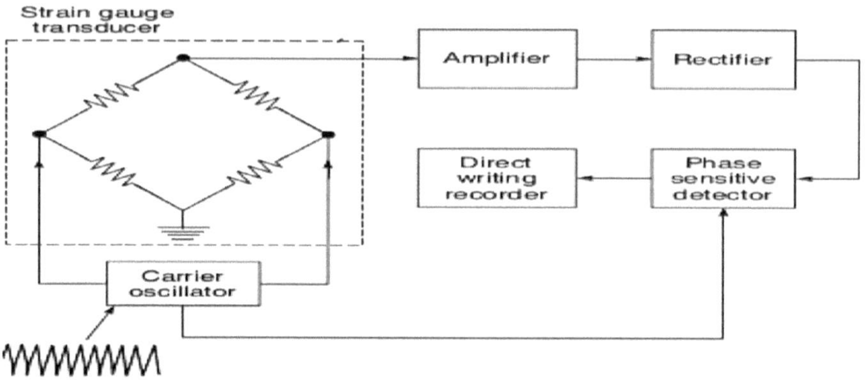

FIGURE 10.1 Block diagram carrier amplifier.

A carrier amplifier is made up of several components, including a carrier oscillator, a bridge balance, a calibration circuit, a high-gain AC amplifier, a phase-sensitive detector, and a DC output amplifier. The block diagram of the carrier amplifier is shown in Figure 10.1 (Fan et al., 2012).

10.3.2 CHOPPER AMPLIFIERS

The block diagram of the chopper amplifier is shown in Figure 10.2. The chopper amplifier amplifies microvolt-level DC signals. The chopper amplifier is used to avoid the drift problem associated with the direct-coupled amplifier. A chopping mechanism is used in the amplifier to transform a slowly fluctuating DC into an AC voltage (a chopper modulator chops the DC into a square wave).

The AC voltage amplitude is proportional to the direct input current and phase dependent on the original signal's polarity. An AC amplifier amplifies the AC square wave, which is then demodulated to produce an

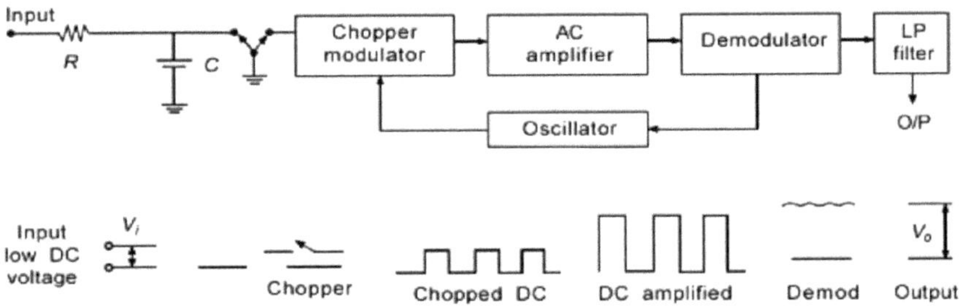

FIGURE 10.2 Block diagram of chopper amplifier.

amplified DC. Both single-ended and differential input chopper amplifiers are offered. In medicine, chopper amplifiers are used to amplify small DC signals of a few microvolts (μV). They are utilized with temperature sensors (thermistors, thermocouples), strain gauges, and other transducers.

10.3.3 ISOLATION AMPLIFIERS

To prevent against leakage currents, isolation amplifiers are utilized. They disrupt the ohmic continuity of electric signals among the amplifier's input as well as output. The block diagram of the isolation amplifier is shown in Figure 10.3. We can utilize one of three isolation methods:

- Optical isolation
- Transformer isolation
- Capacitive isolation

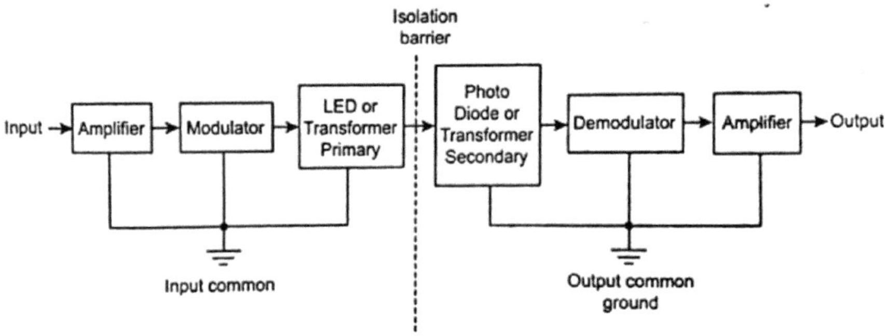

FIGURE 10.3 Block diagram of isolation amplifier.

10.3.3.1 OPTICAL ISOLATION

As shown in Figure 10.4, the light intensity of the LED in the end stage of amplification fluctuates as the input signal changes. This light is coupled to the phototransistor via an optocoupler. This light illuminates a phototransistor. The phototransistor's collector current is proportional to the light intensity. Feedback from the output may be provided for stabilizing purposes. Electrical isolation is used to safeguard patients from electrical dangers. Pacemakers, electrocardiographs, pressure monitors, pressure transducers, and other biomedical devices are designed to electrically segregate the patient's portion linked to the circuit from the section of the circuit linked to the ac power line as well as the ground.

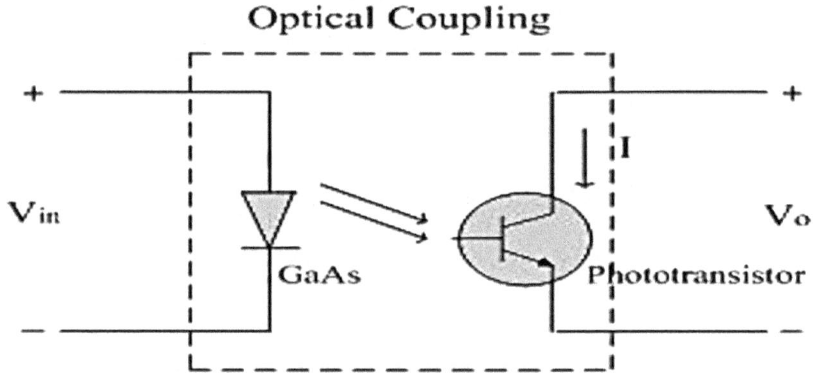

FIGURE 10.4 Block diagram of isolation amplifier.

10.4 DIFFERENTIAL AMPLIFIERS

Differential amplifiers are the most common biomedical amplifiers utilized in the input stage of a biomedical measurement system. The differential amplifier has three input terminals, one of which is set to the reference potential and the other two live as shown in Figure 10.5a. The differential amplifier is used when it is necessary to measure the voltage difference among two locations that change amplitude at different rates and in various patterns. Heart-generated voltages detected by bio-electrodes on the arms and legs, as well as brain-generated voltages detected by bio-electrodes on the scalp, are two examples of signals that must be monitored with a differential amplifier.

10.4.1 ADVANTAGES OF DIFFERENTIAL AMPLIFIERS OVER OTHER ELECTRONIC AMPLIFIERS

- Its capacity to filter out common-mode interferences, which are typically taken up by electrodes from the body along with valuable bioelectric signals.
- It offers good stability besides versatility as a direct-coupled amplifier.
- It achieves excellent stability because it is insensitive to temperature changes, which is a common source of excessive drift in other configurations.
- It is adaptable to a wide range of applications, including those that require floating inputs and outputs as well as those that require grounded inputs as well as outputs.
- Common-mode rejection refers to the differential amplifier's ability to reject common voltages on its two input leads and is to obtain the equivalent response; the ratio of common-mode input to differential input is used. The abbreviation is CMRR.
- CMRR is a critical parameter for differential amplifiers, and it is commonly represented in decibels (dB).
- In biomedical instrumentation systems, the CMRR for the input stage should be as high as possible, allowing only desired signals to flow through the amplifier while unwanted signals are rejected at the pre-amplifier stage.
- A matched pair of transistors in the input stage of the pre-amplifier and a substantial "tail" resistance in the long-tailed pair are often utilized to achieve a high rejection ratio for in-phase signals.
- To minimize the impact of fluctuations in electrode impedances, an input stage amplifier or pre-amplifier with a high input impedance is necessary. It has been demonstrated that a low-input impedance results in significant distortions in data recordings.
- Operation amplifiers are high-gain integrated dc amplifiers with differential input connections and external feedback capabilities that may perform mathematical operations. Integrated circuits are the most common form of these devices.
- Most Op.Amps have a common-mode rejection of between 60 and 90 dB. This might not be adequate to eliminate common-mode noise, which is common in biomedical measurements.

Furthermore, the input impedance is not very high, making it challenging to handle signals from high-impedance sources. Using field-effect transistors in the input differential stage is one technique to boost the Op.Amp's input impedance. Alternatively, using an instrumentation amplifier in the pre-amplifier stage is the best option. However, the differential amplifier is ideally suitable for most biomedical measuring applications; it has the following drawbacks:

- Because the amplifier's input impedance is low, it draws current from the source and loads it to a certain extent.
- In most cases, the amplifier's common-mode rejection ratio (CMMR) is less than 60 dB, which is insufficient in modern biomedical measurement systems.
- The I.Amp, which is a better form of a differential amplifier, overcomes the differential amplifier's limitations. A buffered amplifier is connected to a simple differential amplifier to make an I.Amp.

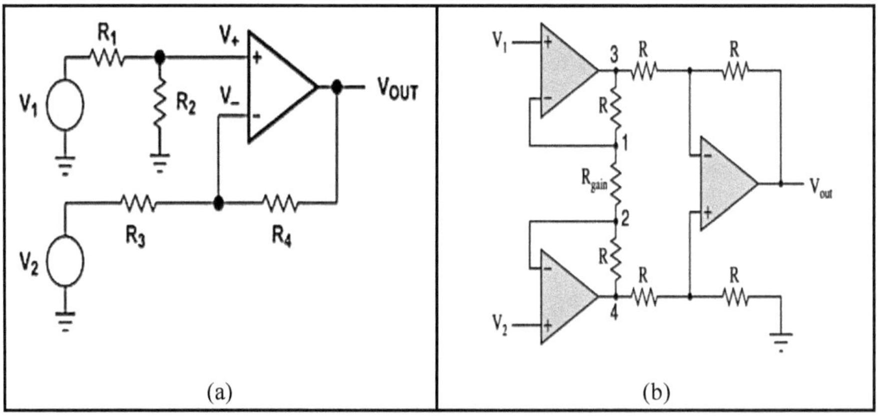

FIGURE 10.5 Schematics of (a) differential amplifier and (b) instrumentational amplifier.

10.5 INSTRUMENTATION AMPLIFIER

An I.Amp is a differential voltage gain device designed for use in environments where precision measurements are challenging to make. It is made up of three Op.Amp's and seven resistors. A buffered amplifier and a basic differential make up the I.Amp. Because a sensor generates a signal among its terminals, the differential amplifier is required for biomedical sensors.

In other cases, however, neither terminal may be connected to the same ground as your measuring circuit, resulting in the terminals being biased at a high potential or riding on a noisy voltage. The differential amplifier corrects this problem by directly measuring the difference between the sensor's terminals. The schematic diagram is shown in Figure 10.5b.

10.5.1 CRITICAL CHARACTERISTICS OF INSTRUMENTATION AMPLIFIERS

- One resistor controls the voltage gain from the differential input (V_1–V_2) to the single-ended output (RG).
- Both inputs have an extremely high input resistance that does not change while the gain is changed.
- Not the common-mode voltage, but the differential between the two input voltages determines the output voltage.

10.5.1.1 IN BIOMEDICAL APPLICATIONS, INSTRUMENTATION AMPLIFIERS ARE PREFERRED

- Their input impedance is very high.
- They have a high ratio of common-mode rejection.
- Currents with a low bias and an offset.
- Low power consumption.
- High slew rate.
- If the source impedance varies, the performance does not degrade as much.
- Independent reference levels for the source and amplifier are possible.

These benefits have led to the widespread adoption of instrumentation amplifiers in the biological system. As a result, many topologies have been proposed to improve signal amplification, while rejecting undesirable common-mode signals.

10.5.2 DIFFERENT INSTRUMENTATIONAL AMPLIFIER TOPOLOGIES

Different topologies have been proposed to improve performance in amplifying signals to compatible levels, whereas rejecting undesired common-mode signals since the I.Amp concept was introduced. The original switched-capacitor I.Amp (Burt and Zhang, 2006), the 3-opamp I.Amp employs voltage feedback, which has become the industry standard (Chow and Wang, 2007) in addition to the recently reported current-feedback I.Amp (Denison et al., 2007) and capacitively coupled I.Amp will all be discussed in the next section.

10.5.2.1 SWITCHED-CAPACITOR INSTRUMENTATIONAL AMPLIFIER

Figure 10.6a depicts the network topology of a switched-capacitor I.Amp. To perform a single operation, two steps are necessary. Phase 1 will store the input voltage in the sampling capacitors $C_{in1,2}$ and the offset of the amplifier A_1 in the offset cancellation capacitors $C_{oc1,2}$. Among the sampling capacitors, $C_{in1,2}$, also the feedback capacitors $C_{fb1,2}$, a charge distribution occurs in phase 2. The input common-mode component is efficiently eliminated since the sample plates of $C_{in1,2}$ is shorted together; also, CMRR equal to 120 dB can be attained with rail-to-rail input common-mode (Burt and Zhang, 2006). On the other hand, the switched-capacitor construction limits the amplifier's performance. The capacitor mismatch limits the gain precision since C_{in}/C_{fb} specifies the amplifier gain. A large sampling capacitor is necessary to keep the I.Amp. Noise at nV/√Hz, resulting in low input impedance. Furthermore, the switches' charge injection, as well as clock feedthrough, cause sampling noise (kT/C), which reduces amplifier precision (Fan et al., 2012).

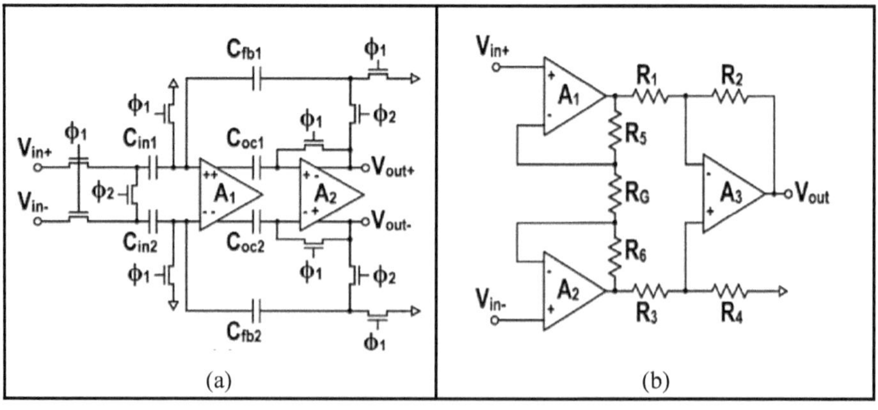

FIGURE 10.6 Topology: (a) switched-capacitor I.Amp and (b) 3-Amp I.Amp.

10.5.2.2 AMPLIFIERS WITH VOLTAGE FEEDBACK

The 3-opamp I.Amp Network topology achieves a constant gain by forming voltage feedback with resistors. The schematic of a classic 3-opamp I.Amp is shown in Figure 10.6b. To buffer the input voltage, the first stage used two Op.Amps, A_1 and A_2. In the second stage, one differential amplifier enhances the differential voltage, whereas rejecting the common-mode voltage. If R_{1-6} is matched, only one gain resistor R_G is required to establish the amplifier gain when using the following equation:

$$V_{out} = (V_{in+} - V_{in-})\left(1 + \frac{2R_5}{R_G}\right)\frac{R_2}{R_1} \quad (10.1)$$

This topology has good linearity as well as high input impedance since the inputs are buffered (Bajoria et al., 2011). A_1 and A_2 clip the input common-mode range since they cannot abide signals beyond the supply rail. Furthermore, laser-trimmed thin-film resistors are necessary for matching R_{1-6} to obtain >80 dB CMRR, which raises the cost (Ivanov, 2012). Furthermore, the 3-opamp I.Amp is not very power efficient because two low-noise, high-gain Op.Amps are required in the first stage.

10.5.2.3 AMPLIFIERS WITH CURRENT FEEDBACK

The current-feedback instrumentation amplifier (CFIAmp) is the most often used topology for precision I.Amps because it provides high CMRR and high input impedance while maintaining a large common-mode input range. Input and output transconductors G_{in} and G_{out} and a feedback G_{fb} make up a standard CFIAmp. The input voltage V_{in} and the feedback voltage V_{fb} are transformed to current via G_{in} and G_{fb}, respectively, as shown in Figure 10.7a. $V_{in}G_{in} = V_{fb}G_{fb}$ is guaranteed by the considerable G_{out} and the feedback loop. $R_{1,2}$ (Kwon et al., 2019) can be used to set the gain by matching G_{in} and G_{fb} in the following equation:

$$V_{out} = (V_{in+} - V_{in-})\left(\frac{R_1 + R_2}{R_2}\right)\frac{G_{in}}{G_{fb}} \quad (10.2)$$

To obtain a high CMRR, the CFIAmp employs isolation and balancing techniques. Because G_{in} has a high output impedance, the input common-mode voltage causes only a little common-mode current, which quickly cancels out at the feedback node. Indirect current feedback isolates the input and output common-mode voltages, resulting in a CMRR of more than 120 dB (Witte et al., 2008). The matching of the input and feedback transconductors G_{in} and G_{fb} determines the gain accuracy of the CFIAmp. Gain precision of 0.1% can be achieved using CFIAmp in most cases. However, three transconductors are required; CFIAmp's high-power consumption prevented its use in low-power designs.

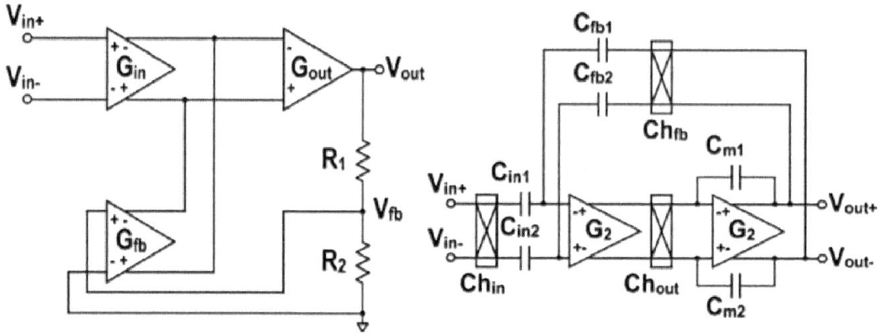

FIGURE 10.7 Topology: (a) Current-feedback I.Amp and (b) capacitively coupled I.Amp.

10.5.2.4 AMPLIFIERS WITH CAPACITIVELY COUPLED CHOPPER

Fundamental network topology and design deliberations of amplifiers with capacitively coupled chopper are discussed below.

10.5.2.4.1 Fundamental Network Topology

Recently, the topology of a capacitively coupled I.Amp with chopper stabilization was stated, particularly useful for biopotential sensing. A capacitively coupled chopper instrumentation amplifier (CCIAmp) comprises an Op.Amp and a capacitive feedback network, as it is shown in Figure 10.7b. C_{in}/C_{fb} controls CCIAmp gain in the same way as switched-capacitor I.Amp does. Using an input chopper Ch_{in} before amplification and an output chopper Ch_{out} after amplification, the input signal is first shifted to high frequencies, then amplified and shifted back, while the amplifier offset and $1/f$ noise are only shifted to high frequencies. An amplifier's offset and $1/f$ noise can be eliminated after filtering. Due to the lack of transconductors in the feedback loop, CCIAmps are more suited to low-power designs. Compared to I.Amp based on the three traditional topologies, a CCIAmp has four main advantages.

1. Rail-to-rail-sensing capability: The use of complementary switches allows a CCIAmp to have a rail-to-rail DC CM input range without the need for a rail-to-rail Op.Amp input stage.
2. High-power efficiency: The Op.Amp noise dominates the noise of a CCIAmp (Denison et al., 2007; Yeager et al., 2010), making it more power-efficient than three-Op.Amp as well as current-feedback I.Amps.
3. High-gain accuracy: Deep submicron technology's precise lithography ensures robust matching between C_{in} and C_{fb}. As a result, high-gain accuracy is achieved without the requirement for trimming.
4. Appropriateness for low-power design: With very large impedances, the capacitive feedback network can be set up, which reduces the feedback network's current consumption, particularly for significant output signals.

10.5.2.4.2 Design Deliberations

Figure 10.7b depicts a block diagram of the planned CCIAmp. It consists of a two-stage Miller-compensated Op.Amp with a transconductance input. G_{M1} and an integrator built around G_{M2}. Around the Op.Amp is a capacitive bridge made up of input capacitors $C_{in1,2}$ as well as feedback capacitors $C_{fb1,2}$. The gain G of the CCIAmp is certain by taking into account the Op.Amp's finite open-loop gain.

$$G = \frac{A_0}{1 + A_0 C_{fb1,2} / C_{in1,2}} \tag{10.3}$$

A_0 denotes the Op.Amp's open-loop gain. For instance, A_0 should be more than 100 dB to ensure a less than 0.1% gain error. A single-stage Miller-compensated Op.Amp would not achieve this. As a result, a Miller-compensated Op.Amp with two stages was adopted. The grouping of $CH_{in1,2}$ as well as $C_{in1,2}$ can be considered as a $1/2 f_{chop} C_{in}$ equivalent input resistor, where f_{chop} is the chopping frequency. This resistor, therefore, determines the input impedance of the CCIAmp. The combination of CH_{fb} and C_{fb} can be thought of as a $1/2f_{chop}C_{in}$ equivalent feedback resistor, where f_{chop} is the chopping frequency. These resistors, therefore, determine the input impedance of the CCIAmp. The combination of CH_{fb} and C_{fb} can be thought of as a $1/2\,f_{chop}C_{fb}$ equivalent feedback resistor that loads the CCIAmp's output stage. CH_{out} upmodulates the offset and $1/f$ noise of G_{M1}, which is then filtered by the integrator built around G_{M2}. The ripple-reduction loop (RRL) described in the next section will suppress the upmodulated offset and $1/f$ noise of G_{M2}, while the gain of G_{M1} will suppress the offset and $1/f$ noise of G_{M2}. High-resistance resistors configured as MOS transistors operating in their subthreshold region correctly bias the DC level at the Op.Amp's input to a reference voltage V_{ref} (Denison et al., 2007). The choppers' operation will produce spikes because the input and output signal voltages constantly charge and discharge the bridge capacitors $C_{in1,2}$ and C_{fb}. The output spikes associated with $C_{fb1,2}$ will be sent to a succeeding ADC and may cause inaccuracy due to the Op.Amp's finite output impedance. The output stage of the CCIAmp Op.Amp must be able to generate currents substantially more extensive than the average DC current necessary to operate the capacitive bridge to limit the duration of these spikes. Smaller feedback capacitors with lower capacitance matching can be used to lessen the amplitude of the spikes. To reduce the spikes, a low-pass filter can be applied after the CCIAmp, but this comes at the cost of increased power consumption and chip space. A better method is to ensure that the following ADC samples the CCIAmp's output only after it has settled ultimately. In fully integrated systems, this is simple to implement.

10.5.2.4.3 Implementation

The CCIAmp's gain is set to 100 in this implementation. The frequency of f_{chop} is set to 5 kHz, more significant than G_{M1}'s $1/f$ noise corner. More charge injection and clock feedthrough will increase f_{chop}, resulting in a greater residual offset (Burt and Zhang, 2006). Resistance is around 8 MΩ without parasitic effects and 800 MΩ with $C_{in1,2}$ = 12 pF. Fringe capacitors were used to build the capacitive bridge (metal–oxide–metal). The Op.Amp is depicted schematically in Figure 10.8. G_{M1} is implemented as a folded-cascode OTA, whereas G_{M2} is implemented as a class A output stage with a large output swing. Despite their relatively high threshold voltages, all of the transistors employed in the CCIAmp are thick-oxide transistors (0.6 V). This is due to the low-gate leakage currents and increased inherent gain of such transistors. Leakage currents can create considerable faults in a low-power design, particularly at the Op.Amp's virtual ground node (Va). The bias resistors have a resistance of roughly 10 GΩ due to noise considerations; Thus, gate leakage from the two PMOS input transistors is sufficient to clip the input voltage. The two-stage Miller-compensated CCIAmp Op.Amp's simulated DC gain is 130 dB, which translates to a gain error of 0.01% for $G = 100$, according to Equation (10.3). Because $C_{in1,2}/C_{fb1,2}$ determines most of the gain, the ultimate gain inaccuracy will be calculated by $C_{in1,2}/C_{fb1,2}$'s spread process and variation, which is predicted to be around 0.1%. The noise of the G_{M1} input stage dominates the noise of the CCIA. To achieve great power efficiency, the input PMOS differential pair is biased in weak inversion.

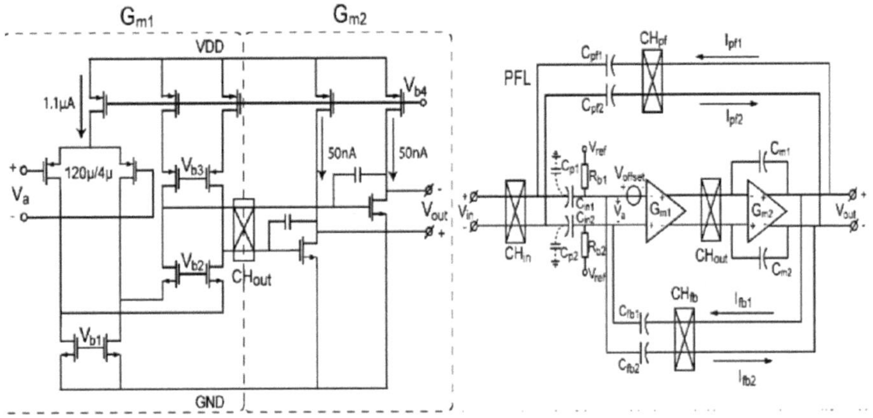

FIGURE 10.8 Schematic of (a) the CCIAmp and (b) the CCIAmp with the positive feedback loop.

It consumes 61% of the total supply current, resulting in a simulated noise voltage density $V_{nOp.Amp}$ of the input stage of 55 nV√Hz. The CCIAmp's input-referred noise is essentially equal to $V_{nOp.Amp}$ (Denison et al., 2007) when $C_{in1,2}/C_{fb1,2} = 100$. Because the Miller capacitor $C_{M1,2}$ (fringe capacitor) is 30 pF, the CCIAmp's unity-gain frequency is 70 kHz. The class A output stage's bias current is set to 2 × 50 nA, enough to drive the capacitive bridge with a 1 V_{pp} output signal. The bias resistors $R_{b1,2}$ are implemented as subthreshold NMOS transistors. Their resistance is tuned to around 10 GΩ to achieve an input noise density of roughly 10 nV√Hz (Denison et al., 2007), which is minimal in comparison to the CCIAmp as a whole.

10.5.2.4.4 Drawback of CCIAmp

The CCIAmp has two significant flaws: (1) limited input impedance, which is mainly dictated by $C_{in1,2}$'s equivalent resistance and f_{chop}; and (2) chopping ripple caused by G_{M1}'s upmodulated offset and $1/f$ noise. A positive feedback loop (PFL) is used to increase the CCIAmp's input impedance. It is made up of a positive feedback path that connects the CCIAmp's input and output. It transforms the output voltage into a current that is fed back into the signal source. The current drawn from the signal source by the switching capacitor resistor created by C_{Hin} and $C_{in1,2}$ is partially compensated by this current, increasing the CCIAmp's input impedance. The upmodulated offset and $1/f$ noise of G_{M1} are primarily responsible for the chopping ripple. A RRL is used to suppress it (Hsiao et al., 2012; Kusuda, 2010). This detects ripple at the CCIAmp output and creates a current to compensate for the offset current of G_{M1}. There will be no output ripple when this current is appropriately adjusted. A DC servo loop (DSL) can be used in biosensing applications when high DC electrode offsets are predicted. The DSL is essentially a negative feedback integrating path. The output of the CCIAmp is integrated, and the resulting signal is sent back to its virtual ground, canceling any DC component at the CCIAmp's output. The DSL functions as a high-pass filter effectively rejecting electrode offset that would otherwise saturate the CCIAmp. The PFL, RRL, and DSL's operating principles and design concerns will be discussed in further depth in the following sections.

10.5.2.4.5 Positive Feedback Loop (PFL)

Working principle and implementation of PFL are discussed below.

10.5.2.4.5.1 Working Principle

Figure 10.8b shows a block schematic of the CCIAmp with a PFL. A chopper CH_{pf} and two feedback capacitors $C_{pf1,2}$ offer positive feedback to the CCIAmp's input in this loop. The PFL creates currents $I_{pf1,2}$ equal to $I_{fb1,2}$ in the ideal scenario. Therefore, no input current is pulled from the signal source, and the CCIAmp's input impedance is infinite. Making $I_{pf1,2}$ and $I_{fb1,2}$ equal, the value of $C_{pf1,2}$ for infinite input impedance can be calculated:

$$\begin{aligned} I_{pf1,2} &= 2\left(V_{out} - V_{in}\right) \times C_{pf1,2} \times f_{chop} \\ &= 2V_{out} \times C_{pf1,2} \times f_{chop} = I_{pf1,2} \\ &\geq C_{pf1,2} = \frac{C_{in1,2}}{G-1} \end{aligned} \quad (10.4)$$

Because the CCIAmp must supply the current running through it, the PFL charges the CCIAmp. 1/2 f_{chop} is the comparable loading resistance. $C_{pf1,2}$ = 800 MΩ. This loading is the same as the $C_{fb1,2}$ negative feedback path.

10.5.2.4.5.2 Implementation

To achieve an infinite input impedance with G = 100, $C_{in1,2}$ = 12 pF, and $C_{fb1,2}$ = 120 fF, $C_{pf1,2}$ must be 121.21 fF (Eq. 10.2). This can be difficult to the layout. Therefore, it is decided to be equal to $C_{fb1,2}$ in this work. The compromised enhanced input impedance of the CCIAmp is then given by

$$Z_{in\_pf} = \frac{V_{in}}{I_{in\_pf}} = \frac{G}{2f_{chop} \times C_{in1,2}} = 100Z_{in} \quad (10.5)$$

I_{in_pf} is the net current pulled from the signal source, where Z_{in} is the actual input impedance, and Z_{in_pf} is the boosted input impedance.

10.5.2.4.5.3 Parasitic Effects

In practice, the parasitic capacitance $C_{p1,2}$ (shown in Figure 10.8b) between $C_{in1,2}$'s bottom plate and the ground will further reduce the input impedance. With a resistance of 1/2 f_{chop}, CH_{in} and $C_{p1,2}$ serve as an equivalent parasitic resistor As per discussion in Section 10.5.2.4.5.2, a PFL dimensioned will not be compensated for the current taken by this register. As a result, the maximum input impedance is limited by this parasitic resistor. $C_{p1,2}$ typically accounts for 10–40% of $C_{in1,2}$ in a normal CMOS process. As a result, a PFL dimensioned according to Equation (10.4) will only raise the input impedance by 2.5× to 10×. The PFL can be built to compensate for the extra current flowing via the parasitic resistor $I_{p1,2}$. The following is how Equation (10.4) can be changed:

$$\begin{aligned} I_{pf_{modi1,2}} &= 2(V_{out} - V_{in}) \times C_{pf1,2_{modi}} \times f_{chop} \\ &= I_{fb1,2} + (V_{in}) \times C_{p1,2} \times f_{chop} = I_{fb1,2} + I_{p1,2} \\ &= C_{pf1,2\_modi} = \frac{C_{in1,2} + C_{p1,2}}{G-1} \end{aligned} \quad (10.6)$$

The modified compensatory current provided by the PFL is $I_{pf\_modi1,2}$, and is the best value for $C_{pf1,2}$. However, because the exact value of $C_{p1,2}$ will be unpredictable in practice, $C_{pf1,2}$ can be made flexible to achieve maximum input impedance.

10.5.2.4.6 Loop of Ripple Reduction

Working principle and implementation of loop of ripple reduction are discussed below.

10.5.2.4.6.1 Working Principle

The offset and $1/f$ noise of the upmodulated G_{M1} cause a ripple at the CCIAmp's output. The ripple at the output is around 10 mV G_{M1} offset, G_{M1} = 13 S, f_{chop} = 5 kHz, and $C_{m1,2}$ = 30 pF.

$$V_{ripple} = \frac{V_{offset} \times G_{m1}}{2f_{chop} \times C_{m1,2}} = \frac{10\,\text{mV} \times 13\,\mu\text{S}}{2 \times 5\,\text{kHz} \times 30\,\text{pF}} = 433\,\text{mV} \quad (10.7)$$

For a 1-V supply, this would require too much clearance and would have to be suppressed. Increasing f_{chop} and $C_{m1,2}$ results in a greater residual offset and more chip area, whereas decreasing G_{M1} results in more noise. There are several successful methods for reducing the ripple. To notch out the chopping ripple, Burt and Zhang (2006) used a switched-capacitor notch filter. This approach uses relatively little energy. However, using a notch filter in the signal route makes frequency correction more difficult. To lessen the ripple in Kusuda (2010), an auto-correction loop is used. This strategy makes the frequency adjustment process more accessible. On the other hand, the loop detects the ripple at a virtual ground node, where it is rather modest, necessitating a relatively high gain.

An AC-linked continuous-time RRL is used in this study (Fan et al., 2012; Wu et al., 2009). Figure 10.9a shows a block diagram of the RRL. Sensing capacitors $C_{s1,2}$, a demodulating chopper CH_{RRL}, an integrator, and a compensating transconductor G_{M4} make up the circuit. $C_{S1,2}$ senses and converts the significant ripple voltage at the amplifier's output into an AC current, which is then integrated by the integrator into a voltage, which G_{M4} then transforms into a current, compensating for G_{M1}'s offset current. At f_{chop}, the RRL forms a notch whose breadth is chosen by variable design factors like $C_{s1,2}$ and G_{M4} (Wu et al., 2009). The critical disadvantage of this method compared to Fan et al. (2012) is that $C_{s1,2}$ burdens the amplifier's output and should thus be kept minimal. The RRL in Fan et al. (2012) and Wu et al. (2009) uses a passive integrator consisting of a current buffer and an integration capacitor. However, the offset of the current buffer causes a second harmonic ripple, which may necessitate a large integration capacitor to filter (Fan et al., 2012). Low f_{chop} makes this more difficult. An auto-zeroed SC integrator can be used to solve this problem. An average auto-zeroed SC integrator, on the other hand, is reset during one phase to record its offset on an auto-zero capacitor. The integrator's output must not be linked to G_{M4} during this phase, or an error-compensating current will be injected into the $CCIA_{mp}$. An auto-zeroed SC integrator with correct output voltage during all phases is offered to solve this problem. Figure 10.9b shows a block diagram of the RRL with such an integrator. Sensing capacitors $C_{s1,2}$, a demodulation chopper CH_{RRL}, integration capacitors $C_{int1,2}$, auto-zero capacitors $C_{az1,2}$, and a single-stage Op.Amp G_{M3} make up the SC integrator. CH_{RRL} is in sync with f_{chop}. The remaining switches (S_1–S_6) are driven at a switching frequency of f_s, which is half of f_{chop}. The RRL can detect a total cycle ripple during phase 1 since f_s has an integration phase 1 and an auto-zero phase 2, each of which incorporates a complete cycle of f_{chop}. Figure 10.9b depicts a timing diagram. $C_{s1,2}$ converts the ripple voltage into an AC current during 1, which is subsequently demodulated by CH_{RRL} and integrated on $C_{int1,2}$. To compensate for G_{M1}'s offset current, G_{M4} converts the voltages on $C_{int1,2}$ into a current. During 2, $C_{S1,2}$ is shorted to ground, preventing the integration of ripple current. The offset of G_{M3} is sampled and saved on $C_{az1,2}$ since it is configured in unity-gain mode. $C_{int1,2}$ is disconnected from G_{M3}'s output during this time, holding the voltage set at the conclusion of the last 1 and linked to G_{M4}'s input. G_{M1} receives the correct compensatory current in both phases as a result of this. The compensating current fully compensates for G_{M1}'s offset current in an ideal scenario, leaving no output ripple in a steady state.

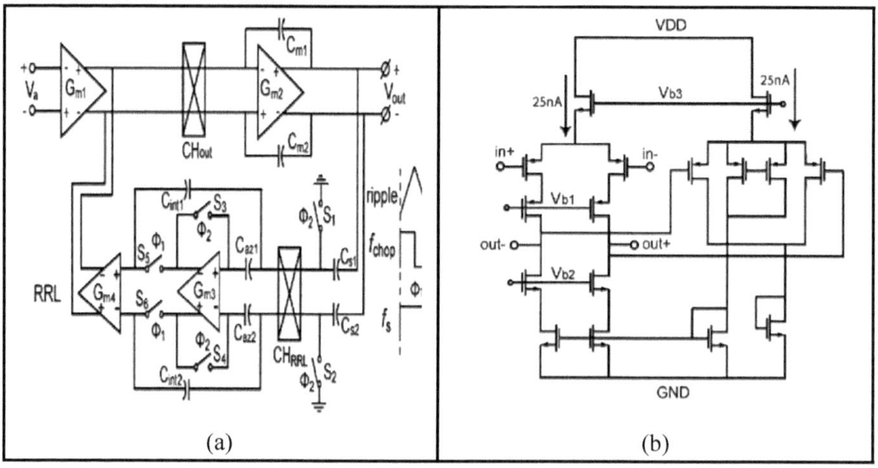

FIGURE 10.9 Schematic of (a) the ripple-reduction loop and (b) ripple-reduction loop switched capacitor integrated Op.Amp.

10.5.2.4.6.2 Implementation

The RRL's unity-gain frequency is determined by the values of $C_{s1,2}$, $C_{int1,2}$, and the transconductance of G_{M4}, which is given by Wu et al. (2009).

$$f_{0RRL} = \frac{G_{m4} C_{s1,2}}{2piC_m C_{int1,2}} \tag{10.8}$$

The RRL's notch width is equivalent to $2f_{0RRL}$. With the CCIAmp's bandwidth set to 700 Hz and f_{chop} set to 5 kHz, f_{0RRL} should be less than 4.3 kHz to keep the signal bandwidth of the CCIAamp. Furthermore, the value of G_{M4} must usually be lower than G_{M1} to reduce the noise of the RRL V_{nRRL}, which is derived using the following equation when applied to the CCIAamp's input.

$$V_{nRRL} = \left(\frac{C_{in1,2} + C_{fb1,2} + C_g}{C_{in1,2}} \right) \frac{\sqrt{\left(V_{ninte}^2 + V_{nGm4}^2\right) G_{m4}}}{G_{m1}} \tag{10.9}$$

where V_{ninte} is the RRL integrator's output voltage noise, and $V_{nG_{M4}}$ is G_{M4}'s input voltage noise. G_{M4} is meant to be 0.65 S, which is 20× smaller than G_{M1}, to make V_{nRRL} minimal compared to G_{M1}'s noise. Using $C_{S1,2}$ = 240 fF, $C_{int1,2}$ = 2.5 pF, and $C_{M1,2}$ = 30 pF, Equation (10.6) calculates f_{0RRL} to be roughly 330 Hz, which is significantly less than 4.3 kHz. This RRL hardly loads the CCIAmp output with $C_{s1,2}$ = 240 fF. To minimize charge injection errors from switch $S_{3,4}$ and preserve chip area, $C_{az1,2}$ was set to 1.4 pF. To achieve significant DC open-loop gain, the G_{M3} uses a telescopic architecture, as shown in Figure 10.9b. The loop gain of the RRL is determined by $A_{G_{M3}}$, which is provided by

$$L(0) = \frac{A_{G_{M3}} G_{M4}}{C_{M1,2} f_{chop}} \tag{10.10}$$

The ripple should ideally be dampened by a factor of $L(0)$. To suppress output ripple by 1000 times and keep the input-referred ripple on the order of a few microvolts, at least 48 dB is required. The telescopic's open-loop gain is simulated to be 76. The G_{M3} requires 50 nA of supply current, which is insignificant when compared to the CCIAamp's total current usage.

10.5.2.4.7 DC Servo Loop

10.5.2.4.7.1 Working Principle and Implementation

When a substantial electrode offset is present, the DSL can be used for biosensing. Although disabling the choppers around the CCIAmp can readily yield a high-pass transfer function (Verma et al., 2010; Yeager et al., 2010), the reduced CMRR owing to feedback capacitor mismatch is undesirable. Chopping is maintained to achieve a high CMRR, and a high-pass transfer function is accomplished by implementing a DSL, as described in Denison et al. (2007). The CCIAmp's restricted bandwidth is automatically granted the low-pass feature, which is greater than the maximum ECG/EEG signal bandwidth (around 100 Hz). Figure 10.10 shows a block diagram of the CCIAmp with such a DSL. The DSL consists of an integrator that amplifies the DC signal at the CCIAmp's output, a chopper that upmodulates the amplified DC signal, and capacitors $CH_{p1,2}$ that feed the upmodulated signal to the virtual ground of the CCIAmp. The integrator will continue to integrate until the signal at the CCIAmp's output is DC free. The DSL generates a high-pass corner f_{hp}, as described in Denison et al. (2007).

$$f_{hp} = \frac{C_{hp1,2}}{C_{fb1,2}} f_{0DSL} \tag{10.11}$$

where f_{0DSL} is the integrator's unity-gain frequency in the DSL. For biosignals such as ECG/EEG signals, F_{hp} is set to 0.5 Hz (Yazicioglu et al., 2008; Verma et al., 2010). The values of $C_{hp1,2}$ are calculated using the equation below:

$$V_{outmax} = \frac{C_{in1,2}}{C_{hp1,2}} V_{eo} \tag{10.12}$$

where V_{eo} is the maximum predicted electrode offset and V_{outmax} is the DSL integrator's maximum output voltage (V_{DSL_OUT}), which in this case equals 1 V. A maximum V_{eo} of 50 mV can be expected for wet electrodes. As a result, $C_{hp1,2}$ is set to 600 fF. f_{0DSL}, on the other hand, is estimated to be 0.1 Hz (Eq. 10.9). With such a low unity-gain frequency, an SC integrator can take up a lot of chip space, which is not ideal for wireless sensor nodes. A considerable time constant (VLT) SC integrator is used in this study to reduce chip area considerably.

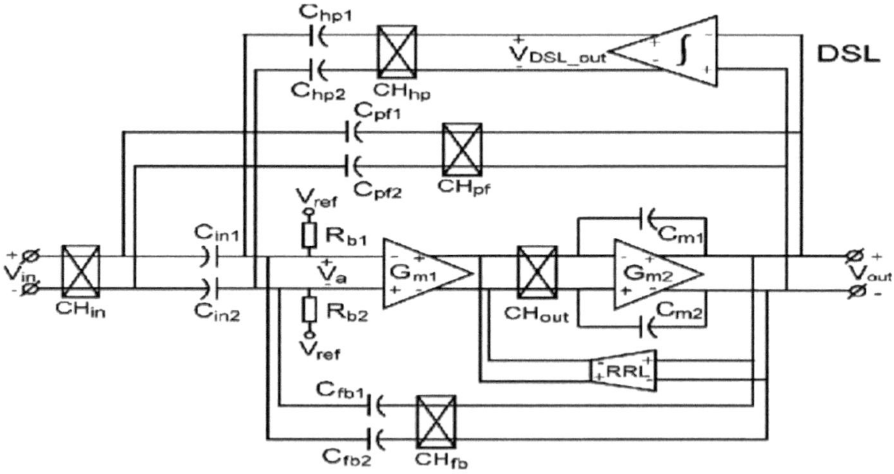

FIGURE 10.10 Schematic of CCIAmp with optional DC servo loop.

10.5.2.4.7.2 Very-Large Time Constant SC Integrator (VLT-SC Integrator)

Figure 10.7 shows a block schematic of the VLT-SC integrator. The integrator consists of an Op.Amp and a capacitor network ($C_{a1,2}$, $C_{A1,2}$, $C_{a'1,2}$, and S_1–S_7) around it. To sample at the zero-crossing point of the

CCIAmp's output ripple, all switches in the capacitor network are powered at a switching frequency f_{sVLT} equal to $2f_{chop}$. Figure 10.10 depicts a timing diagram. When $C_{a1,2} = C_{a'1,2}$, the transfer function of a VLT-SC integrator is provided by the equation:

$$H(Z) = -\frac{Z^{-1/2}}{1-Z^{-1}}\left(\frac{C_{a1,2}}{C_{A1,2}}\right)^2 \quad (10.13)$$

The VLT-SC integrator's unity-gain frequency f_{0VLT} can be calculated by setting (*Z*) to unity.

$$f_{0VLT} = \frac{f_{sVLTC^2_{a1,2}}}{2piC^2_{A1,2}} \quad (10.14)$$

A standard fully differential SC integrator's unity-gain frequency is determined by

$$f_{0stand} = \frac{f_{swiC_{sam}}}{2piC_{inte1,2}} \quad (10.15)$$

The switching frequency for switches S_1–S_4 is f_{swi}. When switching at 2.5 kHz, the VLT-SC integrator employs $C_{a1,2} = C_{a'1,2} = 240$ fF and $C_{A1,2} =$ 15 pF to produce the 0.1-Hz unity-gain frequency computed by Equation (10.9), whereas a regular integrator must need $C_{inte1,2} = 937.5$ pF according to Equation (10.13) to obtain the same unity-gain frequency with the same sampling capacitor! This demonstrates how the VLT-SC integrator saves a lot of space.

10.6 METRICS INVESTIGATION

Table 10.1 summarizes the results of the most recent I.Amp designs. Low cost, low-power, low-noise, and quick startup settling are sought for biomedical applications. The following sections look at several metrics as well as some existing strategies for improving them.

10.6.1 CMRR

With careful layout design and further trimming, the traditional 3-opamp can only attain 80 dB CMRR (Kwon et al., 2019). CFIAmp and

CCIAmp have lately received attention since I.Amp's should have >120 dB CMRR for precise signal acquisition (Wu et al., 2011). CFIAmp beats all other topologies in CMRR because of the isolation and high impedance of the input transconductor. Several strategies can be applied to I.Amp to boost CMRR even more. CMRR can be improved by using laser-trimmed thin-film resistors, but this comes at a cost. Chopping and offset cancellation techniques can be used together to achieve a CMRR of >130 dB (Witte et al., 2008).

10.6.2 INPUT BIAS CURRENT

Input bias current in CMOS transistors is in the pA range, but it varies greatly depending on temperature and technology. Because of the charge injection and clock feedthrough, the input biases current increases dramatically when choppers are used. Given the high input source impedance, a 1-nA input bias current can produce a 100-V offset voltage, which is quite impressive when compared to the I.Amp offset's voltage (Burt and Zhang, 2006). To maintain an acceptable input bias current, designers must keep in mind that the current source must be biased in strong inversion, and the chopping frequency should never exceed a few hundred kHz (100 pA). Using extra coupling capacitors and a switch-driven inverter (Kusuda (2015) proposes an on-chip charge mismatch correction circuit to further minimize the input bias current.

10.6.3 INPUT OFFSET

Chopping is the most common method for lowering the I.Amp offset. In unlike auto-zeroing, which suffers from aliasing and noise folding during sampling, chopping moves the input offset and low-frequency noise to the chopping frequency (tens to hundreds of kHz), while maintaining the broadband noise characteristics reducing flicker noise and voltage drift. The ripple that arises at the output after chopping, on the other hand, is a source of concern, and it must be eliminated using techniques like double sampling, notch filtering, RRL, auto-correction feedback loop, or trimming (Burt and Zhang, 2006). Some research suggests employing an AC-coupled RRL to sense and feedback the modulated ripple at the output via a local feedback loop to cancel the original offset (Fan et al., 2011, 2012; Wu et al., 2009).

10.6.4 GAIN ACCURACY

The degree to which the measured gain matches the predetermined amount is referred to as gain accuracy. Precision I.Amp often requires gain accuracy of 0.1%, and the gain should be insensitive to PVT variation (Bajoria et al., 2011). The amplifier gain is specified differently for different topologies, either through resistance or capacitance ratios. The ratio of the input capacitance to the feedback capacitance determines the gain of both switched-capacitor I.Amp and CCIAmp. Capacitance matching is mainly dictated by the process spread and variation as lithography technology advances. Thus, with no trimming, the gain accuracy of normal switched-capacitor I.Amp and CCIAmp should be around 0.1%, which is adequate for precision I.Amp applications (Wu et al., 2009). A voltage feedback network was developed in the 3-Op.Amp I.Amp technique, and a single resistor controlled the gain. To minimize the gain error to 0.3%, the industry used a laser-trimmed on-chip thin-film resistor. The gain drift with temperature is still significant (tens of ppm/C), and metal film resistors often have a 1% resistance fluctuation (Kwon et al., 2019). The mismatch of the input and feedback transconductors, on the other hand, limits the gain accuracy of CFIAmp. Low-threshold cascode transistors can be utilized in the input stage to improve gain accuracy, but no more than 0.5% matching can be achieved. Another method is to use resistors to apply source degeneration to the input pair and then use resistors to establish the input transconductance with an untrimmed precision of 0.1% (Kwon et al., 2019). In Bajoria et al. (2011), a dynamic element matching technique is developed to improve gain accuracy further at the expense of additional ripple suppression circuits.

10.6.5 NOISE

To assess the performance of different I.Amp designs, the noise efficiency factor (NEF) was created. The input-referred noise V_{rms} of the I.Amp is compared to the thermal noise of a bipolar transistor or MOSFET to define it.

$$\mathrm{NEF} = V_{\mathrm{rms,in}} \sqrt{\frac{2 \times I_{\mathrm{tol}}}{pi \cdot U_T \cdot 4kT \cdot \mathrm{BW}}} = \vartheta \sqrt{\frac{2 \times I_{\mathrm{tol}}}{pi \cdot U_T \cdot 4kT}} \quad (10.16)$$

where I_{tol} denotes the I.Amp supply current, U_{T} denotes the thermal voltage, and BW denotes the I.Amp bandwidth. To negate the bandwidth term, NEF can also be stated by replacing V_{rms} with its noise spectrum ϑ in V/√Hz. Using NEF^2 VDD, a modified metric, power efficiency factor, was proposed to account for the various supply voltages in different designs. To improve noise performance, several I.Amp topologies are presented. The simple two-transistor structure of inverter-based OTA allows for ultralow supply voltage design and minimizes total input noise (Chow and Wang, 2007). The current-reuse technology reduces the NEF by 1.4 by doubling the input transistor transconductance. The NEF was also improved by other strategies such as stacked transistors and partial OTA sharing (Han et al., 2013). The I.Amp bandwidth employed in the sensor node is typically minimal (less than 1 kHz). In general, I.Amp with a smaller gain bandwidth has a smaller NEF. However, as discussed below, and I.Amp with a lower NEF does not necessarily guarantee that it consumes less energy, especially for biomedical applications.

10.6.6 SETTLING TIME

Existing I.Amp (s-level) have a much longer settling time than regular Op.Amps (ns-level) (Ivanov, 2012). The system stability is a significant worry due to the enormous waves generated at chopping frequency and the charge injection in switching, and it takes a long time to settle. As a result, I.Amp has a far smaller bandwidth than ordinary amplifiers. Amplifiers always have a slow-settling ripple near the chopping frequency, especially during startup. I.Amp, on the other hand, operates intermittently in biomedical applications and has a short active duration. T.S.'s settling time should be as short as possible to save energy throughout the startup process.

To reduce settling time, a multipath architecture is presented in Qinwen et al. (2011). Because the ripple reduction Loop generates a notch in the low-frequency path, a frequency compensation network aids in the merging of the two frequency lines, blurring the notch and converting the system to first order. As a result, the overall I.Amp bandwidth has grown dramatically. The suggested CFIA has a settling time of 2.5 s with a 100-mV input step and a 100-pF load. However, the possibility of pole-zero doublets due to layout mismatch may prolong the settling process. Similar techniques were used to produce quick settling (4 s to 0.01%) with a more extensive signal input (4 V step) in a chopped amplifier (Goel and Singh, 2014). Any nonlinear Op.Amp operation, such as saturation or slewing, is detected using a window comparator. The slow low-frequency path will not affect the large-signal settling if the Op.Amp is kept in linear mode. If the current dissipation (1.65 mA) is scaled into A level, the settling time will exceed the ms level. Based on existing I.Amp designs with good noise, gain, and offset performance, future biomedical applications, primarily battery-powered, will require more research into decreasing their startup time.

TABLE 10.1 Summary of Performance and Comparisons of Developed I.Amp.

References	Technology used	Supply voltage	CMRR	Noise	Power dissipation
Martins et al. (1998)	Standard CMOS	± 4.5 V	99 dB	1.4 μV	500 μW
Harrison and Charles (2003)	1.5 μm CMOS	± 2.5 V	≥88 dB	2.2 μV_{rms}	80 μW
Shojaei et al. (2004)	0.35 μm CMOS	± 5 mV	100 dB	0.3 μV/√Hz	9 μW
Shojaei et al. (2004)	AMI 1.5 μm CMOS	3 V	>29 dB	7.8 μV_{rms}	115 μW
Chow and Wang (2007)	UMC 0.18 μm CMOS	1.8 V	167.18 dB	6.29 μV/√H z	3.196 mW
Zhang et al. (2009)	SMIC 0.18 μm CMOS	1.8 V	≥85 dB	–	37.8 μW
Fan et al. (2011)	65 nm CMOS	1 V	134 dB	60 nV/Hz	1.8 μW
Tseng et al. (2012)	0.18 μm CMOS TSMC	0.4–0.8 V	125 dB	–	0.09 mW
Goel and Singh (2014)	0.18 μm CMOS	5 mV	67.7 dB	1.75 pV/√Hz	263 mW
Hsiao et al. (2013)	0.35 μm CMOS	3.3 V	130 dB	–	1 mW
Kusuda (2015)	0.35 μm CMOS	3 V	110 dB	26 nV/√Hz	40.5 μW
Yaul et al. (2017)	0.32 μm CMOS	3.3 V	120 dB	18 nV/√Hz	561 μW
Jeon et al. (2020)	0.35 μm CMOS	16 mV	118 dB	3 μV_{rms}	1.5 μW
Pham et al. (2021)	28 nm CMOS	50 mV	>80 dB	136 nV/√Hz	1 μW

10.7 CONCLUSION

This chapter outlines the importance of the power amplifier in the biomedical measurement system and an essential requirement for the bio-amplifier. A detailed discussion is done on the type of amplifier used in biomedical instrumentation and its characteristics. Among all types, the instrumentational amplifier is most preferred because of its good performance in terms of CMMR, power consumption, cost voltage gain noise, and so on; further, a detailed analytical analysis has been done on the I.Amp. There are structural and performance differences between I.Amp topologies. Specific circuit approaches proposed in the literature are examined together with some standard I.Amp parameters, including gain, offset, noise, and CMRR. In 65-nm CMOS technology, a precise CCIAmp was implemented. In terms of NEF, offset, CMRR, PSRR, and gain accuracy, it delivers cutting-edge results for DC measurements. The adoption of a capacitively coupled chopper architecture results in high-power efficiency. Rather than employing a rail-to-to-rail input stage, it uses a DC CM rail-to-rail input range. The amplifier consumes 1.8 W of power when powered by a 1-V source and has a chip area of 0.1 mm. The CCIAmp can be used for biopotential sensing with an extra DSL and consumes 2.1 W.

KEYWORDS

- **bio amplifier**
- **instrumental amplifier**
- **common mode rejection ratio (CMRR)**
- **complementary metal-oxide semiconductor (CMOS)**
- **field-effect transistor**
- **DC servo loop (DSL)**
- **ripple reduction loop (RRL)**

REFERENCES

Bajoria, S.; Snoeij, M. F.; Schaffer, V.; Ivanov, M. V.; Wang, S.; Makinwa, K. A. A. A 36-V Voltage-to-Current Converter with Dynamic Element Matching and Auto-Calibration for AC Ripple Reduction. In *European Solid-State Circuits Conference*, 2011. DOI: 10.1109/ESSCIRC.2011.6044971.

Burt, R.; Zhang, J. A Micropower Chopper-Stabilized Operational Amplifier Using a SC Notch Filter with Synchronous Integration inside the Continuous-Time Signal Path. *IEEE J. Solid State Circuits* **2006,** *41* (12), 2729–2736. DOI: 10.1109/JSSC.2006.884195.

Chow, H. C.; Wang, J. Y. High CMRR Instrumentation Amplifier for Biomedical Applications. In *2007 9th International Symposium on Signal Processing and Its Applications, ISSPA 2007, Proceedings*, 2007; Vol 2, pp 1–4. DOI: 10.1109/ISSPA.2007.4555532.

Denison, T.; Consoer, K.; Santa, W.; Avestruz, A. T.; Cooley, J.; Kelly, A. A 2 μW 100 nV/rtHz Chopper-Stabilized Instrumentation Amplifier for Chronic Measurement of Neural Field Potentials. *IEEE J. Solid State Circuits* **2007,** *42* (12), 2934–2945. DOI: 10.1109/JSSC.2007.908664.

Fan, Q.; Sebastiano, F.; Huijsing, J. H.; Makinwa, K. A. A. A 1.8 μW 60 nV/√Hz Capacitively Coupled Chopper Instrumentation Amplifier in 65 nm CMOS for Wireless Sensor Nodes. *IEEE J. Solid State Circuits* **2011,** *46* (7), 1534–1543. DOI: 10.1109/JSSC.2011.2143610.

Fan, Q.; Huijsing, J. H.; Makinwa, K. A. A. A 21 nV/√Hz Chopper-Stabilized Multipath Current-Feedback Instrumentation Amplifier with 2 μV Offset. *IEEE J. Solid State Circuits* **2012,** *47* (2), 464–475. DOI: 10.1109/JSSC.2011.2175269.

Goel, A.; Singh, G. Novel High Gain Low Noise CMOS Instrumentation Amplifier for Biomedical Applications. In *Proceedings—2013 International Conference on Machine Intelligence Research and Advancement, ICMIRA 2013*, 2014; pp 392–396. DOI: 10.1109/ICMIRA.2013.83.

Han, D.; Zheng, Y.; Rajkumar, R.; Dawe, G. S.; Je, M. A 0.45 V 100-channel neural-recording IC with sub-μW/Channel Consumption in 0.18 μ CMOS. *IEEE Trans. Biomed. Circuits Syst.* **2013,** *7* (6), 290–292. DOI: 10.1109/TBCAS.2014.2298860.

Harrison, R. R.; Charles, C. A Low-Power Low-Noise CMOS Amplifier for Neural Recording Applications. *IEEE J. Solid State Circuits* **2003,** *38* (6), 958–965. DOI: 10.1109/JSSC.2003.811979.

Hsiao, Y. M.; Shiau, M. S.; Li, K. H.; Hou, J. J.; Hsu, H. S.; Wu, H. C.; Liu, D. G. Design a Bioamplifier with High CMRR. *VLSI Des.* **2013,** *2013*, 1–5. DOI: 10.1155/2013/210265.

Ivanov, E. V. Switched-Capacitor Level-Shifting Technique with Sampling Noise Reduction for Rail-to-Rail Input Range Instrumentation Amplifiers. *IEEE Trans. Circuits Syst. I* **2012,** *59* (12), 2867–2880. DOI: 10.1109/TCSI.2012.2206455.

Jeon, H.; Bang, J. S.; Je, M. A CMRR Enhancement Circuit Employing G-Controllable Output Stages for Capacitively Coupled Instrumentation Amplifiers. *IEEE Trans. Circuits Syst. II* **2020,** *67* (9), 1539–1543. DOI: 10.1109/TCSII.2020.3013009.

Kusuda, Y. Auto Correction Feedback for Ripple Suppression in a Chopper Amplifier. *IEEE J. Solid State Circuits* **2010,** *45* (8), 1436–1445. DOI: 10.1109/JSSC.2010.2048142.

Kusuda, Y. A 60 V Auto-Zero and Chopper Operational Amplifier with 800 kHz Interleaved Clocks and Input Bias Current Trimming. *IEEE J. Solid State Circuits* **2015,** *50* (12), 2804–2813. DOI: 10.1109/JSSC.2015.2456891.

Kwon, Y.; Kim, H.; Kim, J.; Han, K.; You, D.; Heo, H.; Cho, D.; Ko, H. Fully Differential Chopper-Stabilized Multipath Current-Feedback Instrumentation Amplifier with R-2R

DAC Offset Adjustment for Resistive Bridge Sensors. *Appl. Sci.* **2019,** *10* (1), 63. DOI: 10.3390/app10010063.

Martins, R.; Selberherr, S.; Vaz, F. A. A CMOS IC for Portable EEG Acquisition Systems. *IEEE Trans. Instrum. Meas.* **1998,** *47* (5), 1191–1196. DOI: 10.1109/19.746581.

Pham, X. T.; Nguyen, N. T.; Nguyen, V. N.; Lee, J. W. Area and Power-Efficient Capacitively Coupled Chopper Instrumentation Amplifiers in 28 nm CMOS for Multi-Channel Biosensing Applications. *IEEE Access* **2021,** *9*, 86773–86785. DOI: 10.1109/ACCESS.2021.3087737.

Qinwen, F.; Sebastiano, F.; Huijsing, J. H.; Makinwa, K. A. A. A Capacitively Coupled Chopper Instrumentation Amplifier in 65 nm CMOS for Wireless Sensor Nodes. *IEEE J. Solid-State Circuits* **2011,** *46* (7), 1534–1543.

Shojaei-Baghini, M.; Lai, R. K.; Sharma, D. K. An Ultra-Low-Power CMOS Instrumentation Amplifier for Biomedical Applications. In *2004 IEEE International Workshop on Biomedical Circuits and Systems*, 2004; pp 1–4. DOI: 10.1109/BIOCAS.2004.1454082.

Shojaei-Baghini, M.; Lal, R. K.; Sharma, D. K. A Low-Power and Compact Analog CMOS Processing Chip for Portable ECG Recorders. In *2005 IEEE Asian Solid-State Circuits Conference, ASSCC 2005*, 2005; pp 473–476. DOI: 10.1109/ASSCC.2005.251768.

Stage, I. A Sub-μW 36 nV/√Hz Chopper Amplifier for Sensors Using a Noise-Efficient Inverter-Based, 2016; pp 94–96.

Tseng, Y.; Ho, Y.; Kao, S.; Su, C. A 0.09-μW Low Power Front-End Biopotential Amplifier for Biosignal Recording. *IEEE Trans. Biomed. Circuits Syst.* **2012,** *6* (5), 508–516. DOI: 10.1109/TBCAS.2012.2188029.

Verma, N.; Shoeb, A.; Bohorquez, J.; Dawson, J.; Guttag, J.; Chandrakasan, A. P. A Micro-power EEG Acquisition SoC with Integrated Feature Extraction Processor for a Chronic Seizure Detection System. *IEEE J. Solid State Circuits* **2010,** *45* (4), 804–816. DOI: 10.1109/JSSC.2010.2042245.

Witte, J. F.; Huijsing, J. H.; Makinwa, K. A. A. A Current-Feedback Instrumentation Amplifier with 5 μV Offset for Bidirectional High-Side Current-Sensing. *IEEE J. Solid State Circuits* **2008,** *43* (12), 2769–2775. DOI: 10.1109/JSSC.2008.2005695.

Wu, R.; Makinwa, K. A. A.; Huijsing, J. H. A Chopper Current-Feedback Instrumentation Amplifier with a 1 mHz 1/*f* Noise Corner and an AC-Coupled Ripple Reduction Loop. *IEEE J. Solid State Circuits* **2009,** *44* (12), 3232–3243. DOI: 10.1109/JSSC.2009.2032710.

Wu, R.; Huijsing, J. H.; Makinwa, K. A. A. A Current-Feedback Instrumentation Amplifier with a Gain Error Reduction Loop and 0.06% Untrimmed Gain Error. *Dig. Tech. Pap. IEEE Int. Solid State Circuits Conf.* **2011,** *45* (10), 244–246. DOI: 10.1109/ISSCC.2011.5746303.

Yazicioglu, R. F.; Merken, P.; Puers, R.; Van Hoof, C. A 200 μ Weight-Channel EEG Acquisition ASIC for Ambulatory EEG Systems. *IEEE J. Solid State Circuits* **2008,** *43* (12), 3025–3038. DOI: 10.1109/JSSC.2008.2006462.

Yeager, D.; Zhang, F.; Zarrasvand, A.; George, N. T.; Daniel, T.; Otis, B. P. A 9 μA, Addressable Gen2 Sensor Tag for Biosignal Acquisition. *IEEE J. Solid State Circuits* **2010,** *45* (10), 2198–2209. DOI: 10.1109/JSSC.2010.2063930.

Zhang, J.-Y.; Wang, L.; Li, B. Design of Low-Offset Low-Power CMOS Amplifier for Biosensor Application. *J. Biomed. Sci. Eng.* **2009,** *2* (7), 538–542. DOI: 10.4236/jbise.2009.27078.

Index

K

L

M

N

O

P

R

S